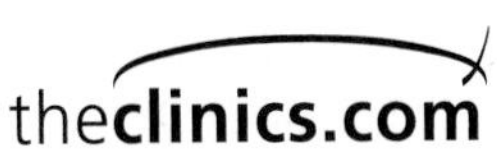

ENDOCRINOLOGY AND METABOLISM CLINICS OF NORTH AMERICA

Cushing's Syndrome

GUEST EDITORS
James W. Findling, MD
Hershel Raff, PhD

June 2005 • Volume 34 • Number 2

SAUNDERS
An Imprint of Elsevier, Inc.
PHILADELPHIA LONDON TORONTO MONTREAL SYDNEY TOKYO

W.B. SAUNDERS COMPANY
A Division of Elsevier Inc.

1600 John F. Kennedy Boulevard • Suite 1800 • Philadelphia, Pennsylvania 19103-2899

http://www.theclinics.com

ENDOCRINOLOGY AND METABOLISM CLINICS OF NORTH AMERICA
June 2005
Editor: Joe Rusko

Volume 34, Number 2
ISSN 0889-8529
ISBN 1-4160-2687-8

Endocrinology and Metabolism Clinics of North America (ISSN 0889-8529) is published quarterly by Elsevier Inc. Corporate and editorial offices: 1600 John F. Kennedy Boulevard, Suite 1800, Philadelphia, PA 19103-2899. Accounting and circulation offices: 6277 Sea Harbor Drive, Orlando, FL 32887-4800. Periodicals postage paid at Orlando, FL 32862, and additional mailing offices. Subscription prices are USD 170 per year for US individuals, USD 279 per year for US institutions, USD 85 per year for US students and residents, USD 210 per year for Canadian individuals, USD 336 per year for Canadian institutions, USD 235 per year for international individuals, USD 336 per year for international institutions and USD 118 per year for Canadian and foreign students/residents. To receive student/resident rate, orders must be accompained by name of affiliated institution, date of term, and the *signature* of program/residency coordinator on institution letterhead. Orders will be billed at individual rate until proof of status is received. Foreign air speed delivery is included in all *Clinics* subscription prices. All prices are subject to change without notice. POSTMASTER: Send address changes to *Endocrinology and Metabolism Clinics of North America*, W.B. Saunders Company, Periodicals Fulfillment, Orlando, FL 32887-4800. **Customer Service: (+1) 800-654-2452 (US). From outside of the US, call (+1) 407-345-4000; e-mail: hhspcs@harcourt.com.**

Reprints. For copies of 100 or more, of articles in this publication, please contact the Commercial Rights Department, Elsevier Inc., 360 Park Avenue South, New York, NY 10010-1710; phone: (+1) 212-633-3813; fax: (+1) 212-462-1935; e-mail: reprints@elsevier.com

Endocrinology and Metabolism Clinics of North America is covered in *Index Medicus, EMBASE/Excerpta Medica, Current Contents/Clinical Medicine, Current Contents/Life Sciences, Science Citation Index, ISI/BIOMED, BIOSIS, and Chemical Abstracts.*

Printed in the United States of America.

GUEST EDITORS

JAMES W. FINDLING, MD, Director, Endocrine–Diabetes Center, St. Luke's Medical Center; and Clinical Professor, Department of Medicine, Medical College of Wisconsin, Milwaukee, Wisconsin

HERSHEL RAFF, PhD, Director, Endocrine Research Laboratory, St. Luke's Medical Center; and Professor, Medicine and Physiology, Medical College of Wisconsin, Milwaukee, Wisconsin

CONTRIBUTORS

ALBERTO ANGELI, MD, Professor and Director, Division of Internal Medicine, University of Turin, Azienda Sanitaria Ospedaliera San Luigi, Orbassano, Italy

WIEBKE ARLT, MD, MRC Senior Clinical Fellow and Senior Lecturer, Division of Medical Sciences, Endocrinology, Institute of Biomedical Research, University of Birmingham, Birmingham, United Kingdom

DAVID C. ARON, MD, MS, Director, Veterans Affairs Health Services Research and Development Center for Quality Improvement Research, Louis Stokes Department of Veterans Affairs Medical Center; and Professor, Medicine, Division of Clinical and Molecular Endocrinology, Department of Medicine, Case Western Reserve University School of Medicine, Cleveland, Ohio

CÉLINE BARD, MD, Associate Professor, Department of Radiology, Hôtel-Dieu du Centre Hospitalier de l'Université de Montréal, Montreal, Quebec, Canada

BEVERLY M.K. BILLER, MD, Associate Professor, Medicine, Harvard Medical School; and Associate Physician, Medicine, Neuroendocrine Unit, Massachusetts General Hospital, Boston, Massachusetts

GIORGIO BORRETTA, MD, Director, Division of Endocrinology, Azienda Ospedaliera Santa Croce e Carle, Cuneo, Italy

YVAN BOULANGER, PhD, Associate Professor, Department of Radiology, Hôpital Saint-Luc du Central Hospitalier de l'Université de Montréal, Montreal, Quebec, Canada

ISABELLE BOURDEAU, MD, Assistant Professor, Division of Endocrinology, Department of Medicine, Hôtel-Dieu du Centre Hospitalier de l'Université de Montréal, Montreal, Quebec, Canada

SILVIA BOVIO, MD, Postdoctoral Fellow, Division of Internal Medicine, University of Turin, Azienda Sanitaria Ospedaliera San Luigi, Orbassano, Italy

HENRI COHEN, PhD, Professor, Cognitive Neuroscience Center, Université du Québec à Montréal, Montreal, Quebec, Canada

ANNAMARIA COLAO, MD, PhD, Dr Prof, Associate Professor, Department of Molecular and Clinical Endocrinology and Oncology, "Federico II" University, Naples, Italy

ANTONGIULIO FAGGIANO, MD, Dr, Student Fellow, Department of Molecular and Clinical Endocrinology and Oncology, "Federico II" University, Naples, Italy

JAMES W. FINDLING, MD, Director, Endocrine–Diabetes Center, St. Luke's Medical Center; and Clinical Professor, Department of Medicine, Medical College of Wisconsin, Milwaukee, Wisconsin

HÉLÈNE FORGET, PhD, Professor, Department of Psychology, Université du Québec en Outaouais, Gatineau, Quebec, Canada

RACHEL L. HOPKINS, MD, Senior Fellow, Division of Endocrinology and Metabolism, Albany Medical College, Albany, New York

LAUREN JACOBSON, PhD, Associate Professor, Center for Neuropharmacology and Neuroscience, Albany Medical College, Albany, New York

ANDRÉ LACROIX, MD, Member, Division of Endocrinology; and Professor and Chairman, Department of Medicine, Hôtel-Dieu du Centre Hospitalier de l'Université de Montréal, Montreal, Quebec, Canada

MATTHEW C. LEINUNG, MD, Associate Professor, Medicine; and Head, Division of Endocrinology and Metabolism, Albany Medical College, Albany, New York

JOHN R. LINDSAY, MD, Clinical Fellow, Reproductive Biology and Medicine Branch, National Institute for Child Health and Human Development, National Institutes of Health, Bethesda, Maryland

GAETANO LOMBARDI, MD, Dr Prof, Full Professor, Department of Molecular and Clinical Endocrinology and Oncology, "Federico II" University, Naples, Italy

BARBARA P. LUKERT, MD, Professor, Medicine, Division of Metabolism, Endocrinology and Genetics, University of Kansas School of Medicine, Kansas City, Kansas

CARL D. MALCHOFF, MD, PhD, Associate Professor, Medicine, Division of Endocrinology, University of Connecticut Health Center, Farmington, Connecticut

DIANA M. MALCHOFF, PhD, Assistant Professor, Medicine, Division of Endocrinology, University of Connecticut Health Center, Farmington, Connecticut

LYNNETTE K. NIEMAN, MD, Senior Investigator, Reproductive Biology and Medicine Branch, National Institute for Child Health and Human Development, National Institutes of Health, Bethesda, Maryland

GIANGIACOMO OSELLA, MD, Staff Physician, Division of Internal Medicine, Unversity of Turin, Azienda Sanitaria Ospedaliera San Luigi, Orbassano, Italy

ANNA PIA, MD, Staff Physician, Division of Endocrinology, Endocrinologia, Azienda Ospedaliera Santa Croce e Carle, Cuneo, Italy

ROSARIO PIVONELLO, MD, PhD, Dr, Research Fellow, Department of Molecular and Clinical Endocrinology and Oncology, "Federico II" University, Naples, Italy

HERSHEL RAFF, PhD, Director, Endocrine Research Laboratory, St. Luke's Medical Center; and Professor, Medicine and Physiology, Medical College of Wisconsin, Milwaukee, Wisconsin

GIUSEPPE REIMONDO, MD, Research Fellow, Division of Internal Medicine, University of Turin, Azienda Sanitaria Ospedaliera San Luigi, Orbassano, Italy

JOSEPH L. SHAKER, MD, Clinical Professor, Medicine, Endocrine–Diabetes Center, St. Luke's Medical Center, University of Wisconsin School of Medicine, Milwaukee, Wisconsin

PAUL M. STEWART, MD, Professor, Division of Medical Sciences, Endocrinology, Institute of Biomedical Research, University of Birmingham, Birmingham, United Kingdom

BROOKE SWEARINGEN, MD, Associate Professor, Surgery, (Neurosurgery), Harvard Medical School; and Associate Visiting Neurosurgeon, Department of Neurosurgery, Massachusetts General Hospital, Boston, Massachusetts

MASSIMO TERZOLO, MD, Associate Professor, Division of Internal Medicine, University of Turin, Azienda Sanitaria Ospedaliera San Luigi, Orbassano, Italy

GEOFFREY B. THOMPSON, MD, Professor, Surgery, Mayo Clinic College of Medicine; and Vice-Chair, Department of Surgery, Mayo Clinic, Rochester, Minnesota

ANDREA L. UTZ, MD, PhD, Harvard Medical School; and Clinical and Research Fellow in Medicine (Endocrinology), Neuroendocrine Unit, Massachusetts General Hospital, Boston, Massachusetts

MARY LEE VANCE, MD, Professor, Medicine and Neurosurgery, University of Virginia Health System, Charlottesville, Virginia

WILLIAM F. YOUNG, Jr, MD, Professor, Medicine, Mayo Clinic College of Medicine; and Vice-Chair, Divisions of Endocrinology, Diabetes, Metabolism, Nutrition, and Internal Medicine, Mayo Clinic, Rochester, Minnesota

CONTENTS

FORTHCOMING ISSUES

September 2005

Pediatric Endocrinology
Joseph I. Wolfsdorf, MD, *Guest Editor*

RECENT ISSUES

March 2005

Type 2 Diabetes and Cardiovascular Disease
Daniel Einhorn, MD, and Julio Rosenstock, MD, *Guest Editors*

December 2004

Menopause and Hormone Replacement Therapy
Nanette Santoro, MD, and
Judi Lee Chervenak, MD, *Guest Editors*

September 2004

Metabolic Syndrome: Part II
Scott M. Grundy, MD, PhD, *Guest Editor*

June 2004

Metabolic Syndrome: Part I
Scott M. Grundy, MD, PhD, *Guest Editor*

March 2004

Type I Diabetes
Peter A. Gottlieb, MD, *Guest Editor*

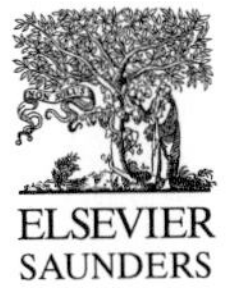

ELSEVIER
SAUNDERS

Endocrinol Metab Clin N Am
34 (2005) xiii–xv

ENDOCRINOLOGY
AND METABOLISM
CLINICS
OF NORTH AMERICA

Preface

Cushing's Syndrome

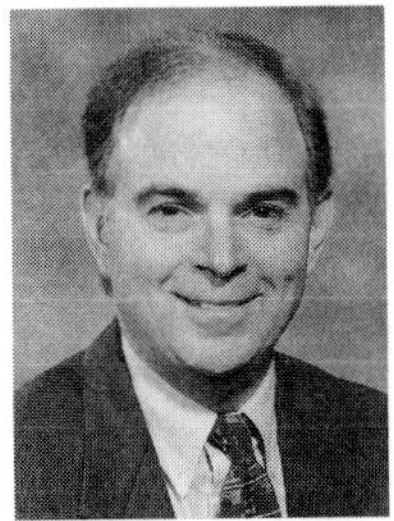

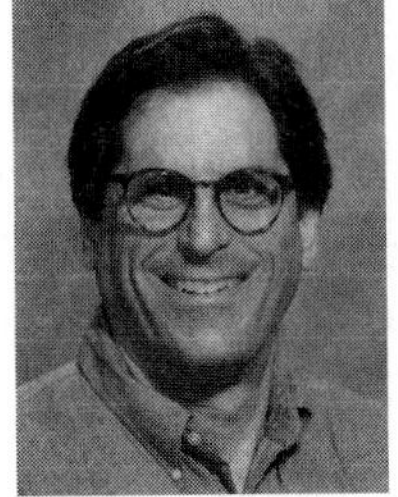

James W. Findling, MD Hershel Raff, PhD
Guest Editors

The diagnosis and management of Cushing's syndrome is the most challenging problem in clinical endocrinology. It has been over a decade since *Endocrinology and Metabolism Clinics of North America* devoted an issue to this enigmatic disorder. Much has changed since 1994. The recognition of subclinical hypercortisolism, particularly in patients who have incidentally discovered adrenal adenomas, has provided clinicians with a sobering lesson on just how difficult it may be to distinguish this syndrome from the very common metabolic syndrome with its Cushing's phenotype. More importantly, screening studies of high-risk populations (eg, poorly controlled diabetes mellitus) has found a surprisingly high percentage (2%–5%) of patients who have endogenous hypercortisolism. It is also now clearer that biochemical studies previously thought to represent the gold standard for diagnosis are much less sensitive than previously thought, thereby mandating a new diagnostic approach (eg, late-night salivary cortisol). In addition, during the past decade, there has been increasing recognition of the importance of 11β-hydroxysteroid dehydrogenase (11β-HSD) as a regulator of glucocorticoid action in many tissues. There also is an increased appreciation for the adverse effects of glucocorticoids on the central nervous system, an understanding of the pathophysiology of the bilateral nodular adrenal hyperplasia, and recognition of laparoscopic adrenalectomy as a safer approach to adrenal surgery. This issue captures, for the clinician, an update of the physiology of the hypothalamic-pituitary-adrenal axis and the characteristics, evaluation, and treatment of patients who have spontaneous Cushing's syndrome.

0889-8529/05/$ - see front matter
doi:10.1016/j.ecl.2005.01.015 *endo.theclinics.com*

The first article serves as prologue. In it, Dr. Aron reviews the history of Dr. Cushing and his initial descriptions of Cushing's syndrome and disease.

The next three articles focus on the basic principles of the hypothalamic–pituitary–adrenal axis. Dr. Jacobson reviews the physiologic control of the hypothalamic–pituitary–adrenocortical axis including stress-induced corticotropin (ACTH) release, glucocorticoid negative feedback, and the interaction with immune and metabolic status. Drs. Arlt and Stewart then describe the synthesis, metabolism, and action of endogenous cortisol and focus on the regulation of steroid binding to the glucocorticoid and mineralocorticoid receptors, with particular attention to the 11β-HSD story. The basic principles section concludes with the evaluation of glucocorticoid resistance and hypersensitivity by Drs. Malchoff and Malchoff. Particularly fascinating is the focus on mutations and polymorphisms of the glucocorticoid receptor.

The next section is devoted to a comprehensive description of the features of Cushing's syndrome. In the first article of this group, Drs. Pivonello, Faggiano, Lombardi, and Colao address the risk of cardiovascular disease in Cushing's syndrome and its relation to the metabolic syndrome. Drs. Shaker and Lukert then address the role of glucocorticoids in the development of metabolic bone disease in endogenous and exogenous Cushing's syndrome. Although effects of glucocorticoid excess on the central nervous system has been described before, the article of Drs. Bourdeau et al go into much more detail on cognitive function and neurologic findings using new, more sophisticated analytical tools. In the final article of this section, Drs. Hopkins and Leinung address the difficult issue of glucocorticoid withdrawal and provide a logical sequence to follow when weaning patients from glucocorticoid therapy.

The final section addresses the diagnosis and treatment of Cushing's syndrome. A new approach using nighttime salivary cortisol to screen patients for even the subtlest signs of Cushing's syndrome is described. Drs. Lindsay and Nieman follow this up with biochemical and radiologic approaches to the differential diagnosis of Cushing's syndrome. With the advent of new methods to visualize the adrenal glands comes the increase in incidentally discovered adrenal lesions in patients who either have mild or no symptoms of glucocorticoid excess. Drs. Terzolo et al provide a comprehensive analysis of this emerging problem. Drs. Lacroix and Bourdeau then describe the recent descriptions of aberrant receptor expression causing bilateral, nodular adrenal hyperplasia. Once the diagnosis of Cushing's disease is made with petrosal sinus sampling, the most common curative approach is to perform pituitary surgery to remove the ACTH-secreting microadenoma. Drs. Utz et al describe this delicate pituitary surgery and make suggestions for postoperative management. If pituitary surgery is unsuccessful, some have advocated the use of pituitary radiotherapy. Dr. Vance describes the logic behind this approach and provides important warnings about the potential for adverse effects. Finally, Drs. Young and

Thompson provide a systematic analysis of the surgical approach for adrenal Cushing's focusing on the most modern, laparoscopic adrenalectomy.

We anticipate that the next issue of the *Endocrinology and Metabolism Clinics of North America* devoted to Cushing's syndrome (in approximately 2015) will provide clinicians with even a better understanding of the biologic importance of mild cortisol excess. It is probable that more sensitive and specific diagnostic tools that have not yet been considered will be available. We also hope that there will be new therapeutic agents, not only specifically targeting ACTH-secreting neoplasms, but also providing a means to simply and safely attenuate excessive cortisol production from the adrenal glands. Regardless of the progress that may be forthcoming in the next decade, one thing we have said on numerous occasions will surely still be true: If you have never missed the diagnosis of Cushing's syndrome or been humbled by trying to established its cause, then you should refer your patients who have suspected hypercortisolism to someone who has.

James W. Findling, MD
Director, Endocrine–Diabetes Center
St. Luke's Medical Center
2801 West KK River Parkway
Suite 245
Milwaukee, WI 53215, USA

E-mail address: james.findling@aurora.org

Hershel Raff, PhD
Director, Endocrine Research Laboratory
St. Luke's Medical Center
2801 West KK River Parkway
Suite 245
Milwaukee, WI 53215, USA

E-mail address: hraff@mcw.edu

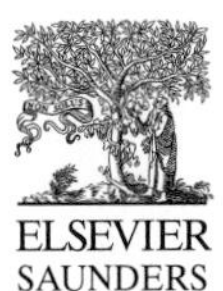
ELSEVIER
SAUNDERS

Endocrinol Metab Clin N Am
34 (2005) 257–269

ENDOCRINOLOGY
AND METABOLISM
CLINICS
OF NORTH AMERICA

Cushing's Syndrome from Bedside to Bench and Back: A Historical Perspective

David C. Aron, MD, MS[a,b,*]

[a] *Veterans Affairs Health Services Research and Development Center for Quality Improvement Research, Louis Stokes Department of Veterans Affairs Medical Center, 10701 East Boulevard, Education Office 14 (W), Cleveland, OH 44106, USA*

[b] *Division of Clinical and Molecular Endocrinology, Department of Medicine, Case Western Reserve University School of Medicine, 10900 Euclid Avenue, Cleveland, OH 44106, USA*

In this time of enormous and rapid scientific advance in biomedicine, it seems quaint to review historical aspects of a disorder described nearly a century ago whose problems in diagnosis and treatment have to a large extent been solved. In addition to the intrinsic value of the study of history, however, there are lessons for medical advancement that have broader implications for how research is supported and how physicians are trained. For those interested in a detailed chronology of the events in the advance of knowledge of pituitary and adrenal anatomy, physiology, biochemistry, and pathophysiology, there are standard works and recent reviews [1–5]. The author's approach will be somewhat different, focusing on the development of Cushing's syndrome as a clinical entity, a process that has moved from bedside to bench and back again [6].

The description and elucidation of Cushing's syndrome has paralleled developments in medicine. Initially, there was a clinical description consisting of a complex of signs and symptoms that were recognized as sufficiently different from other disease entities or syndromes to merit a new designation. This clinical entity or syndrome represents a recurrent pattern that stands out as a unit and has to do with disease—disturbed physiologic function. As such, this concept has to do essentially with the practice of medicine [7]. As knowledge accumulates, it helps to understand the condition, how it came

* Veterans Affairs Health Services Research and Development Center for Quality Improvement Research, Louis Stokes Department of Veterans Affairs Medical Center, 10701 East Boulevard, Education Office 14 (W), Cleveland, OH 44106.

E-mail address: david.aron@med.va.gov

0889-8529/05/$ - see front matter. Published by Elsevier Inc.
doi:10.1016/j.ecl.2005.01.011

into being, how it relates to various other factors, and various other states (ie, it provides an explanation for a set of symptoms). With time it may prove valuable in the care of the patient and might also force modification of the original concept of the clinical entity [6,7]. Although theories to explain the pattern (the science of medicine) may change, the clinical entity bridges the gap between theories (eg, Cushing's syndrome caused by hyperpituitarism versus hyperadrenalism). Theories may broaden or narrow that clinical entity. For example, Cushing's syndrome is now considered to represent a spectrum from full-blown Cushing's syndrome as it was described initially to a state of subclinical autonomous cortisol hypersecretion manifested solely by glucose intolerance or obesity. The clinical entity is the persistent thread among the shifting theories and offers a way to examine development of biomedical knowledge in ways that have implications for today.

In 1960, Liddle and Shute [6] described three periods in the evolution of Cushing's syndrome as a clinical entity: description of the clinical syndrome, explanation of the syndrome as hypercortisolisin, and delineation of three causes of hypercortisolism. They recognized that this evolution was continuing to include the identification of atypical forms (eg, micronodular and macronodular adrenal hyperplasia and ectopic corticotrophin-releasing hormone [CRH] syndrome), as well as to understand better the pathophysiology underlying the symptoms, including their molecular basis. This article focuses on the first two periods. The main actor in each of these periods represents the synergistic effects of clinical and experimental expertise; each of these individuals was a consummate clinician-investigator who combined his knowledge and skills from each of these domains.

Harvey Cushing's interest in the pituitary, and the clinical description of the syndrome

Knowledge of the physiologic role of the adrenals and the pituitary began with recognition of clinical disorders. Bartolomeo Eustachius is the first person known to have described the adrenal glands, which in 1563 he termed the "glandulae renibus incumbents," and his drawing in the *Opuscula Anatomica* is the first known representation. Virtually nothing was known about their function until the mid–19th century, a fact confirmed by Thomas Addison's statement that, "at the present moment, the function of the suprarenal capsules, and the influence they exercise in the general economy, are almost or altogether unknown" [1,4]. In this 1855 work, he described a series of patients who have various adrenal lesions—tuberculosis, metastases, and atrophy—some of whom clearly suffered from adrenal insufficiency. Addison's interest in the adrenals began with his observation of adrenal abnormalities in a form of fatal anemia (pernicious anemia) [1–4], and his clinical description has not been matched since. Shortly thereafter, Charles Brown-Sequard performed adrenalectomies and sham operations on dogs (a controlled study) and demonstrated that the adrenals were indispensable to life. Tumors of the adrenal had been recognized at least since the 18th century and were associated with various symptoms, particularly virilization. Individual cases also had been described that fit the clinical picture of Cushing's syndrome.

The pituitary gland was recognized earlier than the adrenals. Galen, the court physician to the Roman Emperor Marcus Aurelius (3rd century CE), recognized the existence of the pituitary gland, and the conception of the pituitary as a phlegm gland was attributed to him; the pituitary was thus named (*pituita* is Latin for "phlegm"). Andreas Vesaluis, the pioneering Flemish anatomist, named the structure *glandula pituitam cerebri excepiens* ("in the little phlegm acorn drawn out of the brain"). This was consistent with the Galenic concept of a structure necessary to eliminate waste products or residues generated in the brain. The English anatomist Richard Lower suggested in his 1672 *Dissertatio de Origine Catarrhi* what might today be considered an endocrine function of the pituitary: "for whatever Serum is separated into the ventricles of the brain and tissues out of them through the Infundibulum to the Glandula pituitaria distills not upon the Palate but is poured again into the blood and mixed with it" [1,5].

By the turn of the 20th century, apart from the clinical description of acromegaly and its association with a pituitary tumor, little was known. In fact, in his classic monograph entitled "The Pituitary Body and Its Disorders," Cushing (Fig. 1) contrasted the progress in investigation of the functions of the thyroid and adrenal glands: "The other glands have notably lagged behind, with the pituitary body at the tail of the procession. For though this structure was added to the group of so-called ductless glands by Liegeois some fifty years ago, its inaccessibility has been sufficient

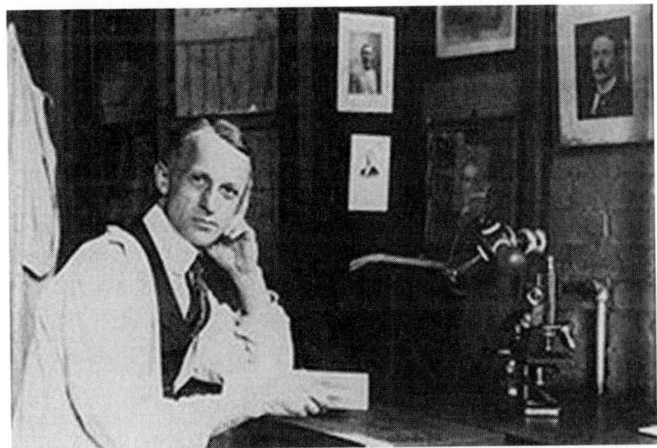

Fig. 1. Harvey Cushing (1868–1939). (*From* Named Professorships, Deanships, and Directorships. John Hopkins University; with permission. Available at: http://webapps.jhu.edu/namedprofessorships/professorshipdetail.cfm?professorshipID = 125. Accessed on February 9, 2005.)

to discourage investigation even were there no other difficulties to be encountered" [8].

Harvey Cushing's interest in the pituitary gland may find its origin in a misdiagnosed case [9–11]. In 1901, Harvey Cushing returned to the United States from a European tour and began to develop his surgical career. Among his first cases was a sexually immature 14-year-old obese girl seeking treatment for progressive visual loss and headache. He was unable to localize the lesion clinically and rather than perform an exploratory craniotomy, he performed palliative decompressions. Although the headache improved, the girl's vision deteriorated. Cushing then explored the posterior fossa in the hopes of finding a cerebeller tumor, but to no avail and the girl died postoperatively of pneumonia. An autopsy revealed a pituitary cystic tumor. The misdiagnosis was made worse because Cushing recently had spent time learning about brain tumor localization in the laboratory of one of the leading neurologists of the day, Charles Sherrington, and several months after this case, he learned of a similar case from someone who had studied with him in the same laboratory, Alfred Frohlich. Frohlich described a case of adiposogenital dystrophy in a boy who had a pituitary tumor and sent a reprint to Cushing. Frohlich not only made the correct diagnosis, but also convinced a surgeon to operate. It may have been wounded pride and intellectual interest in an intriguing case that set Cushing on a course to study the functions and disorders of the pituitary gland.

Cushing recognized the importance of clinical issues pointing the way in research. In his 1914 Weir Mitchell Lecture, Cushing [12] emphasized the importance of tumors in the process of clarifying the function of an endocrine gland:

> "It may be recalled that much of our knowledge of pituitary disorders has revolved around the question of tumor—using the term in a comprehensive sense. It was the presence of a tumor which first led Marie, and subsequently Frohlich, to couple with this comparatively obscure gland the syndromes which bear their names. And for the most of us to-day manifestations of tumor continue to be a necessary guidepost, so that those who venture to predict pituitary disease in their absence do so with misgivings and merely on the ground that similar constitutional symptoms have been known to arise in conjunction with a growth."

Cushing's skill as neurosurgeon and his development of new techniques gave him an advantage over other experimental physiologists. When pituitary disorders were first being diagnosed, neurosurgery as a subspecialty did not exist. The daunting prospect of surgery on the pituitary in the years following Marie's description of acromegaly is given in a 1896 textbook of head and neck surgery cited by Johnson [1]:

> "Where the growth lies in contact with the base of the skull, that is, springs from the inferior surface of the brain, conservation would pronounce the word inaccessible. This warning, however, is quite unneeded by the genes

audax omnia perpeti; for example, by such as announce that they think operations forthe removal of tumors from the base of the brain are feasible; such daring characterized a specialist in cerebral surgery, whom the writer heard say that he believed it possible to so open the skull and lift up the brain as to catch a view of the foramen magnum. The reader may ask, Did he mean this of the living subject?"

Cushing's first approach to the pituitary by way of the extracranial route took place in 1909, and an excellent surgical result was achieved. He remarked, however, that "surgeons, however, cannot afford to enter into this new field too precipitously, not simply by reason of the peculiar inaccessibility of the gland—for operative resources will overcome these difficulties—but principally on account of the present uncertainties in regard to its physiological properties" [13]. By 1912, Cushing had achieved some excellent surgical outcomes, but he looked toward a different future [8]:

"It is conceivable that the day is not far distant when our present methods of dealing with hypophyseal enlargements, with scalpel, rongeur and curette—new as these measures actually are and brilliant as the results may often be—will seem utterly crude and antiquated, for it is quite probable that surgery will, in the end, come to play a less, rather than a more important, role in ductless gland maladies. This Utopia, however, will be reached only when a sufficient understanding of the underlying aetiological agencies enables us to make more precocious diagnoses."

Using his neurosurgical skills, Cushing was able to show in dogs that complete pituitary removal was lethal and concluded that the pituitary was essential to life. Although he was less successful in dissecting out the anterior and posterior lobes of the pituitary individually, he did show that partial destruction of the anterior pituitary was associated with the development of a Frohlich-syndrome. Cushing also described the transient, hypertrophic effects of hypophysectomies on the thyroid, adrenal cortex, and gonads. Although unable to account for these effects, they suggested a relationship between the adenohypophysis and its target glands. Cushing also knew that acidophil tumors of the pituitary were associated with acromegaly. Although unable to prove it, Cushing, based on a clinical response to partial tumor resection in a patient who had acromegaly, speculated that the acidophilic cells of the pituitary made a growth-promoting factor that could account for the disordered growth.

Although a researcher, Cushing was also a consummate clinician and sought to apply his knowledge in the clinic. Here is where he met Minnie G, one of his first patients who had what Cushing called a "polyglandular syndrome," indicating that secondary functional alterations in members of the ductless gland series occurred whenever the activity of one of the glands becomes primarily deranged, and that it was difficult to tell which of the structures is primarily at fault. In retrospect, however, she clearly suffered from hypercortisolism (Fig. 2). Her case, described in detail in the 1912

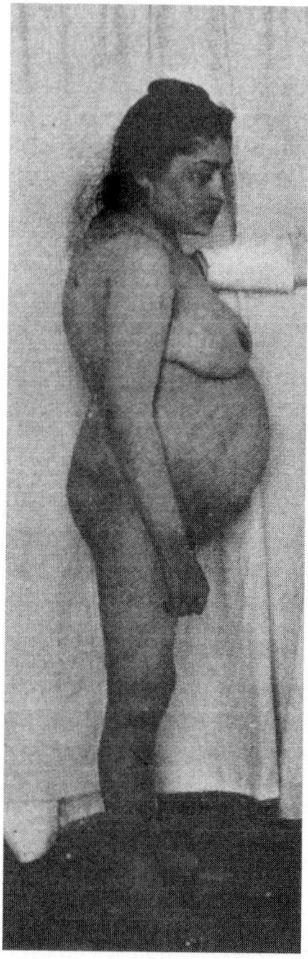

Fig. 2. Minnie G: a patient who had Cushing's syndrome. (*From* Cushing H. The pituitary body and its disorders. Philadelphia: J.B. Lippincott; 1912; with permission.)

book [8], ends with the tantalizing statement: "An exploration of the adrenals is under consideration."

This was never undertaken, however. Cushing commented that in addition to skeletal undergrowth, adiposity, and sexual dystrophy on the one hand and painful and tender adiposis with asthenia and psychic disturbances on the other, the case is an instance of the combination of intracranial pressure symptoms with amenorrhrea, adiposity, and low physical stature—a syndrome that might well be caused by hypophyseal deficiency. But here, however, the similarity to the cases of hypopituitarism ended. He went on to write that a symptom-complex of this type has been described in association with certified adrenal lesions, which makes it seem that the adiposo-genital syndrome may occur with derangements of other of the ductless glands than the hypophysis itself, and believed that one might soon recognize the consequences of hyperadrenalism.

Cushing continued his clinical practice and laboratory investigation, accumulating twelve cases that formed the basis of his classic 1932 paper [14]. Shortly thereafter, Bishop and Close gave the syndrome the eponym *Cushing's syndrome*. Although aware of the occurrence of adrenal hyperplasia in some cases, Cushing nevertheless held to the view that the pituitary was the primary problem, with the main factor being a basophil adenoma of the pituitary gland, a finding in two of the patients. He wrote [14]:

> "While there is every reason to concede, therefore, that a disorder of somewhat similar aspect may occur in association with pineal, with gonadal, or with adrenal tumors, the fact that the peculiar polyglandular syndrome which pains have been taken herein conservatively to describe, may accompany a basophil adenoma in the absence of any apparent alteration in the adrenal cortex other than a possible secondary hyperplasia, will give pathologists reason in the future more carefully to scrutinize the anterior-pituitary for lesions of similar composition."

He believed that hypersecretion of gonadotropin, which, along with growth hormone, was one of the two pituitary factors known, might be the factor responsible, but he could not produce this experimentally. Collip's discovery of adrenocorticotropic hormone (ACTH) would open another path for investigation. Cushing's success owed to his keen powers of observation, skills as an experimentalist, and serendipity in his ability to relate disease syndromes to an overproduction or to an absence of secretory products of the pituitary [11]. Although he set a high standard for other clinician-investigators to follow, one who met and exceeded this standard was Fuller Albright.

Fuller Albright and the identification of the common factor underlying Cushing's syndrome

Fuller Albright (Fig. 3) was considered the preeminent clinical and investigative endocrinologist of his day by many of his contemporaries, and his 1944 address to the American Society for Clinical Investigation is a classic [15,16]. Schwartz noted that in a brief introductory note to his bibliography, Albright wrote, "in my opinion, my contributions divide themselves into two groups: (a) clinical descriptions and (b) elucidations of pathological physiology." In category (a), he, along with his students and associates, described de novo or made definitive contributions to the delineation of an astonishing 14 major syndromes over 20 years [16]. In category (b), not only did he excel in the area of calcium metabolism for which he is best known, but also in the area of adrenal function (and others).

The importance of Cushing's syndrome in Albright's work is reflected in a diagram annotated by Felix Kolb, one of his students (and one of the

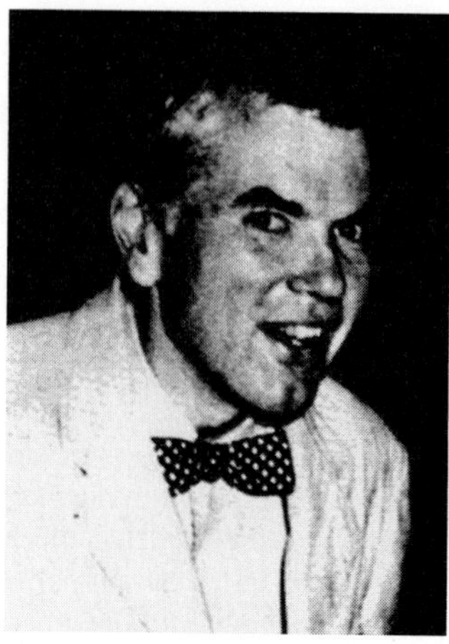

Fig. 3. Fuller Albright (1900–1969). (*From* Biographical memoirs. Vol. 48. National Academy of Sciences; 1976; with permission. Available at: http://books.nap.edu/books/0309023491/html/2.html. Accessed on February 9, 2005.)

author's teachers). A picture of a patient who had Cushing's syndrome is prominently displayed on Albright's diagram of the "do's" and "do not's" of clinical investigation (Fig. 4). In addition, among the most heavily cited life sciences papers between 1945 and 1954 was Albright's Harvey 1942–3 Lectures on Cushing's Syndrome [17]. Here, Albright described the logical progression of his hypotheses and his moving from bench to bedside and back [18]. His investigations stemmed from clinical observation. He wrote [18]:

> "To be absolutely accurate, one should probably confine the term 'Cushing's Syndrome' to those individuals who present a certain striking clinical picture (vide infra) associated with a basophile tumor of the pituitary. However, the author will use the term to refer to patients with the clinical picture regardless of the etiology. From a clinical point of view, the syndrome is so striking that it seems almost certain that all individuals with it have some common denominator as regards the etiology."

His first attempt was to see whether this symptom complex could not be explained entirely on the basis of an hypergluconeogenesis coupled with a resistance to glucose oxidation resulting from an hyperadrenocorticism. Because this hypothesis should lead not only to too much sugar but also to too little protein, it might likewise explain the deficiency in tissues, notably the weakness of the muscles, the osteoporosis, the thin skin, and the easy bruisability. It also might explain the obesity. If the disorder does not involve a change in the total energy output but merely a change in the proportions of carbohydrates, fats, and proteins in the metabolic mixture,

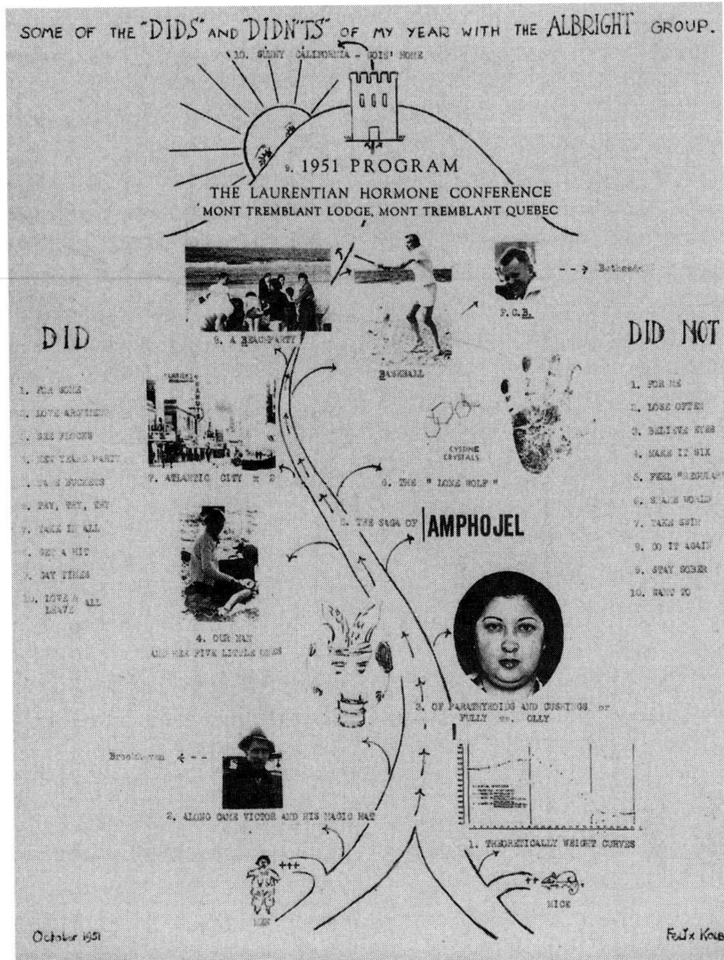

Fig. 4. Some "did's" and "didn'ts" from the author's year with the Albright group. 1951 cartoon by Felix Kolb, MD. Background diagram from Albright's Presidential Address to the American Society of Clinical Investigation. Note the picture of a patient who had Cushing's syndrome. (*From* Kolb F. Lessons learned from Fuller Albright. In: Kolb F, editor. In honor of Fuller Albright: father of modern endocrinology. The Endocrinologist 2000;(Suppl):132; with permission.)

one would expect the increased burning of protein to result in decreased burning and hence storage of fats.

Albright, however, quickly saw problems with this hypothesis. He found it somewhat disconcerting that patients who had Cushing's syndrome were never found to be in markedly negative nitrogen balance before therapy was instituted; indeed, most had been in slightly positive nitrogen balance. Moreover, patients who have hypoinsulin diabetes mellitus, in whom the diabetes mellitus is not under control, do not develop a clinical picture like Cushing's syndrome despite the markedly increased conversion of proteins into sugars that must happen in that condition. Finally, his hypothesis predicted that patients who had Cushing's syndrome be resistant to ketosis, which they were not.

Abandoning that hypothesis, he tested another one, positing a fundamental disturbance in the ability to burn fat. Another of his meticulous metabolic studies, however, showed that not to be the case. Albright wrote, "When it came to looking around for a new hypothesis, the one certain fact *from a clinical point of view* was that the patients with Cushing's Syndrome were suffering from deficiency of tissues (emphasis added)."

Because the evidence presented made clear that the disorder was not an excessive breakdown of tissue, the alternative thesis suggested itself; namely, that there was a difficulty in synthesis of tissue. It still seemed possible that the fundamental disorder was a hyperadrenocorticism with respect to the *S* hormone, but that this hormone, instead of converting proteins and hence tissues into sugar, inhibits the production of tissue. As aptly put by Dr. E.C. Reifenstein, Jr., the hormone is antianabolic rather than catabolic. Although Albright was aware of no data that did not harmonize with this new theory, he believed that such data undoubtedly would be forthcoming and that a new hypothesis or a further modification of the present one would be necessary [18]. The issue was not settled in the literature for several years, but Albright had identified hyperadrenalism as the factor common to patients who have Cushing's syndrome, whether they had basophilic adenomas of the pituitary, adrenal tumors, or adrenal hyperplasia. Like Harvey Cushing, Fuller Albright's success resulted largely from the combination of clinical and experimental expertise and the synergy of rigorous logic and knowledge-based intuition [16].

With time, various causes of hypercortisolism were delineated: (1) autonomous secretion of cortisol by an adrenocortical neoplasm, (2) hypersecretion of cortisol in response to excessive secretion of ACTH by the pituitary gland, and (3) hypersecretion of cortisol in response to ectopic ACTH. This occurred against a background of rapid advance in laboratory techniques to measure the relevant hormones and elucidate the pathophysiology of the hypothalamic–pituitary–adrenal axis. Tests were developed to distinguish among these types of hypercortisolism and other types were described (eg, micronodular adrenal hyperplasia and ectopic CRH syndrome). Developments in diagnosis and corresponding advances in imaging techniques and therapy continue, making it possible to correct hypercortisolism in most patients. Over this period, endocrinology has changed, discarding such dogma as one gene-one hormone, one cell-one hormone, one hormone-one receptor, and one hormone- uniform predictable therapeutic response in all patients, among others [19]. Better diagnostic tests are being developed to shorten the time from onset of disease to diagnosis and to learn about the molecular basis of cortisol action and pathogenesis of tumors.

Summary

Biomedical research is a complex network of processes and events. Much interest has been placed on distinctions between basic and clinical research or between basic and applied research. The dividing line between basic and applied biomedicine is elusive at best, however [10]. Similarly, there has been an emphasis on the process of going from bench to bedside rather than vice versa [10]. Among the many reasons for this is the culture of academic medicine in which the ethos is the value of the discovery of new knowledge over all else and the merit of the hard science of molecular biology as opposed to any other type of endeavor [20]. For example, Alvin Feinstein [21] writing about the decline of pathophysiologic research stated, "...prestige was least for studies of therapeutic interventions in patient care, and rose as the research went to explication of organ-system pathophysiology, to physiology, and eventually to molecular mechanisms of biology. Being inversely proportional to the structural size of the object under investigation, prestige increased as the investigated material became smaller, from intact organism, to organ, and eventually to infracellular structures and cell-free extracts." The history of Cushing's syndrome illustrates the synergy between clinicians and researchers, particularly as personified in the same individual.

The problems in linking experimental science and clinical practice are not new [22]. Harvey Cushing also played an active role to solidify the links. These efforts took place against a background surprisingly relevant to contemporary issues. In a letter to Harvard Medical School Dean David Esall (7 March 1925), Cushing [23] wrote, "If the pre-clinical departments succeed in driving the clinician out of the school entirely, instead of encouraging him to work there, it will be one more source of estrangement between those departments which deal with patients and those which do not." Addressing the dedication of the William H. Welch Medical Library of the Johns Hopkins University School of Medicine in 1929, he commented on the progressive decentralization of medical schools and the increasing specialization of preclinical and clinical departments, saying [24]:

> "More and more the preclinical chairs at most of our schools have come to be occupied by men whose scientific interests may be quite unrelated to anything that obviously has to do with Medicine, some of whom I, indeed, confess to a feeling that by engaging in problems that have an evident bearing on the healing art they lose caste among their fellows. They have come to have their own societies, separate journals of publication, a scientific lingo foreign to other ears, and are rarely seen in meetings of medical practitioners, with whom they have wholly lost contact."

Similarly, Fuller Albright described the split personality of members of the American Society for Clinical Investigation. In his 1944 Presidential Address [18] he said that a member is "one trying to ride two horses—attempting to be an investigator and a clinician at one and the same time... this rider of two horses, however, must remember that there are two horses;

he must avoid the danger on one side that he, as a clinician, be swamped with patients and the equal danger on the other side that he, an investigator, be segregated entirely from the bedside." Amid the large initiatives to foster translational research (ie, moving from bench to bedside), it would be well to recognize that the interplay, from bedside to bench and back in multiple iterations, was brought us to the point where one can successfully treat individuals afflicted with the group of disorders called "Cushing's syndrome." Only the continued interplay will allow further progress.

References

[1] Rolleston HD. The endocrine organs in health and disease. London: Oxford Univ. Press; 1936.
[2] Medvei VC. A history of endocrinology. Lancaster (UK): MTP Press; 1982.
[3] Welbourne RB. The history of endocrine surgery. New York: Praeger; 1990.
[4] Lindholm J. Cushing's syndrome: historical aspects. Pituitary 2000;3:97–104.
[5] Aron DC. The path to the soul: Harvey Cushing and surgery on the pituitary and its environs in 1916. Perspect Biol Med 1994;37:1551–60.
[6] Liddle GW, Shute AM. The evolution of Cushing's syndrome as a clinical entity. Adv Intern Med 1969;15:155–75.
[7] King LS. Medical thinking. A historical preface. Princeton (NJ): Princeton University Press; 1982.
[8] Cushing H. The pituitary body and its disorders. Philadelphia: J.B. Lippincott; 1912.
[9] Fulton JF. Harvey Cushing: a biography. Springfield (IL): Charles C Thomas; 1946.
[10] Swazey JP, Reeds K. Today's medicine, tomorrow's science. Essays on paths of discovery in the biomedical sciences. DHEW Publication No. (NIH) 78–244. US Department of Health, Education, and Welfare Public Health Service National Institutes of Health [1978]. Available at: http://newman.baruch.cuny.edu/digital/2001/swazey_reeds_1978/default.htm. Accessed February 9, 2005.
[11] Savitz SI. Cushing's contributions to neuroscience, part 2: Cushing and several dwarfs. Neuroscientist 2001;7:469–73.
[12] Cushing H. The Weir Mitchell Lecture. Surgical experiences with pituitary disorders. JAMA 1914;63:1515–25.
[13] Cushing H. Partial hypophysectomy for acromegaly with remarks on the function of the hypophysis. Ann Surg 1909;50:1002–17.
[14] Cushing H. The basophil adenomas of the pituitary body and their clinical manifestations (pituitary basophilism). Johns Hopkins Hospital Bull 1932;50:137–95.
[15] Albright F. Presidential Address to the American Society for Clinical Investigation, Atlantic City, New Jersey, May 8, 1944. Some of the "do's" and "do-not's" of clinical investigation. J Clin Invest 1944;23:921–6.
[16] Schwartz TB. How to learn from patients: Fuller Albright's exploration of adrenal function. Ann Intern Med 1995;123:225–9.
[17] Garfield G. Essays of an information scientist: creativity, delayed recognition, and other essays. Current Contents 1989;12:3–10.
[18] Albright F. Cushing's syndrome: its pathology and physiology, its relationship to the adreno-genital syndrome, and its connection with the problem of the reaction of the body to injurious agents. Harvey Lect 1942–1943 1943;38:123–86.
[19] Bouillon R. The changing face of endocrinology. Karger Gazette 2003;16:1–3.

[20] Aron DC, Headrick LA. Educating physicians ready to improve care and safety is no accident: it requires a systematic approach. Qual Saf Health Care 2002;11:168–73.
[21] Feinstein AR. Basic biomedical science and the destruction of the pathophysiologic bridge from bench to bedside. Am J Med 1999;107:461–7.
[22] Nathan DG. Careers in translational clinical research—historical perspectives, future challenges. JAMA 2002;287:2424–7.
[23] Tilney NL. Harvey Cushing and the surgical research laboratory. Surg Gyn Obstet 1980;151: 263–70.
[24] Cushing H. The binding influence of a library on a subdividing profession in the medical career and other papers. Boston: Little Brown & Co.; 1940.

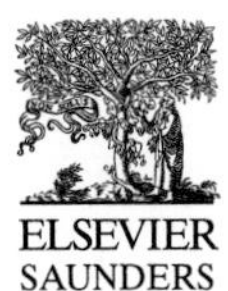
ELSEVIER
SAUNDERS

Endocrinol Metab Clin N Am
34 (2005) 271–292

ENDOCRINOLOGY
AND METABOLISM
CLINICS
OF NORTH AMERICA

Hypothalamic–Pituitary–Adrenocortical Axis Regulation

Lauren Jacobson, PhD

Center for Neuropharmacology and Neuroscience, Albany Medical College, MC-136, Albany, NY 12208, USA

The hypothalamic–pituitary–adrenocortical (HPA) axis is a classic neuroendocrine system subserving control of adrenocortical glucocorticoid secretion by the brain. As covered elsewhere in this issue, glucocorticoids have a variety of effects on peripheral tissues that can roughly be categorized as prioritizing energy use and distribution toward overcoming the homeostatic challenge posed by stress. These actions include effects on metabolism, cardiovascular tone, and immune reactivity [1]. Glucocorticoids also have complex and seemingly contradictory effects on mood and cognition that can be viewed as increasing the positive and negative salience of external stimuli [2–4]. These effects dictate tight control of glucocorticoid secretion, not only to be able to respond appropriately to stress, but also to minimize the deleterious effects of glucocorticoid excess. This article discusses the mechanisms by which glucocorticoids are normally controlled and the pathophysiological significance of defects in these control mechanisms (Fig. 1).

Components of the hypothalamic–pituitary–adrenocortical axis

The adrenal cortex

The zona fasciculata cells of the adrenal cortex synthesize and secrete glucocorticoids in response to corticotropin (ACTH) secreted by corticotroph cells of the anterior pituitary. Cortisol is the main glucocorticoid produced by the human adrenal cortex; in rodents, which do not express 17α-hydroxylase, corticosterone is the only adrenal glucocorticoid [5]. ACTH stimulates adrenocortical steroidogenesis and secretion by means of the

E-mail address: jacobsl@mail.amc.edu

0889-8529/05/$ - see front matter
doi:10.1016/j.ecl.2005.01.003 ***endo.theclinics.com***

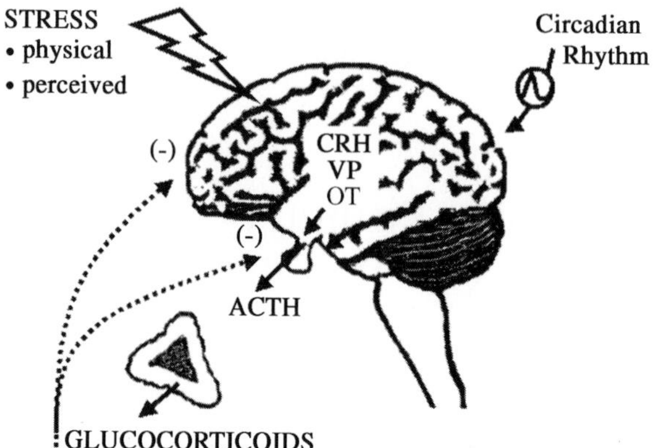

Fig. 1. Major stimulatory (*solid lines*) and inhibitory regulators (*dotted lines*) of the HPA axis. Glucocorticoid secretion by the adrenal cortex is stimulated by ACTH from corticotroph cells of the anterior pituitary. ACTH, in turn, is regulated by multiple hypothalamic factors. Corticotropin-releasing hormone (CRH), in combination with vasopressin (VP) and oxytocin (OT), stimulates ACTH release. Hypothalamic ACTH-releasing factor neurons are regulated by afferent pathways conveying sensory and cognitive information. HPA activity increases in response to stress and in a circadian rhythm paralleling the activity cycle. Glucocorticoids ultimately regulate their own secretion by feedback inhibition of stress-induced and circadian HPA activity. The brain, which expresses both glucocorticoid receptors and high-affinity mineralocorticoid receptors, is most sensitive to glucocorticoid negative feedback. Sustained elevations in glucocorticoids also can inhibit ACTH secretion by means of glucocorticoid receptors in the anterior pituitary. Other factors, including immune and metabolic signals, may provide additional feedback control by regulating and being regulated by glucocorticoids.

G protein-coupled melanocortin-2 receptor [6]. As its name implies, ACTH is also critical for trophic support of the adrenal cortex. In the absence of ACTH, the adrenal cortex undergoes apoptosis and loses secretory capacity [7]. Conversely, chronic ACTH stimulation causes an increase in size, cell number, and secretory activity of the zona fasiculata [5]. This effect accounts for the increased adrenal size or ACTH sensitivity sometimes observed in pituitary-dependent Cushing's syndrome or in depressed patients exhibiting HPA hyperactivity [8–10]. The proliferative effect of ACTH recently has been proposed to be due to increased vascularization and paracrine growth factor secretion in the adrenal cortex, rather than to direct stimulation of adrenocortical cells; non-ACTH fragments of the pro-opiomelanocortin (POMC) precursor molecule also may be involved [7,11,12].

Glucocorticoid secretion depends on ACTH levels and on adrenal nerves. Maximal glucocorticoid secretion occurs at relatively low plasma levels of ACTH. When the duration of ACTH-induced glucocorticoid secretion is taken into account, however, total integrated glucocorticoid secretion is directly related to ACTH over an approximately 100-fold range of plasma ACTH concentrations [13]. Splanchnic nerve innervation of the adrenal also influences adrenocortical responsiveness to ACTH in a complex manner that depends on the circadian cycle and the nature of the stimulus. Splanchnic nerve activity may be inhibitory at the trough of the circadian rhythm, while enhancing glucocorticoid secretion at the circadian peak or during stress [14]. Thus, while adrenocortical glucocorticoid secretion is tied closely to the stimulatory signal it receives, it can be difficult to infer hypothalamic–pituitary activity from limited glucocorticoid measurements, particularly under stimulated conditions.

The corticotroph

The corticotroph cells of the anterior pituitary produce ACTH by selective proteolytic processing of POMC. This cleavage, performed by prohormone convertase 1, results in the production and secretion of an N-terminal peptide, $ACTH_{1\text{-}39}$, and β-lipotropin [15]. The corticotroph does not produce α-melanocyte–stimulating hormone (α-MSH). Unlike other POMC-expressing cells, such as the melanotrophs of the neurointermediate lobe and the POMC neurons of the arcuate hypothalamus, corticotrophs do not express the prohormone convertase 2 enzyme necessary to cleave α-MSH from the ACTH molecule [15].

Corticotrophs are controlled by several stimulatory hypothalamic factors. Of these, the 41 amino acid corticotropin-releasing hormone (CRH) is the most potent. CRH increases ACTH secretion and *POMC* gene expression in corticotrophs through the G protein-coupled CRH receptor-1 [16–18]. Vasopressin and oxytocin, two related 9 amino acid peptides, typically play accessory roles to CRH in regulating ACTH secretion. Vasopressin and oxytocin have only weak ACTH-releasing activity on their own, but in combination with CRH, each evokes greater ACTH secretion than can be attributed to the additive effects of each individual hormone [19–21]. CRH also has the most consistent effects to stimulate *POMC* gene expression [16]. Evidence to date indicates that both vasopressin and oxytocin stimulate ACTH secretion through the V1b vasopressin receptor, also known as the V3 receptor [22,23].

Unlike the adrenocortical dependence on ACTH, corticotrophs do not require CRH for trophic support. Corticotrophs appear developmentally before hypothalamic CRH expression and appear normal in CRH and CRH receptor-1 knockout mice [17,18,24], although the POMC precursor may not be processed fully in the absence of CRH [25]. Appropriate developmental and hormonal regulation of *POMC* gene expression is conferred by trans-acting factors binding within the proximal 450 bp of the POMC promoter [26,27]. One of these factors, TPit, has been shown to be required to prevent differentiation of corticotrophs into other pituitary cell types; mutations in TPit occur in a high percentage of patients who have isolated ACTH deficiency [28,29].

ACTH-releasing factor neurons

This article focuses on CRH, vasopressin, and oxytocin as hypothalamic ACTH secretagogues. Epinephrine also has been measured at elevated levels in portal blood and may play a role in stress-induced ACTH secretion. However, epinephrine is unlikely to originate from hypothalamic neurons, and its role in ACTH regulation in humans is uncertain [30].

Hypophysiotrophic CRH neurons are contained within the medial paraventricular hypothalamus (PVN) [31–33]. Vasopressin is expressed by magnocellular neurons of the PVN, magnocellular neurons of the supraoptic nucleus (SON), and by CRH neurons in the parvocellular PVN [33]. Oxytocin is expressed by magnocellular neurons of the PVN and SON, in neurons that are largely (except during lactation) different from those expressing vasopressin [34]. The terms, magnocellular and parvocellular will respectively be used here to distinguish between PVN vasopressin neurons projecting to the posterior pituitary and those regulating ACTH through projections to the external zone of the median eminence. These divisions, however, may be less anatomically distinct in other species such as the mouse [33].

This neuroanatomical distribution notwithstanding, expression of CRH, vasopressin, and oxytocin exhibits some plasticity. Many CRH neurons express vasopressin under basal conditions and upregulate vasopressin in response to stimulation [33]. Cosecretion of vasopressin and CRH would enhance ACTH when these neurons are activated [33]. Oxytocin neurons also express low levels of CRH basally and much higher levels after chronic osmotic stimuli [35]. Both vasopressin expression by CRH neurons and induction of CRH in oxytocin neurons are inhibited by glucocorticoids [33,34]. This glucocorticoid dependence makes it likely that the plasticity in ACTH secretagogue expression contributes to maintaining appropriate glucocorticoid levels.

The PVN also has prominent descending projections that express CRH, vasopressin, and oxytocin. At least in the rat, these fibers originate from PVN regions that are topographically distinct from those for neuroendocrine neurons [35–37]. Descending PVN projections terminate monosynaptically in virtually all of the brainstem and spinal cord areas containing parasympathetic and sympathetic preganglionic neurons [37]. Although not formally part of the neuroendocrine HPA axis, these projections have the potential to influence adrenocortical activity indirectly by influencing activity of the adrenal sympathetic innervation.

Glucocorticoid feedback

Glucocorticoid feedback inhibition occurs in several time domains, referred to as fast, delayed (or intermediate), and slow feedback [38]. As the first two of these domains refer specifically to inhibition of stimulated HPA activity, mechanisms for this inhibition are discussed in the sections on circadian and stress-induced HPA activity. Slow feedback, reflecting chronic exposure to glucocorticoids over days or weeks, affects both basal and stimulated hypothalamic–pituitary activity. Removal of normal glucocorticoid feedback by surgical or chemical adrenalectomy increases plasma ACTH, anterior pituitary *POMC* gene expression, and the secretion and gene expression of *CRH* and *vasopressin* in neurons of the parvocellular PVN [5,33,39–44]. Posterior pituitary vasopressin is also responsive to glucocorticoid levels in dogs and humans [45]. Treatment of adrenalectomized rodents with fixed levels of corticosterone normalizes basal hypothalamic–pituitary activity when glucocorticoid levels approximate the normal circadian mean. When chronic glucocorticoid exposure of adrenalectomized or intact subjects exceeds the 24-hour mean, the capacity of the HPA axis to respond to stimulation, and ultimately to maintain basal activity, is suppressed [46]. Sustained high levels of glucocorticoids, as may occur in Cushing's patients, or in patients given immunosuppressive steroid therapy, inhibit ACTH and its antiapoptotic effects on the adrenal cortex. Depending on the duration and level of glucocorticoid exposure, the resulting adrenal insufficiency can take up to a year to reverse and poses a significant risk of morbidity and mortality [47].

Two receptors mediate the effects of endogenous adrenal glucocorticoids, the higher affinity, low-capacity mineralocorticoid receptor (MR, or type I), and the lower affinity, high-capacity glucocorticoid receptor (GR, or type II). MR expression is restricted to peripheral aldosterone targets such as kidney and colon, and to a limited number of brain regions. GR is expressed widely in many peripheral tissues and brain regions [48]. MR in peripheral target tissues is normally protected from binding adrenal glucocorticoids by the action of type 2 11β-hydroxysteroid dehydrogenase, which converts cortisol or corticosterone to their inactive 11-dehydro forms [49].

By virtue of having higher levels of MR, the brain is more sensitive than the corticotroph to glucocorticoid feedback. Although some MRs are present in the anterior pituitary, both ligand binding and functional pharmacology studies indicate that GR effects predominate in the pituitary [50–52], while inhibition of the brain–pituitary unit displays characteristics of MR regulation [53–55]. Comparison of brain and pituitary sensitivity to feedback in rats with PVN or sham lesions indicates that without hypophysiotrophic input, ACTH fails to respond to the removal of glucocorticoid feedback. Supraphysiologic glucocorticoid levels (ie, in excess of the normal daily mean) also are required to inhibit CRH-induced ACTH secretion in PVN-lesioned rats [56]. Adrenalectomy-induced increases in ACTH are also lacking in the CRH knockout mouse [25]. Thus, brain input is required for appropriate ACTH responses to changes in glucocorticoid feedback. GR-mediated feedback inhibition at the pituitary only occurs at chronic glucocorticoid levels that incur adverse peripheral effects [5].

Like the corticotroph, however, the PVN and the rest of the hypothalamus also only express GR [48,57]. MR expression is highest in the hippocampus and septum, with moderate levels in the amygdala, cranial nerve nuclei, and autonomic relays such as the nucleus of the solitary tract (NTS) and nucleus ambiguus [50,58]. These expression patterns suggest that MR-dependent inhibition of hypothalamic activity is mediated by extra-hypothalamic sites.

Glucocorticoid receptors expressed in many brain nuclei, including most regions of MR expression [48,57]. Colocalization of MR and GR has been shown in hippocampal CA1 and CA2 pyramidal neurons [59]. This overlap between GR and MR expression may be significant, because heterodimerization between MR and GR has unique effects on gene expression in vitro [60]. Given the widespread expression of GR in hindbrain and forebrain sources of afferents to the PVN [48,57], GR-mediated feedback is also likely to occur at multiple sites proximal to the CRH neuron. Support for this possibility comes from the inhibitory effects on HPA activity of localized steroid implants [61–64]. As might be predicted from the undesirable effects of chronic GR occupancy, these inhibitory effects are limited to stimulated HPA activity, and are discussed as they relate to circadian- or stress-induced HPA function.

Circadian hypothalamic–pituitary–adrenocortical activity

Glucocorticoid levels in the unstressed state vary in a circadian rhythm. This rhythm anticipates circadian rhythms in activity, with peak glucocorticoid levels occurring in the 2- to 4-hour window around waking, and nadir levels occurring in a similar time frame around sleep onset. In humans, who are normally diurnally active, peak glucocorticoids occur in the early morning, while trough levels occur around 11 pm [65]. In nocturnally active rodents, this cycle is reversed.

Central control of the circadian rhythm in hypothalamic–pituitary–adrenocortical activity

Increased glucocorticoid secretion at the circadian peak depends on increased hypothalamic–pituitary activity and on increased sensitivity of the adrenal cortex to ACTH [5,66]. There is negligible hypothalamic drive for glucocorticoid secretion at the circadian nadir, and glucocorticoids may be virtually undetectable at this time [5]. The circadian rhythm in HPA activity occurs in the absence of light cues and depends on the hypothalamic suprachiasmatic nucleus (SCN). The SCN has a net effect to stimulate peak hypothalamic–pituitary activity [67]; there also may be an inhibitory influence on adrenocortical activity at the circadian nadir [68,69]. Food intake also serves as a pattern generator for HPA activity that is both independent of the SCN, and, if dissociated from normal activity and light cycle cues, capable of overriding SCN control [66,70]. The ventromedial hypothalamus (VMH) is an important, although possibly not the only, mediator of food-entrained HPA activity [70]. These SCN- and feeding-dependent mechanisms may explain why rhythms in hypothalamic *CRH* gene expression do not fully predict those of pituitary-adrenal activity [42,71], and why diurnal variations in adrenocortical activity do not require cyclic variations in CRH [72].

Glucocorticoid feedback control of the circadian rhythm in hypothalamic–pituitary–adrenocortical activity

Hypothalamic–pituitary activity exhibits circadian rhythmicity in the absence of glucocorticoids, but the set-point and amplitude of this rhythm are highly sensitive to feedback inhibition. Feedback inhibition provides precisely timed and controlled glucocorticoid levels over an approximately 200-fold range. The low levels of corticosterone necessary to normalize circadian nadir ACTH secretion in adrenalectomized rodents suggest that feedback regulation at this time of day is mediated by MR [5,39,42,73]. This prediction is borne out by elevations in basal ACTH and glucocorticoids after acute administration of MR, but not GR, antagonists [39,54,55]. MR knockout mice also have been reported to have significantly elevated circadian nadir glucocorticoid levels [74]. Although some investigators have reported that 24-hour mean corticosterone levels also normalize *CRH* and *vasopressin* expression [44], this has not been a consistent finding [39,40,42]. Dissociation between *ACTH* secretagogue gene expression and plasma ACTH, which reflects secretagogue release, further suggests that inhibition of ACTH-releasing factor secretion occurs proximal to the hypophysiotrophic neurons themselves [5].

Appropriate regulation of circadian peak HPA activity requires GR and MR occupancy. This effect is consistent with the predicted capacity of GR to bind the higher levels of glucocorticoids secreted during this period. Central drive for these higher glucocorticoid levels is revealed when adrenal steroid synthesis is impaired [75,76] or blocked by adrenalectomy and low-level glucocorticoid replacement. Under these conditions, marked increases in plasma ACTH, anterior pituitary *POMC* mRNA, and parvocellular PVN *CRH* and *vasopressin* gene expression occur at the circadian peak [5, 39,42,44]. Chronic GR blockade by systemic administration of the glucocorticoid antagonist RU 486 also only disinhibits HPA activity at the circadian peak [77,78]. Brain sites for GR-mediated feedback of circadian activity have not been investigated extensively. Implants of RU 486 over the NTS, however, have been found to increase circadian peak glucocorticoid levels selectively [64], consistent with the peak-specific effects of systemic RU 486 [77,78].

Mineralocorticoid receptor occupancy also is required to control circadian peak HPA axis activity. Acute and chronic administration of MR antagonists has been shown to increase circadian peak and trough levels of HPA axis activity in rodents and people [39,54,55]. It also has been suggested that MR binding capacity is greater than initially estimated [79], implying that MR may regulate stimulated HPA activity not only by establishing the baseline set-point, but also by mediating effects of stimulus-induced glucocorticoid secretion. MR inhibition of peak and trough HPA activity ultimately ensures that peripheral glucocorticoid effects, which are mediated exclusively by GR, are limited to the minimum necessary for physiological benefit [46].

The high levels of MR and GR in the hippocampus [48] have made them attractive candidates to mediate feedback regulation of circadian HPA activity. Although not all studies support this idea [63], the studies that have shown effects of hippocampal manipulations have been relatively consistent. Lesions of the hippocampus or its main projection pathway, the fornix, have been reported to disinhibit HPA activity at the circadian nadir, while hippocampal corticosterone implants inhibit circadian nadir levels of plasma ACTH in adrenalectomized rats [63]. More localized lesions of the ventral subiculum, or of its projections in the lateral fornix, can recapitulate the increases in plasma ACTH and PVN *CRH* gene expression predicted from loss of glucocorticoid feedback at the circadian nadir [63]. The ventral subiculum receives input from the MR-expressing CA1 region of the hippocampus [48,80,81] and projects to inhibitory γ-aminobutyric acid (GABA)ergic neurons in the peri-PVN that impinge on CRH neurons [63,80,81]. Collectively, these data suggest a mechanism by which the hippocampus might inhibit circadian HPA activity.

Pathophysiology of altered circadian hypothalamic–pituitary–adrenocortical activity

Maintaining low glucocorticoid concentrations for the 4 to 6 hours of the circadian nadir is important for avoiding the effects of glucocorticoid excess on peripheral tissues. Peripheral glucocorticoid effects have often been termed "permissive" to recognize that they do not require increases in glucocorticoids at the time of stress, or to the levels observed during stress, to confer the protective effects of glucocorticoids on survival. This term is somewhat misleading, as it implies that glucocorticoid levels are of secondary importance, as long as some glucocorticoids are present. In fact, deviations from the set-points defined by the circadian rhythm have a marked impact on the regulation of HPA function and other glucocorticoid-sensitive endpoints. Rats given corticosterone implants that elevate circadian trough glucocorticoid levels inhibit their endogenous adrenocortical activity to keep 24-hour mean glucocorticoid levels constant. Despite similar 24-hour mean concentrations, however, rats with significantly elevated circadian trough levels of corticosterone show evidence of insulin resistance and immune suppression [46].

The consequences of inadequate glucocorticoid secretion at the circadian peak are less well-defined. In adrenalectomized rats, providing glucocorticoid replacement in a circadian pattern rather than at a constant level allows more efficient termination of ACTH responses to stress [82]. These results suggest that activation of the HPA axis is sensitive to prior levels of GR occupancy achieved during routine, unstressed HPA activity. Increased cortisol responses to stress also have been correlated with diminished amplitude of the circadian rhythm in humans [83].

Circadian HPA activity is disrupted in healthy individuals by shifts in the activity cycle, sleep deprivation, and aging. The lack of synchrony between glucocorticoid secretion and environmental cues has been suggested to contribute to the discomforts of shift work and jet lag [65,84]. Sleep debt elevates circadian nadir glucocorticoid levels and is associated with decreased glucose tolerance [65]. Thus, as in rats, there is evidence in humans that slight increments in baseline glucocorticoid secretion have significant metabolic effects. Circadian trough glucocorticoid levels also increase during normal human aging [85]; this process could contribute to the age-related weight gain and visceral fat deposition that has been identified as a major mortality and morbidity risk [86].

Several pathological states alter the circadian rhythm in glucocorticoids. Primary among these are Cushing's syndrome and mood disorders. A high proportion of depressed patients show evidence of elevated basal cortisol secretion [87]. Some of these patients experience psychiatric improvement after treatments that interfere with glucocorticoid synthesis or receptor binding [88–90], suggesting that increased glucocorticoid secretion may be contributing to, and not just reflecting, disease pathology.

Stress-induced hypothalamic–pituitary–adrenocortical activity

Stress is any actual or perceived threat to well-being. Although originally dubbed a nonspecific response by Selye [91] because of its reliability, stress-induced HPA activity is a highly specific process, mediated by stressor-specific afferent inputs to the hypothalamus and transduced into an endocrine signal by specific combinations of hypothalamic ACTH-releasing factors. These features in turn produce a pituitary-adrenal response that is related directly to stimulus intensity [5].

Afferent pathways for stress-induced hypothalamic–pituitary–adrenocortical activity

As thoughtfully refined and enunciated by Herman et al, there are compelling arguments that neural coding of the HPA response depends on stressor modality [63]. A physical stressor, defined as a situation posing a real threat of tissue damage or death if uncorrected, typically stimulates HPA activity by means of defined somatosensory, viscerosensory, or osmosensory afferent pathways. Most of these projections arise from the brainstem or diencephalon [63]. Selective lesions have been used to demonstrate the dependence of HPA responses to hemorrhage, hypoglycemia, hypoxia, and systemic interleukin (IL)-1β administration on projections from the NTS and ventrolateral medulla [35,92–94]. These areas serve as relays for baroreceptor, chemoreceptor, and vagal afferents and play a role in brain glucose sensing [94–96]. The dependence on medullary projections is stimulus-specific, because lesions impairing responses to osmotic stimuli do not have generalized effects on medulla-dependent stressors [35].

In contrast, stressors with a predominantly psychological component, in which the individual is subjectively, but not objectively, in danger, have been proposed to depend less on primary sensory relays and more heavily on the forebrain [63]. This proposal is based on the failure of medullary lesions to affect hypothalamic responses to the predominantly psychological stress of footshock [97], and on the ability of prefrontal cortex and ventral subiculum lesions to selectively disinhibit HPA responses to the psychological stress of restraint [62,63]. In contrast, prefrontal cortex and ventral subiculum lesions did not affect HPA responses to the physical stimulus of ether inhalation [62,63]. Prefrontal cortex lesions also did not alter circadian variations in pituitary–adrenal activity [62], suggesting that pathways engaged by restraint stress are distinct from those for circadian cues. Similar distinctions have been put forward for the respective roles of the central and medial nuclei of the amygdala in stimulating HPA responses to physical and psychological stimuli [63].

Nevertheless, exceptions to these distinctions are emerging. Ventral subiculum lesions were recently found to inhibit glucocorticoid responses to hypoxia [98], suggesting that physical stressors are not uniformly independent of forebrain control. Conversely, activation of CRH neurons by restraint is decreased by medullary lesions, indicating that a primarily psychological stressor is not fully independent of lower order ascending inputs [99]. These complexities suggest that stressors may be multi-modal and dependent on unique neurocircuitries.

Corticotropin secretagogue responses to stress

Stress-related afferent impulses are translated by the hypothalamus into specific combinations of ACTH secretagogues. Although all approaches to assessing secretion of CRH, vasopressin, and oxytocin have limitations, consensus nonetheless has emerged regarding the roles of these ACTH-releasing factors in HPA responses to stress. Consistent with the strong dependence of ACTH secretion on CRH, PVN CRH neurons exhibit some degree of activation in response to all stressors, whether this activation is determined by assay of portal blood CRH, CRH depletion from nerve terminals in the external median eminence, increases in *CRH* gene expression, or induction of the neuronal activity marker, Fos, in CRH neurons [33,35,63,100].

In contrast with the general stress-induced activation of CRH neurons, coding of stressor modality is accomplished by the involvement of vasopressin and oxytocin. A variety of physical stressors, including hypoglycemia, hemorrhage, immune stimuli, and ether inhalation, activate parvocellular PVN neurons expressing vasopressin and CRH [33,101]. PVN oxytocin neurons also may be recruited by physical stressors, with or without vasopressin involvement [35,100,102]. Where the relative involvement of vasopressin and oxytocin has been investigated, however, psychological stresses typically engage PVN oxytocin selectively over vasopressin neurons [103–105].

Stressors with osmotic or nausea-inducing components involve a strong, but not exclusive, contribution from neurohypophysial vasopressin and oxytocin; this contribution is demonstrable as decreased plasma ACTH in rats in which magnocellular neuron activity is inhibited by hyponatremia. In contrast, responses to hypoglycemia and novelty are unimpaired by suppressing neurohypophysial function [106]. These results suggest that the vasopressin and oxytocin involved in the latter responses [33,105] are derived from adenohypophysially-relevant PVN projections to the median eminence. In summary, multi-factorial combinations of CRH with vasopressin and oxytocin dictate ACTH responses to stress, with a bias toward combinations of CRH and oxytocin in psychological stress. Stress-specific contributions from magnocellular vasopressin and oxytocin neurons may further diversify ACTH responses to the same hormones.

Feedback regulation of hypothalamic–pituitary–adrenocortical responses to stress

Stress-induced HPA activity is subject to fast and delayed feedback. Fast feedback, evident within seconds of a stimulus, does not require protein synthesis, depends on the rate of increase in glucocorticoids, and is probably limited to inhibition of neuronal activity at the level of surface receptor signaling [5,38]. Glucocorticoids have recently been shown to inhibit PVN neuron excitability by means of retrograde endocannabinoid inhibition of presynaptic glutamate release. Glucocorticoid effects were rapid and could be demonstrated with cell-impermeant glucocorticoid conjugates, suggesting that this mechanism might contribute to fast feedback [107].

Delayed or intermediate feedback occurs within 30 minutes to hours, requires new protein synthesis, and can affect either corticotroph [108] or hypothalamic [38,109] responses to stimulation. At the level of the pituitary, vasopressin-induced ACTH secretion is less sensitive to intermediate glucocorticoid feedback [110]; this resistance could enhance the synergistic effect of vasopressin on CRH-induced ACTH release. At the level of the hypothalamus, CRH and vasopressin neurons are sensitive to glucocorticoid levels during stress. Clamping glucocorticoids around the 24-hour mean increases the amplitude of responses, while acute or chronic administration of higher levels inhibits responses [45,100,101,111,112]. Careful temporal tracking of parvocellular *CRH* and *vasopressin* gene transcription after ether stress indicates that the vasopressin is more likely to be inhibited effectively by glucocorticoids during stress [101]. It is unknown whether this feedback mechanism generalizes to other stresses, or whether it obviates the glucocorticoid-resistant effects of vasopressin on ACTH secretion. Hypothalamic oxytocin secretion appears to be insensitive to glucocorticoid inhibition [43,113], which could enhance ACTH responses to psychological or other stressors involving oxytocin neurons.

Brain sites potentially mediating feedback inhibition of HPA responses to stress have recently been reviewed in detail [63]. PVN infusion of the GR antagonist RU 486 enhances glucocorticoid responses to swim stress, indicating that the high level of PVN GR expression is relevant to feedback control of stress-induced HPA activity [114]. There is also compelling but incomplete evidence to suggest that the hippocampus and prefrontal cortex are involved in mediating glucocorticoid feedback inhibition of HPA responses to stress [63]. Particularly for the prefrontal cortex, feedback actions of glucocorticoids appear to be limited to inhibition of responses to psychological stress [62]. Although the amygdala also expresses high levels of GR and some MR [48], effects of lesions and steroid implants indicate that this region primarily mediates stimulatory drive, rather than corticosteroid-dependent inhibition, during stress [61,63]. Other corticosteroid receptor-expressing regions, notably the NTS, have also failed to show steroid-dependent changes in activity during stress [104]. GR- or MR-expressing neurons in these regions may be selectively responsive to specific stresses, or may, as has been shown for the hippocampus and amygdala [3,4], subserve functions unrelated to endocrine feedback [48,63].

Chronic stress

Chronic stress produces a state in which HPA axis responsiveness is preserved in spite of elevations in glucocorticoids. Whereas HPA responses to a repeated stress may be progressively inhibited (habituated), responses to a novel stimulus are enhanced (facilitated) [115]. Habituation and facilitation are respectively adaptive in minimizing the effects of excess glucocorticoid exposure while preserving adrenocortical function, which otherwise would be suppressed by habituation- and glucocorticoid-induced inhibition of ACTH secretion. Facilitation does not appear to depend on the physical or psychological modality of the stressors [115]. Increased expression of vasopressin in CRH neurons during chronic stress has been suggested to contribute to maintaining HPA responsivity during chronic stress [33,116], although additional, nonvasopressin-expressing CRH neurons also may be involved [117]. Chronic variable stress also alters expression of GABA-synthesizing enzymes in local, PVN-projecting neurons, which could provide stimulus-selective gating of afferent inputs to hypophysiotrophic neurons [118].

Additional control occurs through the posterior paraventricular thalamus, which has been shown to regulate changes in HPA activity during chronic stress. Lesions of this region reveal enhanced HPA responsiveness to stress and decreased sensitivity to glucocorticoid feedback that occur only in chronically stressed rats [119,120]. Thus, the paraventricular thalamus contributes to habituation of HPA activity during chronic stress by maintaining sensitivity to glucocorticoid feedback and by suppressing the facilitative effects of chronic stress.

As with acute stress, MR and GR appear to be involved in the effects of chronic stress on HPA activity. MR, but not GR, antagonism has been shown to prevent HPA habituation during repeated restraint stress [121]. However, the enhancing effects of chronic stress on responses to a novel stimulus are most apparent at corticosterone levels that substantially occupy GR suggesting a positive feedback effect [122,123]. This apparent GR-mediated, facilitative effect can be mimicked by central infusions of corticosterone that occupy GR in adrenalectomized rats. Unlike the inhibitory effects of peripheral elevations in corticosterone, central corticosterone increased basal and restraint-induced ACTH in adrenalectomized rats [124]. This unique facilitative action has been proposed to depend on the inhibitory effects of chronic stress on metabolic balance [115].

Pathophysiology of the hypothalamic–pituitary–adrenocortical stress response

The inability to initiate or appropriately terminate HPA responses to stress is maladaptive. The clinical consequences of inappropriate stress reactivity are recognized best in depression. Stress can precipitate depressive episodes in vulnerable individuals, and most depressed patients exhibit elevated HPA activity reminiscent of that in chronic stress [125,126]. Fast feedback, which specifically affects stimulated HPA activity [38], has been reported to be defective in depression [127]. As discussed previously, reversing abnormal HPA activity has been suggested not only to depend on, but possibly to be required for, successful treatment [128].

More subtle deviations in stress-induced HPA activity may still contribute to health problems. Symptoms of the metabolic X syndrome (visceral obesity, hypertension, type 2 diabetes) have considerable overlap with Cushingoid features [129]. In otherwise normal men, these features cosegregate with increased cortisol responses to subjectively reported stress [83], suggesting that HPA over-reactivity ultimately might contribute to metabolic dysregulation.

Other regulators of hypothalamic–pituitary–adrenocortical activity

Cytokines

Cytokines, including the interleukins, interferons, colony-stimulating factors, and tumor necrosis factor, are soluble molecules that are produced by immune cells and function as chemotactic, growth, and differentiation factors. Like hormones, cytokines circulate in blood and have direct effects on several endocrine tissues. Receptors for several cytokines have been identified in the adrenal, anterior pituitary, and brain [130]. Most cytokines stimulate HPA activity; these effects probably account for early observations that infectious stimuli could elicit adrenocortical activity in rodents in which either the PVN or the pituitary had been ablated [5]. Increased cytokines, particularly IL-6, have also been measured during nonimmune stimuli such as restraint [131]. Although the significance of this effect is unclear, IL-6 recently has been shown to contribute significantly to adrenocortical activity [132]. Cytokine signaling therefore may have an even more general role in endocrine function than previously appreciated. From an immune perspective, cytokine stimulation of glucocorticoid secretion is adaptive in promoting catabolism to supply the metabolic demands of antimicrobial or wound healing defenses, in supporting the acute phase response, and in preventing potentially fatal overactivation of the immune response [1]. In this latter respect, glucocorticoids exert negative feedback on a neuroimmune axis, as originally envisaged by Blalock and Besedovsky [130].

Leptin

The adipocyte hormone leptin has emerged as a major regulator of neuroendocrine function. Produced in proportion to fat mass, leptin indicates whether energy stores are sufficient to support energy-expensive endocrine functions, such as reproduction, or whether energy-conserving measures are required. During starvation, decreases in leptin stimulate increases in HPA activity [133]. Elevated cortisol in anorexia nervosa and in highly trained athletes probably results from leptin deficit induced by food restriction or intensive energy expenditure [134–137]. Leptin has an overall inhibitory effect on HPA activity [133], which can be viewed as suppressing the appetite-stimulating effects of glucocorticoids that would be appropriate during starvation. Leptin is capable of inhibiting adrenalectomy-induced increases in *CRH* gene expression in a manner that is additive with that of glucocorticoids [138]. Because glucocorticoids, in combination with insulin, also promote fat deposition and leptin expression the expression of leptin [139], leptin inhibition of HPA activity may represent a metabolic–neuroendocrine feedback loop, whereby leptin signals to the brain that glucocorticoid levels are sufficient for adequate fat storage.

Summary

As befits a system essential for survival, the HPA axis exhibits considerable plasticity at every level. The adrenal cortex is capable of marked changes in growth, activity, and sensitivity. The corticotroph exhibits differential responses to different combinations of multiple hypothalamic secretagogues. Control of CRH, vasopressin, and oxytocin is encoded by stimulus-specific afferent input to the hypothalamus, with relatively direct primary sensory inputs but more indirect input from higher forebrain structures involved in cognitive or affective processing. Chronic stimulation of the HPA axis alters the complement of ACTH secretagogues expressed by selected hypophysiotrophic neurons and activates pathways required for appropriate habituation and maintenance of HPA activity. All of these functions are ultimately controlled by glucocorticoid feedback, which normally functions to provide the minimum amount of glucocorticoid exposure for maximum physiological benefit. Even slight deviations above the relatively low 24-hour mean glucocorticoid levels incur pathological consequences. Additional nuances of control are afforded by reciprocal regulation between glucocorticoids and the immune and metabolic systems. These inter-relationships suggest that feedback regulation of the HPA axis may be expanded beyond glucocorticoids to include effector molecules for each of the physiological functions that glucocorticoids control.

References

[1] Sapolsky RM, Romero LM, Munck AU. How do glucocorticoids influence stress responses? Integrating permissive, suppressive, stimulatory, and preparative actions. Endocr Rev 2000;21:55–89.

[2] Brown ES, Khan DA, Nejtek VA. The psychiatric side effects of corticosteroids. Ann Allergy Asthma Immunol 1999;83:495–504.

[3] McGaugh JL. Memory consolidation and the amygdala: a systems perspective. Trends Neurosci 2002;25:456–61.

[4] McGaugh JL, Roozendaal B. Role of adrenal stress hormones in forming lasting memories in the brain. Curr Opin Neurobiol 2002;12:205–12.

[5] Dallman MF, Akana SF, Cascio CS, et al. Regulation of ACTH secretion: variations on a theme of B. Rec Prog Horm Res 1987;43:113–73.

[6] Mountjoy KG, Robbins LS, Mortrud MT, et al. The cloning of a family of genes that encode the melanocortin receptors. Science 1992;257:1248–51.

[7] Thomas M, Keramidas M, Monchaux E, et al. Dual hormonal regulation of endocrine tissue mass and vasculature by adrenocorticotropin in the adrenal cortex. Endocrinology 2004;145:4320–9.

[8] Amsterdam JD, Maislin G, Droba M, et al. The ACTH stimulation test before and after clinical recovery from depression. Psychiatry Res 1987;20:325–36.

[9] Doppman JL. Adrenal imaging. In: DeGroot LJ, Jameson JL, DeGroot LJ, et al, editors. Endocrinology. 4th edition. Philadelphia: WB Saunders; 2001. p. 1747–66.

[10] Rubin RT, Phillips JJ, Sadow TF, et al. Adrenal gland volume in major depression. Increase during the depressive episode and decrease with successful treatment. Arch Gen Psychol 1995;52:213–8.

[11] Bicknell AB, Lowry PJ. Adrenal growth is controlled by expression of specific pro-opiomelanocortin serine protease in the outer adrenal cortex. Endocr Res 2002;28:589–95.

[12] Yaswen L, Diehl N, Brennan MB, et al. Obesity in the mouse model of pro-opiomelanocortin deficiency responds to peripheral melanocortin. Nat Med 1999;5: 1066–70.

[13] Keller-Wood ME, Shinsako J, Dallman MF. Integral as well as proportional adrenal responses to ACTH. Am J Physiol 1983;245:R53–9.

[14] Engeland WC. Functional innervation of the adrenal gland by the splanchnic nerve. Horm Metab Res 1998;30:311–4.

[15] Seidah NG, Benjannet S, Hamelin J, et al. The subtilisin/kexin family of precursor convertases: emphasis on PC1, PC2/7B2, POMC and the novel enzyme SKI-1. Ann N Y Acad Sci 1999;885:57–74.

[16] Levin N, Roberts JL. Positive regulation of proopiomelanocortin gene expression in corticotropes and melanotropes. Front Neuroendocrinol 1991;12:1–22.

[17] Smith GW, Aubry JM, Dellu F, et al. Corticotropin releasing factor receptor 1-deficient mice display decreased anxiety, impaired stress response, and aberrant neuroendocrine development. Neuron 1998;20:1093–102.

[18] Timpl P, Spanagel R, Sillaber I, et al. Impaired stress response and reduced anxiety in mice lacking a functional corticotropin-releasing hormone receptor 1. Nat Genet 1998;19:162–6.

[19] Link H, Dayanithi G, Fohr KJ, et al. Oxytocin at physiological concentrations evokes adrenocorticotropin (ACTH) release from corticotrophs by increasing intracellular free calcium mobilized mainly from intracellular stores. Oxytocin displays synergistic or additive effects on ACTH-releasing factor or arginine vasopressin-induced ACTH secretion, respectively. Endocrinology 1992;130:2183–91.

[20] Liu JH, Muse K, Contreras P, et al. Augmentation of ACTH-releasing activity of synthetic corticotropin releasing factor (CRF) by vasopressin in women. J Clin Endocrinol Metab 1983;57:1087–9.

[21] Vale WW, Vaughan J, Smith M, et al. Effects of synthetic ovine corticotropin-releasing factor, glucocorticoids, catecholamines, neurohypophysial peptides, and other substances on cultured corticotrophic cells. Endocrinology 1983;13:1121–30.

[22] Schlosser SF, Almeida OF, Patchev VK, et al. Oxytocin-stimulated release of adrenocorticotropin from the rat pituitary is mediated by arginine vasopressin receptors of the V1b type. Endocrinology 1994;135:2058–63.

[23] Tanoue A, Ito S, Honda K, Oshikawa S, et al. The vasopressin V1b receptor critically regulates hypothalamic-pituitary-adrenal axis activity under both stress and resting conditions. J Clin Invest 2004;113:302–9.

[24] Venihaki M, Majzoub JA. Animal models of CRH deficiency. Front Neuroendocrinol 1999;20:122–45.

[25] Muglia LJ, Jacobson L, Luedke CE, et al. Corticotropin-releasing hormone links pituitary adrenocorticotropin gene expression and release during adrenal insufficiency. J Clin Invest 2000;105:1269–77.

[26] Liu B, Hammer GD, Rubinstein M, et al. Identification of DNA elements cooperatively activating proopiomelanocortin gene expression in the pituitary glands of transgenic mice. Mol Cell Biol 1992;12:3978–90.

[27] Phillips A, Lesage S, Gingras R, et al. Novel dimeric Nur77 signaling mechanism in endocrine and lymphoid cells. Mol Cell Biol 1997;17:5946–51.

[28] Pulichino AM, Vallette-Kasic S, Couture C, et al. Human and mouse TPIT gene mutations cause early onset pituitary ACTH deficiency. Genes Dev 2003;17:711–6.

[29] Pulichino AM, Vallette-Kasic S, Tsai JPY, et al. Tpit determines alternate fates during pituitary cell differentiation. Genes Dev 2003;17:738–47.

[30] Plotsky PM, Cunningham ET, Widmaier EP. Catecholaminergic modulation of corticotropin-releasing factor and adrenocorticotropin secretion. Endocr Rev 1989;10:437–58.

[31] Mouri T, Itoi K, Takahashi K, et al. Colocalization of corticotropin-releasing factor and vasopressin in the paraventricular nucleus of the human hypothalamus. Neuroendocrinology 1993;57:34–9.

[32] Raadsheer FC, Sluiter AA, Ravid R, et al. Localization of corticotropin-releasing hormone (CRH) neurons in the paraventricular nucleus of the human hypothalamus: age-dependent colocalization with vasopressin. Brain Res 1993;615:50–62.

[33] Whitnall MH. Regulation of the hypothalamic corticotropin-releasing hormone neurosecretory system. Prog Neurobiology 1993;40:573–629.

[34] Gainer H, Yamashita M, Fields RL, et al. The magnocellular neuronal phenotype: cell-specific gene expression in the hypothalamo-neurohypophysial system. Prog Brain Res 2002;139:1–14.
[35] Sawchenko PE, Brown ER, Chan RK, et al. The paraventricular nucleus of the hypothalamus and the functional neuroanatomy of visceromotor responses to stress. Prog Brain Res 1996;107:201–22.
[36] Dohanics J, Kovacs KJ, Makara GB. Oxytocinergic neurons in rat hypothalamus: dexamethasone-reversible increases in their corticotropin-releasing factor 1–41 immunoreactivity in response to osmotic stimulation. Neuroendocrinology 1990;51:515–22.
[37] Palkovits M. Interconnections between the neuroendocrine hypothalamus and the central autonomic system. Front Neuroendocrinol 1999;20:270–95.
[38] Keller-Wood ME, Dallman MF. Corticosteroid inhibition of ACTH secretion. Endocr Rev 1984;5:1–24.
[39] Bradbury MJ, Akana SF, Dallman MF. Roles of type I and II corticosteroid receptors in regulation of basal activity in the hypothalamo-pituitary-adrenal axis during the diurnal trough and the peak: evidence for a nonadditive effect of combined receptor occupation. Endocrinology 1994;34:1286–96.
[40] Herman JP. In situ hybridization analysis of vasopressin gene transcription in the paraventricular and supraoptic nuclei of the rat: regulation by stress and glucocorticoids. J Comp Neurol 1995;363:15–27.
[41] Herman JP, Schafer MK, Thompson RC, et al. Rapid regulation of corticotropin-releasing hormone gene transcription in vivo. Mol Endocrinol 1992;6:1061–9.
[42] Kwak SP, Morano MI, Young EA, et al. Diurnal CRH mRNA rhythm in the hypothalamus: decreased expression in the evening is not dependent on endogenous glucocorticoids. Neuroendocrinology 1993;57:96–105.
[43] Plotsky PM, Sawchenko PE. Hypophysial-portal plasma levels, median eminence content, and immunohistochemical staining of corticotropin-releasing factor, arginine vasopressin, and oxytocin after pharmacological adrenalectomy. Endocrinology 1987; 120:1361–9.
[44] Watts AG, Tanimura S, Sanchez-Watts G. Corticotropin-releasing hormone and arginine vasopressin gene transcription in the hypothalamic paraventricular nucleus of unstressed rats: daily rhythms and their interactions with corticosterone. Endocrinology 2004;145: 529–40.
[45] Raff H. Glucocorticoid inhibition of neurohypophysial vasopressin secretion. Am J Physiol 1987;252:R635–44.
[46] Dallman MF, Akana SF, Bhatnagar S, et al. Bottomed out: metabolic significance of the circadian trough in glucocorticoid concentrations. Int J Obes 2000;24(Suppl 2):S40–6.
[47] Axelrod L. Perioperative management of patients treated with glucocorticoids. Endocrinol Metab Clin N Am 2003;32:367–83.
[48] DeKloet ER, Vreugdenhil E, Oitzl MS, et al. Brain corticosteroid receptor balance in health and disease. Endocr Rev 1998;19:269–301.
[49] Seckl JR. 11b-hydroxysteroid dehydrogenase in the brain: a novel regulator of glucocorticoid action? Front Neuroendocrinol 1997;18:49–99.
[50] Arriza JL, Simerly RB, Swanson LW, et al. The neuronal mineralocorticoid receptor as a mediator of glucocorticoid response. Neuron 1988;1:887–900.
[51] DeKloet R, Wallach G, McEwen BS. Differences in corticosterone and dexamethasone binding to rat brain and pituitary. Endocrinology 1975;96:598–609.
[52] Spencer RL, Young EA, Choo PH, et al. Adrenal steroid type I and type II receptor binding: estimates of in vivo receptor number, occupancy, and activation with varying level of steroid. Brain Res 1990;514:37–48.
[53] Dallman MF, Levin N, Cascio CS, et al. Pharmacological evidence that inhibition of diurnal adrenocorticotropin secretion by corticosteroids is mediated via type I corticosterone-preferring receptors. Endocrinology 1989;124:2844–50.

[54] Spencer RL, Kim PJ, Kalman BA, et al. Evidence for mineralocorticoid receptor facilitation of glucocorticoid receptor-dependent regulation of hypothalamic-pituitary-adrenal axis activity. Endocrinology 1998;139:2718–26.
[55] Young EA, Lopez JF, Murphy-Weinberg V, et al. The role of mineralocorticoid receptors in hypothalamic-pituitary-adrenal axis regulation in humans. J Clin Endocrinol Metab 1998;83:3339–45.
[56] Levin N, Shinsako J, Dallman MF. Corticosterone acts on the brain to inhibit adrenalectomy-induced adrenocorticotropin secretion. Endocrinology 1988;122:694–701.
[57] Aaronson M, Fuxe K, Dong Y. Localization of glucocorticoid receptor mRNA in male rat brain by in situ hybridization. Proc Natl Acad Sci U S A 1988;85:9331–5.
[58] Duncan GE, Stumpf WE. A combined autoradiographic and immunocytochemical study of 3H-corticosterone target neurons and catecholamine neurons in rat and mouse lower brain stem. Neuroendocrinology 1985;40:262–71.
[59] VanSteensel B, VanBinnedijk EP, Hornsby CD, et al. Partial colocalization of glucocorticoid and mineralocorticoid receptors in discrete compartments in nuclei of rat hippocampus neurons. J Cell Sci 1996;109:787–92.
[60] Trapp T, Rupprecht R, Castren M, et al. Heterodimerization between mineralocorticoid and glucocorticoid receptor: a new principle of glucocorticoid action in the CNS. Neuron 1994;13:1457–62.
[61] Akana SF, Chu A, Soriano L, et al. Corticosterone exerts site-specific and state-dependent effects in the prefrontal cortex and amygdala on regulation of adrenocorticotropic hormone, insulin and fat depots. J Neuroendocrinol 2001;13:625–37.
[62] Diorio D, Viau V, Meaney MJ. The role of the medial prefrontal cortex (cingulate gyrus) in the regulation of hypothalamic-pituitary-adrenal responses to stress. J Neurosci 1993; 13:3839–47.
[63] Herman JP, Figueiredo H, Mueller NK, et al. Central mechanisms of stress integration: hierarchical circuitry controlling hypothalamo-pituitary-adrenocortical responsiveness. Front Neuroendocrinol 2003;24:151–80.
[64] Scheuer DA, Bechtold AG, Shank SS, et al. Glucocorticoids act in the dorsal hindbrain to increase arterial pressure. Am J Physiol 2004;286:H458–67.
[65] VanCauter E, Copinschi G, Turek FW. Endocrine and other biologic rhythms. In: DeGroot LJ, Jameson JL, DeGroot LJ, et al, editors. Endocrinology. Philadelphia: WB Saunders; 2001. p. 235–56.
[66] Dallman MF. Viewing the ventromedial hypothalamus from the adrenal gland. Am J Physiol 1984;246(1 Pt 2):R1–12.
[67] Cascio CS, Shinsako J, Dallman MF. The suprachiasmatic nuclei stimulate evening ACTH secretion in the rat. Brain Res 1987;423:173–8.
[68] Buijs RM, Hermes MHLJ, Kalsbeek A. The suprachiasmatic-paraventricular nucleus interactions: a bridge to the neuroendocrine and autonomic nervous system. Prog Brain Res 1998;119:365–82.
[69] Jasper MS, Engeland WC. Splanchnicotomy increases adrenal sensitivity to ACTH in nonstressed rats. Am J Physiol 1997;273:E363–8.
[70] Choi S, Wong LS, Yamat C, et al. Hypothalamic ventromedial nuclei amplify circadian rhythms: do they contain a food-entrained endogenous oscillator? J Neurosci 1998;18: 3843–52.
[71] Kwak SP, Young EA, Morano I, et al. Diurnal corticotropin-releasing hormone mRNA variation in the hypothalamus exhibits a rhythm distinct from that of plasma corticosterone. Neuroendocrinology 1992;55:74–83.
[72] Muglia LJ, Jacobson L, Weninger SC, et al. Impaired diurnal adrenal rhythmicity restored by constant infusion of corticotropin-releasing hormone in CRH-deficient mice. J Clin Invest 1997;99:2923–9.
[73] Jacobson L. Glucocorticoid replacement, but not CRH deficiency, prevents adrenalectomy-induced anorexia in mice. Endocrinology 1999;140:310–7.

[74] Gass P, Kretz O, Wolfer DP, et al. Genetic disruption of mineralocorticoid receptor leads to impaired neurogenesis and granule cell degeneration in the hippocampus of adult mice. EMBO Rep 2000;1:447–51.
[75] Akana SF, Shinsako J, Dallman MF. Closed-loop feedback control of the nyctohemeral rise in adrenocortical system function. Fed Proc 1985;44:177–81.
[76] Wajnrajch MP, New MI. Defects of adrenal steroidogenesis. In: DeGroot LJ, Jameson JL, DeGroot LJ, et al, editors. Endocrinology. 4th edition. Philadelphia: WB Saunders; 2001. p. 1721–39.
[77] Bertagna X, Bertagna C, Luton JP, et al. The new steroid analog RU 486 inhibits glucocorticoid action in man. J Clin Endocrinol Metab 1984;59:25–8.
[78] Gaillard RC, Riondel A, Muller AF, et al. RU 486: a steroid with antiglucocorticoid activity that only disinhibits the human pituitary-adrenal system at a specific time of day. Proc Natl Acad Sci U S A 1984;81:3879–82.
[79] Kalman BA, Spencer RL. Rapid corticosteroid-dependent regulation of mineralocorticoid receptor protein expression in rat brain. Endocrinology 2002;143:4184–95.
[80] Canteras NS, Swanson LW. Projections of the ventral subiculum to the amygdala, septum and hippocampus. J Comp Neurol 1992;324:180–94.
[81] Cullinan WE, Herman JP, Watson SJ. Ventral subicular interaction with the hypothalamic paraventricular nucleus: evidence for a relay in the bed nucleus of the stria terminalis. J Comp Neurol 1993;332:1–20.
[82] Jacobson L, Akana SF, Cascio CS, et al. Circadian variations in plasma corticosterone permit normal termination of ACTH responses to stress. Endocrinology 1988;122:1343–8.
[83] Rosmond R, Dallman MF, Bjorntorp P. Stress-related cortisol secretion in men: relationships with abdominal obesity and endocrine, metabolic and hemodynamic abnormalities. J Clin Endocrinol Metab 1998;83:1853–9.
[84] Czeisler C, Johnson MP, Duffy JF, et al. Exposure to bright light and darkness to treat physiologic maladaptations to night work. N Engl J Med 1990;322:1253–9.
[85] VanCauter E, Leproult R, Kupfer DJ. Effects of gender and age on the levels and circadian rhythmicity of plasma cortisol. J Clin Endocrinol Metab 1996;81:2468–73.
[86] Shaper AG, Wannamethee SG, Walker M. Body weight: implications for the prevention of coronary heart disease, stroke and diabetes mellitus in a cohort study of middle-aged men. BMJ 1997;314:1311–7.
[87] Clayton PJ. Depression subtyping: treatment implications. J Clin Psychiatry 1998;59(Suppl 16):5–12.
[88] Belanoff JK, Rothschild AJ, Cassidy F, et al. An open-label trial of C-1073 (Mifepristone) for psychotic major depression. Biol Psychiatry 2002;52:386–92.
[89] Thakore JH, Dinan TG. Cortisol synthesis inhibition: a new treatment strategy for the clinical and endocrine manifestations of depression. Biol Psychiatry 1995;37:364–8.
[90] Wolkowitz OM, Reus VI. Treatment of depression with antiglucocorticoid drugs. Psychosom Med 1999;61:698–711.
[91] Selye H. Thymus and adrenals in the response of the organism to injuries and intoxications. Br J Exp Pathol 1936;17:234–48.
[92] Darlington DN, Shinsako J, Dallman MF. Medullary lesions eliminate ACTH responses to hypotensive hemorrhage. Am J Physiol 1986;251:R106–15.
[93] Ritter S, Watts AG, Dinh TT, Sanchez-Watts G, et al. Immunotoxin lesion of hypothalamically projecting norepinephrine and epinephrine neurons differentially affects circadian and stressor-stimulated corticosterone secretion. Endocrinology 2003;144: 1357–67.
[94] Smith DW, Butler KM, Day TA. Role of ventrolateral medulla catecholamine cells in hypothalamic neuroendocrine cell responses to systemic hypoxia. J Neurosci 1995;15: 7979–88.
[95] Grill H, Kaplan JM. The neuroanatomical axis for control of energy balance. Front Neuroendocrinol 2002;23:2–40.

[96] terHorst GJ, deBoer P, Luiten PGM, et al. Ascending projections from the solitary tract nucleus to the hypothalamus: a phaseolus vulgaris lectin tracing study in the rat. Neuroscience 1989;31:785–97.
[97] Li H-Y, Ericsson A, Sawchenko PE. Distinct mechanisms underlie activation of hypothalamic neurosecretory neurons and their medullary catecholaminergic afferents in categorically distinct stress paradigms. Proc Natl Acad Sci U S A 1996;93:2359–64.
[98] Mueller NK, Dolgas CM, Herman JP. Stressor-selective role of the ventral subiculum in regulation of neuroendocrine stress responses. Endocrinology 2004;145:3763–8.
[99] Dayas CV, Buller KM, Day TA. Medullary neurones regulate hypothalamic corticotropin-releasing factor cell responses to an emotional stressor. Neuroscience 2001;105:707–19.
[100] Plotsky PM. Hypophyseotrophic regulation of adenohypophyseal adrenocorticotropin secretion. Fed Proc 1985;44:207–13.
[101] Kovacs KJ, Foldes A, Sawchenko PE. Glucocorticoid negative feedback selectively targets vasopressin transcription in parvocellular neurosecretory neurons. J Neurosci 2000;20: 3843–52.
[102] Watts AG, Sanchez-Watts G. Physiological regulation of peptide messenger RNA colocalization in rat hypothalamic paraventricular medial parvicellular neurons. J Comp Neurol 1995;352:501–14.
[103] Dayas CV, Butler KM, Day TA. Neuroendocrine responses to an emotional stressor: evidence for involvement of the medial but not the central amygdala. Eur J Neurosci 1999; 11:2312–22.
[104] Li H-Y, Sawchenko PE. Hypothalamic effector neurons and extended circuitries activated in neurogenic stress: a comparison of footshock effects exerted acutely, chronically, and in animals with controlled glucocorticoid levels. J Comp Neurol 1998;393:244–66.
[105] Romero LM, Sapolsky RM. Patterns of adrenocorticotropin secretagogue release with hypoglycemia, novelty, and restraint after colchicine blockade of axonal transport. Endocrinology 1992;132:199–204.
[106] Dohanics J, Hoffman GE, Verbalis JG. Hyponatremia-induced inhibition of magnocellular neurons causes stressor-selective impairment of stimulated adrenocorticotropin secretion in rats. Endocrinology 1991;128:331–40.
[107] Di S, Malcher-Lopes R, Halmos KC, et al. Nongenomic glucocorticoid inhibition via endocannabinoid release in the hypothalamus: a fast feedback mechanism. J Neurosci 2003; 23:4850–7.
[108] Widmaier EP, Dallman MF. The effects of corticotropin-releasing factor on adrenocorticotropin secretion from perifused pituitaries in vitro: rapid inhibition by glucocorticoids. Endocrinology 1984;115:2368–74.
[109] Plotsky PM, Vale WW. Hemorrhage-induced secretion of corticotropin-releasing factor-like immunoreactivity into the rat hypophysial portal circulation and its inhibition by glucocorticoids. Endocrinology 1984;114:164–9.
[110] Bilezikjian LM, Blount AL, Vale WW. The cellular actions of vasopressin on corticotrophs of the anterior pituitary: resistance to glucocorticoid action. Mol Endocrinol 1987;1:451–8.
[111] Imaki T, Xiao-Quan W, Shibasaki T, et al. Stress-induced activation of neuronal activity and corticotropin-releasing factor gene expression in the paraventricular nucleus is modulated by glucocorticoids in rats. J Clin Invest 1995;96:231–8.
[112] Tanimura S, Watts AG. Corticosterone modulation of ACTH secretagogue gene expression in the paraventricular nucleus. Peptides 2001;22:775–83.
[113] Young WS, Mezey E, Siegel RE. Vasopressin and oxytocin mRNAs in adrenalectomized and Brattleboro rats: analysis by quantitative in situ hybridization histochemistry. Brain Res 1986;387:231–41.
[114] DeKloet ER, DeKock S, Schild V, et al. Antiglucocorticoid RU 38486 attenuates retention of a behavior and disinhibits the hypothalamic-pituitary-adrenal axis at different brain sites. Neuroendocrinology 1988;47:109–15.

[115] Dallman MF, Akana SF, Strack AM, et al. Chronic stress-induced effects of corticosterone on brain: direct and indirect. Ann N Y Acad Sci 2004;1018:141–50.
[116] Harbuz MS, Conde GL, Marti O, et al. The hypothalamic-pituitary-adrenal axis in autoimmunity. Ann N Y Acad Sci 1997;823:214–24.
[117] Viau V, Sawchenko PE. Hypophysiotropic neurons of the paraventricular nucleus respond in spatially, temporally, and phenotypically differentiated manners to acute vs. repeated restraint stress. J Comp Neurol 2002;445:293–307.
[118] Bowers G, Cullinan WE, Herman JP. Region-specific regulation of glutamic acid decarboxylase (GAD) mRNA expression in central stress circuits. J Neurosci 1998;18: 5938–47.
[119] Bhatnagar S, Huber R, Nowak N, et al. Lesions of the posteriod paraventricular thalamus block habituation of hypothalamic-pituitary-adrenal responses to repeated restraint. J Neuroendocrinol 2002;14:403–10.
[120] Jaferi A, Nowak N, Bhatnagar S. Negative feedback functions in chronically stressed rats: role of the posterior paraventricular thalamus. Physiol Behav 2003;78:365–73.
[121] Cole MA, Kalman BA, Pace TWW, et al. Selective blockade of the mineralocorticoid receptor impairs hypothalamic-pituitary-adrenal axis expression of habituation. J Neuroendocrinol 2000;12:1034–42.
[122] Akana SF, Dallman MF. Chronic cold in adrenalectomized, corticosterone (B)-treated rats: facilitated corticotropin responses to acute restraint emerge as B increases. Endocrinology 1997;138:3249–58.
[123] Akana SF, Dallman MF, Bradbury MJ, et al. Feedback and facilitation in the adrenocortical system: unmasking facilitation by partial inhibition of the glucocorticoid response to prior stress. Endocrinology 1992;131:57–68.
[124] Laugero KD, Gomez F, Manalo S, et al. Corticosterone infused intracerebroventricularly inhibits energy storage and stimulates the hypothalamo-pituitary axis in adrenalectomized rats drinking sucrose. Endocrinology 2002;143:4552–62.
[125] Caspi A, Sugden K, Moffitt TE, et al. Influence of life stress on depression: moderation by a polymorphism in the 5-HTT gene. Science 2003;301:386–9.
[126] Holsboer F. The rationale for corticotropin-releasing hormone receptor (CRH-R) antagonists to treat depression and anxiety. J Psychiatr Research 1999;33:181–214.
[127] Young EA, Haskett RF, Murphy-Weinberg V, et al. Loss of glucocorticoid fast feedback in depression. Arch Gen Psychiatry 1991;48:693–9.
[128] Zobel AW, Nickel T, Sonntag A, et al. Cortisol response in the combined dexamethasone/ CRH test as predictor of relapse in patients with remitted depression: a prospective study. J Psychiatr Res 2001;35:83–94.
[129] Seckl JR, Morton NM, Chapman KE, et al. Glucocorticoids and 11beta-hydroxysteroid dehydrogenase in adipose tissue. Recent Prog Horm Res 2004;59:359–93.
[130] Turnbull AV, Rivier C. Regulation of the hypothalamic-pituitary-adrenal axis by cytokines: actions and mechanisms of action. Physiol Rev 1999;79:1–71.
[131] Jacobson L, Muglia LJ, Weninger SC, et al. CRH deficiency impairs but does not block pituitary-adrenal responses to diverse stressors. Neuroendocrinology 2000;71:79–87.
[132] Bethin KE, Vogt SK, Muglia LJ. Interleukin-6 is an essential, corticotropin-releasing hormone-independent stimulator of the adrenal axis during immune stimulation. Proc Natl Acad Sci U S A 2000;97:9317–22.
[133] Ahima RS, Saper CB, Flier JS, et al. Leptin regulation of neuroendocrine systems. Front Neuroendocrinol 2000;21:263–307.
[134] Bailer UF, Kaye WH. A review of neuropeptide and neuroendocrine dysregulation in anorexia and bulimia nervosa. Curr Drug Targets CNS Neurol Disord 2003;2:53–9.
[135] Laughlin GA, Yen SSC. Nutritional and endocrine-metabolic aberrations in amenorrheic athletes. J Clin Endocrinol Metab 1996;81:4301–9.
[136] Licinio J, Wong ML, Gold PW. The hypothalamic-pituitary-adrenal axis in anorexia nervosa. Psychiatry Res 1996;62:75–83.

[137] Warren MP, Goodman LR. Exercise-induced endocrine pathologies. J Endocrinol Invest 2003;26:873–8.
[138] Arvaniti K, Huang Q, Richard D. Effects of leptin and corticosterone on the expression of corticotropin-releasing hormone, agout-related protein, and proopiomelanocortin in the brain of ob/ob mouse. Neuroendocrinology 2001;73:227–36.
[139] Solano JM, Jacobson L. Glucocorticoids reverse leptin effects on food intake and body fat in mice without increasing NPY mRNA. Am J Physiol 1999;277:E708–16.

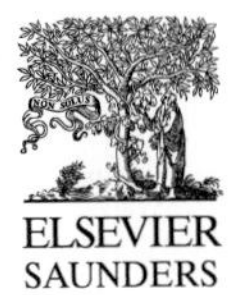
ELSEVIER
SAUNDERS

Endocrinol Metab Clin N Am
34 (2005) 293–313

ENDOCRINOLOGY
AND METABOLISM
CLINICS
OF NORTH AMERICA

Adrenal Corticosteroid Biosynthesis, Metabolism, and Action

Wiebke Arlt, MD, Paul M. Stewart, MD*

Division of Medical Sciences, Endocrinology, Institute of Biomedical Research, University of Birmingham, Wolfson Drive, Room 238, Birmingham, B15 2TT, UK

Adrenal corticosteroids are essential for life, and an appreciation of the mechanisms underpinning their synthesis, secretion, and mode of action in normal physiology is essential if the physician is to diagnose and treat patients who have Cushing's syndromes effectively. In each case, there have been clinically significant advances in the knowledge base over recent years, notably in the understanding of steroidogenesis, cortisol action, and metabolism.

Adrenal steroids and steroidogenesis

Three main types of hormone are produced by the adrenal cortex: glucocorticoids (cortisol, corticosterone), mineralocorticoids (aldosterone, deoxycorticosterone), and sex steroids (mainly the androgen precursors dehydroepiandrosterone [DHEA] and androstenedione). Cholesterol is the precursor for all adrenal steroidogenesis. The principal source of this cholesterol is provided from the circulation in the form of low-density lipoprotein (LDL) cholesterol [1]. Uptake is by specific cell surface LDL receptors present on adrenal tissue; LDL then is internalized by means of receptor-mediated endocytosis. The resulting vesicles fuse with lysozymes, and free cholesterol is produced following hydrolysis. Cholesterol also can be generated de novo within the adrenal cortex from acetyl coenzyme A [2], and there is evidence that the adrenal can use high-density lipoprotein (HDL) cholesterol following uptake through a putative HDL receptor, SR-B1 [3].

This work was supported by the Wellcome Trust (Programme Grant to Dr. Stewart) and the Medical Research Council (Senior Clinical Fellowship to Dr. Arlt).

* Corresponding author.

E-mail address: p.m.stewart@bham.ac.uk (P.M. Stewart).

doi:10.1016/j.ecl.2005.01.002

endo.theclinics.com

The biochemical pathways involved in adrenal steroidogenesis are shown in Fig. 1. The initial hormone-dependent rate-limiting step is the transport of intracellular cholesterol from the outer to inner mitochondrial membrane for conversion to pregnenolone by cytochrome P450scc. Human experiments of nature have confirmed the importance of a 30-kd protein, steroidogenic acute regulatory protein (StAR), in mediating this effect. StAR is induced by an increase in intracellular cAMP following binding of corticotropin (ACTH) to its cognate receptor providing the first important rate-limiting step in adrenal steroidogenesis [4]. Other transporters including the peripheral benzodiazepine-like receptor may be involved.

Steroidogenesis involves the concerted action of several enzymes, all of which have been cloned and characterized. Cholesterol side chain cleavage enzyme and the CYP11B enzymes are localized to the mitochondria and require an electron shuttle system provided through adrenodoxin/adrenodoxin reductase to oxidize/hydroxylate steroids [5]. P450c17, exerting 17α-hydroxylase and 17,20 lyase activity, and P450c21, exerting 21-hydroxylase activity, are localized to the endoplasmic reticulum (ER). Like all microsomal P450 enzymes, they require electron transfer from nicotinamide adenosine dinucleotide phosphate (NADPH) by the enzyme P450 oxidoreductase. In addition, 17,20 lyase activity of P450c17 is dependent upon the flavoprotein cytochrome b_5 that functions as an allosteric facilitator of P450c17 and P450 oxidoreductase interaction [6]. Mutations in the genes

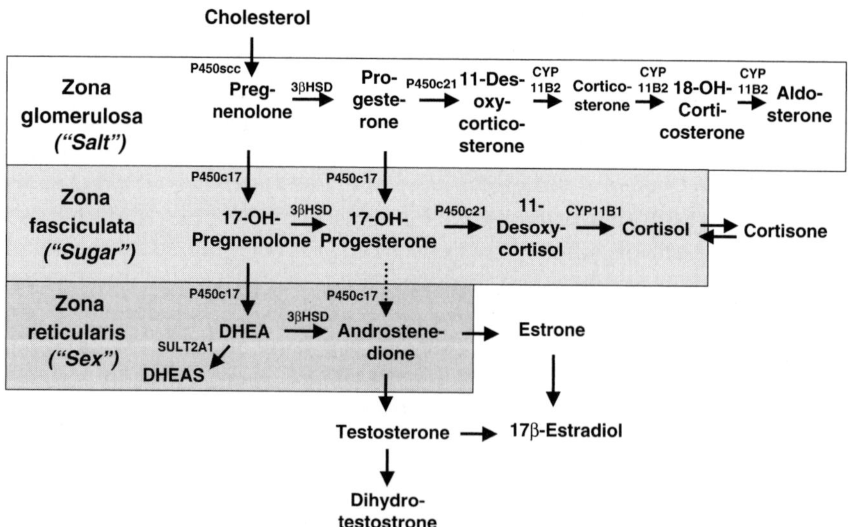

Fig. 1. Steroidogenesis in the human adrenal. Following the StAR-mediated uptake of cholesterol into mitochondria within adrenocortical cells, aldosterone, cortisol, and adrenal androgen precursors are synthesized through the coordinated action of a series of steroidogenic enzymes in a zone-specific fashion.

encoding these enzymes result in human disease [7–13], so some understanding of the underlying pathways and steroid precursors is required.

After uptake of cholesterol to the mitochondrion, cholesterol is cleaved by the P450 cholesterol side chain cleavage enzyme (P450scc) to form pregnenolone [14]. In the cytoplasm, pregnenolone is converted to progesterone by the type II isozyme of 3β-hydroxysteroid dehydrogenase (3β-HSD) [15]. Progesterone is hydroxylated to 17OH-progesterone through the activity of P450c17, encoded by the *CYP17A1* gene. 17-Hydroxylation is an essential prerequisite for glucocorticoid synthesis, and the zona glomerulosa does not express P450c17. P450c17 also possesses 17,20 lyase activity, which results in the production of the C19 adrenal androgen precursors, dehydroepiandrosterone and androstenedione [16]. In people, however, 17-OH progesterone is not an efficient substrate for P450c17, and under physiologic conditions, there is negligible conversion of 17-OH progesterone to androstenedione. Thus, adrenal androstenedione secretion is dependant upon the conversion of dehydroepiandrosterone to androstenedione by 3β-HSD. This enzyme also will convert 17-OH pregnenolone to 17-OH progesterone, but the preferred substrate is pregnenolone.

21-Hydroxylation of either progesterone (zona glomerulosa) or 17-OH-progesterone (zona fasciculata) is performed by the product of the *CYP21A2* gene, P450c21, which exerts 21-hydroxylase activity to yield deoxycorticosterone or 11-deoxycortisol, respectively [17]. The final step in cortisol biosynthesis takes place in the mitochondria and involves the conversion of 11-deoxycortisol to cortisol by the enzyme 11β-hydroxylase, encoded by the *CYP11B1* gene [18]. In the zona glomerulosa, 11β-hydroxylase also may convert deoxycorticosterone to corticosterone. The enzyme aldosterone synthase, encoded by *CYP11B2* also may carry out this reaction, however. In addition, it is required for the conversion of corticosterone to aldosterone by means of the intermediate 18-OH corticosterone [19,20].

Regulation of adrenal steroidogenesis

Zonal specific steroidogenesis in the adrenal cortex

Glucocorticoids are secreted in relatively high amounts (cortisol 10–20 mg/d) from the zona fasciculata under the control of ACTH, while mineralocorticoids are secreted in low amounts (aldosterone 100–150 μg/d) from the zona glomerulosa under the principal control of angiotensin II. As a class, adrenal androgens (DHEA, dehydroepiandrosterone sulfate [DHEAS], and androstenedione) are the most abundant steroids secreted from the adult adrenal gland (>20 mg/d). In each case, this is facilitated through expression of steroidogenic enzymes in a specific zonal manner. The zona glomerulosa cannot synthesize cortisol, because it does not express *CYP17*. In contrast, aldosterone secretion is confined to the outer zona glomerulosa through the restricted expression of *CYP11B2*. Although *CYP11B1* and *CYP11B2* share 95% homology, the 5′ promoter sequences differ and permit regulation of the final steps in glucocorticoid and mineralocorticoid biosynthesis by ACTH and angiotensin II, respectively. DHEA is generated by 17,20 lyase activity of P450c17 in the adrenal zona reticularis, which shows ample expression of cytochrome b5, the required cofactor for 17,20 lyase activity [21]. DHEA is converted by the DHEA sulfotransferase (SULT2A1) to form DHEAS, the major secretory product of adrenal steroidogenesis [22].

In the fetal adrenal, steroidogenesis occurs primarily within the inner fetal zone. Because of a relative lack of 3β-HSD and high DHEA sulfotransferase activity, the principal steroidogenic products are DHEA and DHEAS which are then aromatized by placental trophoblast to estrogens. Thus most maternal estrogen across pregnancy is, indirectly, fetally-derived [23].

Classical endocrine feedback loops are in place to control the secretion of glucocorticoids, whereby cortisol inhibits the secretion of both corticotrophin releasing factor and ACTH from the hypothalamus and pituitary, respectively.

Regulation of mineralocorticoid secretion by the renin–angiotensin–aldosterone system

Aldosterone is secreted from the zona glomerulosa under the control of three principal secretagogues: angiotensin II, potassium, and to a lesser extent ACTH. Other factors, notably somatostatin, heparin, atrial natriuretic factor, and dopamine, can inhibit aldosterone synthesis directly. The secretion of aldosterone and its intermediary 18-hydroxylated metabolites is restricted to the zona glomerulosa because of the zonal-specific expression of aldosterone synthase (*CYP11B2*) [24]. Corticosterone and deoxycorticosterone, while synthesized in both the zona fasciculata and glomerulosa, can act as mineralocorticoids, and this becomes significant in some clinical disease, notably some forms of congenital adrenal hyperplasia and adrenal tumors. Similarly, it is established that cortisol can act as a mineralocorticoid in the setting of impaired metabolism to cortisone performed by the enzyme 11β-hydroxysteroid dehydrogenase type 2.

Angiotensinogen, an α_2-globulin synthesized within the liver, is cleaved by renin to form angiotensin I. Angiotensin I then is converted to angiotensin II by angiotensin-converting enzyme (ACE) in lung and many other peripheral tissues. Angiotensin I has no apparent biologic activity, but angiotensin II is a potent stimulator of aldosterone secretion and is a potent vasoconstrictor. The rate-limiting step in the renin–angiotensin–aldosterone system (RAS) is the secretion of renin, which also is controlled through a negative feedback loop [25]. Renin is secreted from juxtaglomerular epithelial cells within the macula densa of the renal tubule in response to underlying renal arteriolar pressure, oncotic pressure, and sympathetic drive. Thus, low perfusion pressure or low tubular fluid sodium content as seen in hemorrhage, renal artery stenosis, dehydration, or salt loss increases renin secretion. Conversely, secretion is suppressed following a high-salt diet and by factors that increase blood pressure. Autoregulation therefore is maintained, because the increase in renin secretion stimulates angiotensin II and aldosterone production; the concomitant increase in blood pressure and renal sodium retention results in feedback–inhibition of renin secretion. Hypokalemia increases, and hyperkalemia decreases renin secretion; in addition, potassium exerts a direct effect upon the adrenal cortex to increase aldosterone secretion. The sensitivity of the RAS to changes in circulating potassium is high, with changes in potassium concentrations of only 0.1 to 0.5 mmol/L producing marked changes in aldosterone concentrations. Potassium concentrations also determine sensitivity of the aldosterone response to a given infusion of angiotensin II, with high potassium intake increasing responsiveness [26].

Angiotensin II and potassium stimulate aldosterone secretion principally by increasing the transcription of *CYP11B2* in the adrenal zona glomerulosa through common intracellular signaling pathways. Cyclic AMP response elements in the 5′ region of the *CYP11B2* gene are activated following an increase in intracellular calcium ion (Ca^{2+}) and activation of calmodulin kinases. The potassium effect is mediated through membrane depolarization and opening of calcium channels, and the AII effect follows binding of angiotensin II to the surface AT_1 receptor and activation of phospholipase C [24].

The effect of ACTH upon aldosterone secretion is modest and differs in the acute and chronic situation. An acute bolus of ACTH will increase aldosterone secretion, principally by stimulating the early pathways of adrenal steroidogenesis, but circulating levels increase by no more than 10% to 20% above baseline values. ACTH has no effect upon *CYP11B2* gene transcription or enzyme activity. Chronic continual ACTH stimulation has either no effect or an inhibitory effect on aldosterone production, possibly because of receptor down-regulation or suppression of angiotensin II–stimulated secretion caused by a mineralocorticoid effect of cortisol, deoxycorticosterone, or corticosterone.

Adrenal androgen secretion

The adult adrenal secretes approximately 4 mg per day of DHEA, 7 to 15 mg per day of DHEAS, and 1.5 mg per day of androstenedione. DHEA is the crucial sex steroid precursor and only acts androgenic or estrogenic following conversion by the activities of 3β-HSD, a superfamily of 17β-HSD isozymes and aromatase, expressed in peripheral target tissues. This is of clinical importance in many diseases [27]. In women, more than 50% of active androgens are generated by peripheral conversion from DHEA [28]. In men, this contribution is much smaller because of the testicular production of androgens, but adrenal androgen excess even in males may be of clinical significance, notably in patients with congenital adrenal hyperplasia. There is a clear gender difference in DHEAS concentrations, with lower concentrations in adult women compared with men [29]. In people and in some nonhuman primates the secretion of DHEAS shows a characteristic pattern throughout the life cycle. DHEAS is secreted in high quantities by the fetal zone of the adrenal cortex, leading to high circulating DHEAS levels at birth. As the fetal zone involutes, a sharp fall in serum DHEAS to almost nondetectable levels is observed postpartum. DHEAS levels remain very low until they gradually increase between the sixth and 10th years of age, owing to increasing DHEA production by the zona reticularis, a phenomenon termed adrenarche [30,31]. DHEAS concentrations peak during the third decade, followed by a steady decline with advancing age so that levels during the eighth and ninth decade are only 10% to 20% of those in young adults [32]. This decline has been termed adrenopause in spite of unchanged or even increased cortisol secretion [33]. The age-related decline in DHEAS levels shows high interindividual variability, and the decline is associated with a reduction in size of the zona reticularis [34].

Corticotropin stimulates adrenal androgen secretion, which may explain why DHEA and androstenedione demonstrate a similar diurnal rhythm to cortisol. Serum DHEAS does not vary throughout the day, most likely because of its longer half-life. The diurnal rhythm and the pulse amplitude of DHEA secretion show an age-associated attenuation [35]. Moreover, the ACTH-induced increase in DHEA secretion is reduced in elderly subjects [36], whereas the cortisol response to an ACTH challenge is constant or even increased. There are many discrepancies between adrenal androgen and glucocorticoid secretion, however, including the age-specific variation of DHEA secretion, which has led to the suggestion of an additional cortical androgen-stimulating hormone (CASH). Many putative CASHs have been proposed, including proopiomelanocortin derivatives such as joining peptide, prolactin, and insulinlike growth factor 1 (IGF-1), but conclusive proof is lacking. Characteristically, adrenal androgen secretion appears stimulated in ACTH-dependent Cushing's disease, while it is suppressed in the case of adrenal glucocorticoid excess.

Corticosteroid hormone action

Receptors and gene transcription

Both cortisol and aldosterone exert their effects following uptake of free hormone from the circulation and binding to intracellular receptors, termed the glucocorticoid and mineralocorticoid receptors (GR and MR) [37–39]. These are both members of the thyroid/steroid hormone receptor superfamily of transcription factors comprising a C-terminal ligand binding domain, a central DNA binding domain interacting with specific DNA sequences on target genes, and an N-terminal hypervariable region. Splice variants have been described in both cases [40,41], although there is only a single gene encoding the GR and MR.

Glucocorticoid hormone action has been studied in some detail. The binding of steroid to the GRα in the cytosol results in activation of the steroid receptor complex through a process that involves the dissociation of heat shock proteins (HSP 90 and HSP 70) [42]. Following translocation to the nucleus, gene transcription is stimulated or repressed following binding of dimerized GR/ligand complexes to specific DNA sequences (glucocorticoid response elements [GREs]) in the promoter regions of target genes [43]. The GRβ variant may act as a dominant negative regulator of GRα transactivation [40]. The GRγ variant has an additional amino acid within the DNA binding domain of the receptor protein that may reduce GR transactivation [40]. Naturally occurring mutations in the GR (as seen in patients who have glucocorticoid resistance) and in vitro-generated GR mutants have highlighted critical regions of the receptor responsible for binding and transactivation [44,45]. In addition, however, numerous others factors are required (coactivators, corepressors [46]) that may confer tissue specificity of response. In keeping with the diverse array of tissue-specific cortisol action, many hundred glucocorticoid-responsive genes have been identified.

In contrast to the diverse actions of glucocorticoids, mineralocorticoids have been considered to have a more restricted role, principally to stimulate epithelial sodium transport in the distal nephron, distal colon, and salivary glands. Aldosterone binds to the MR, principally in the cytosol (though there is evidence for expression of the unliganded MR in the nucleus), followed by translocation of the hormone-receptor complex to the nucleus. MR and GR share considerable homology, 57% in the steroid-binding domain and 94% in the DNA binding domain. It is perhaps not surprising therefore that there is promiscuity of ligand binding with aldosterone (and the synthetic mineralocorticoid fludrocortisone) binding to the GR and cortisol binding to the MR. For the MR, this is particularly impressive. In vitro, the MR has the same inherent affinity for aldosterone, corticosterone, and cortisol [47]. Specificity upon the MR is conferred through the prereceptor metabolism of cortisol by means of 11β-hydroxysteroid dehydrogenase type 2 (*11β-HSD2*), which inactivates cortisol and corticosterone to inactive 11-keto metabolites, enabling aldosterone to bind to the MR [48,49] (Fig. 2).

Mineralocorticoid receptor-induced epithelial sodium conductance is mediated by the apical sodium channel (comprising three subunits: α, β, and γ) and the α_1 and β_1 subunits of the basolateral Na^+K^+ATPase through transcriptional regulation of an aldosterone-induced gene, serum and glucocorticoid-induced kinase (*sgk*) [50,51]. In addition, recent data have

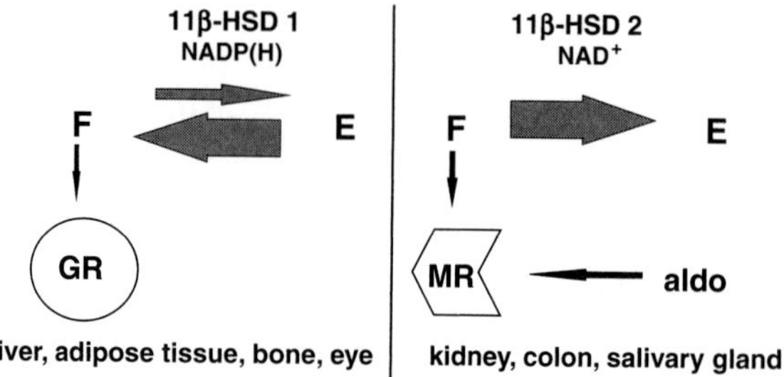

Fig. 2. Schematic role of 11β-HSDs in regulating corticosteroid hormone action at the prereceptor level. 11β-HSD2 in the kidney inactivates cortisol (F) to cortisone (E), enabling aldosterone to bind to the MR in vivo. By contrast, in GR-expressing tissues, 11β-HSD1 principally converts inactive E to F, thereby augmenting GR hormone action.

pointed to an extended cardiovascular role for aldosterone and the MR in inducing cardiac fibrosis and vascular inflammation [52,53], although the exact signaling mechanisms have yet to be determined.

For both glucocorticoids and mineralocorticoids, there is accumulating evidence for so-called nongenomic effects involving hormone response obviating the genomic GR or MR. Responses have been reported within seconds/minutes of exposure to corticosteroids and are thought to be mediated by as yet, uncharacterized membrane-coupled receptors [54].

Cortisol-binding globulin and corticosteroid hormone metabolism

Over 90% of circulating cortisol is bound, predominantly to the α_2-globulin, cortisol-binding globulin (CBG) [55]. This 383 amino acid protein is synthesized in the liver and binds cortisol with high affinity. Affinity for synthetic corticosteroids (except prednisolone, which has an affinity for CBG, approximately 50% of that of cortisol) is negligible. Circulating CBG concentrations are approximately 700 nmol/L; levels are increased by estrogens and in some patients who have chronic active hepatitis but reduced by glucocorticoids and in patients who have cirrhosis, nephrosis, and hyperthyroidism. The estrogen effect can be marked, with levels increasing two- to threefold across pregnancy. This also should be considered when measuring plasma total cortisol in pregnancy and in women taking estrogens. Inherited abnormalities in CBG synthesis are much rarer than those described for thyroid-binding globulin but include patients who have elevated CBG, partial and complete deficiency of CBG, or CBG variants with reduced affinity for cortisol. In each case, alterations in CBG concentrations change total circulating cortisol concentrations accordingly, but free cortisol concentrations are normal. Only this free circulating fraction is available for transport into tissues for biologic activity. The excretion of free cortisol through the kidneys is termed urinary free cortisol (UFF) and represents only 1% of the total cortisol secretion rate.

The circulating half-life of cortisol varies between 70 and 120 minutes. Cortisol is metabolized through many routes (Fig. 3), but the major routes comprise the interconversion of cortisol (Kendall's compound F) to cortisone (compound E) through the activity of 11β-hydroxysteroid dehydrogenases or reduction of the C4-5 double bond by either 5β-reductase or 5α-reductase to yield respectively 5β-tetrahydrocortisol (THF) or 5α-THF (allo-THF). In normal subjects, the 5β metabolites predominate (5β:5α-THF 2:1). THF, allo-THF and tetrahydrocortisone (THE) are conjugated rapidly with glucuronic acid and excreted in the urine. Downstream, cleavage of THF and THE to the C19 steroids 11-hydroxy- or 11-oxo-androsterone or etiocholanolone can occur. Alternatively, reduction of the 20-oxo group by 20α- or 20β-hydroxysteroid dehydrogenase yields α and β cortols and cortolones, respectively, with subsequent oxidation at the C21 position to form the extremely polar metabolites, cortolic, and cortolonic acids. Hydroxylation at C6 to form 6β-hydroxycortisol is described, as is reduction of the C20 position, which may occur without A ring reduction giving rise to 20α- and 20β-hydroxycortisol.

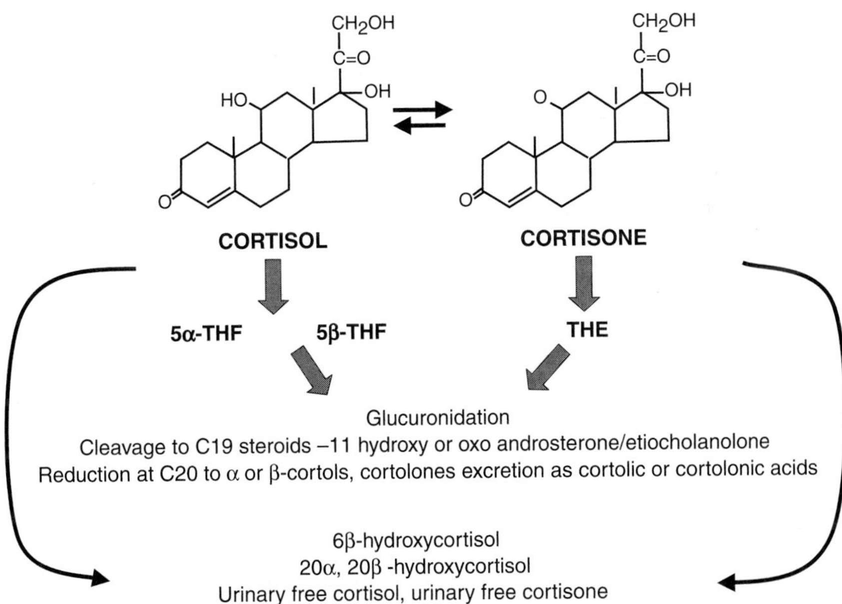

Fig. 3. The principal pathways of cortisol metabolism. Interconversion of hormonally active cortisol to inactive cortisone is catalyzed by two isozymes of 11β-HSD, 11β-HSD1 principally converting cortisone to cortisol and 11β-HSD2 the reverse. A ring reduction is undertaken by 5β or 5β-reductase and 3β-HDSs to yield tetrahydro metabolites (THF, 5β-THF, and THE) that in turn are conjugated with glucuronic acid or cleared to 11-hydroxy/oxo-androsterone or -etiocholoanolone.

Approximately 50% of secreted cortisol appears in the urine as THF, allo-THF, and THE; 25% appears as cortols/cortolones. Ten percent appears as C19 steroids, and 10% appears as cortolic/cortolonic acids. The remaining metabolites are free, unconjugated steroids (cortisol, cortisone, and 6β- and 20α/20β-metabolites of F and E). Hyperthyroidism results in increased cortisol metabolism and clearance and hypothyroidism in the converse, principally because of an effect of thyroid hormone upon hepatic 11β-HSD and 5α/5β-reductases [56]. IGF-1 increases cortisol clearance by inhibiting hepatic 11β-HSD (conversion of cortisone to cortisol) [57]. 6β-Hydroxylation is normally a minor pathway, but cortisol itself and some drugs such as rifampicin induce 6β-hydroxylase and increase clearance [58].

Aldosterone also is metabolized in the liver and kidneys. In the liver, it undergoes tetrahydro reduction and is excreted in the urine as a 3-glucuronide tetrahydroaldosterone derivative. Glucuronide conjugation at the 18 position, however, occurs directly in the kidney, as does 3α and 5α/5β metabolism of the free steroid [59]. Because of the aldehyde group at the C18 position, aldosterone is not metabolized by 11β-HSD. Hepatic aldosterone clearance is reduced in patients who have cirrhosis, ascites, and severe congestive heart failure.

11β-Hydroxysteroid dehydrogenases

Quantitatively, the interconversion of cortisol to cortisone by 11β-hydroxysteroid dehydrogenases (11β-HSD) is the most important cortisol metabolizing pathway [60,61] (Fig. 3). Over the last 10 years, however, 11β-HSD also has emerged as novel factor in the tissue-specific analysis of corticosteroid hormone action, and one that now offers future therapeutic potential. Two distinct 11β-HSD isozymes have been reported. The NAD-dependent dehydrogenase, 11β-HSD2, is coexpressed with the MR in the kidney, colon, and salivary gland and inactivates cortisol to cortisone, thereby enabling aldosterone to bind to the MR in vivo [48,49]. If this enzyme-protective mechanism is impaired, cortisol is able to act as a mineralocorticoid; this explains an inherited form of endocrine hypertension (apparent mineralocorticoid excess) [60] and the hypertension seen in patients who have excessive licorice ingestion and possibly those who have salt-sensitive forms of essential hypertension [62]. Cushing's disease of the kidney reflects a state of local cortisol excess brought about by means of impaired metabolism by 11β-HSD2 despite normal circulating cortisol concentrations.

By contrast, 11β-HSD1 is an NADP(H)-dependent enzyme expressed principally in liver and visceral adipose tissue, but also in brain, bone, gonad, muscle, and other GR-expressing tissues, including the eye [61]. The enzyme is bidirectional, but in intact hepatocytes and adipocytes, oxo-reductase activity and thus the generation of F from E predominates [63,64] (see Fig. 2). This has important metabolic consequences, enhancing GR-dependant hepatic gluconeogenesis and glucose output and adipocyte differentiation, respectively. Therefore, there is great interest in the role of 11β-HSD1 in the pathogenesis and future treatment of patients who have the metabolic syndrome [61]. The enzyme that supplies NADPH to 11β-HSD1 within the endoplasmic reticulum, thereby conferring 11-oxo-reductase activity upon it, is hexose-6-phosphate dehydrogenase (H6PDH). Combined mutations in the genes encoding 11β-HSD1 and H6PDH explain the molecular basis for the putative 11β-HSD1 deficient state, cortisone reductase deficiency, an inherited form of polycystic ovary syndrome [65].

Thus at a prereceptor level, the expression and activity of 11β-HSDs offer a tissue-specific regulator of mineralocorticoid and glucocorticoid hormone action. This is important not only for the activity of endogenous steroids, cortisol and cortisone, but also the synthetic pharmacologic counterparts, prednisolone and prednisone [66].

Effects of glucocorticoids

Carbohydrate, protein, and lipid metabolism

Glucocorticoids increase blood glucose concentrations through their action on glycogen, protein, and lipid metabolism (Fig. 4). In the liver,

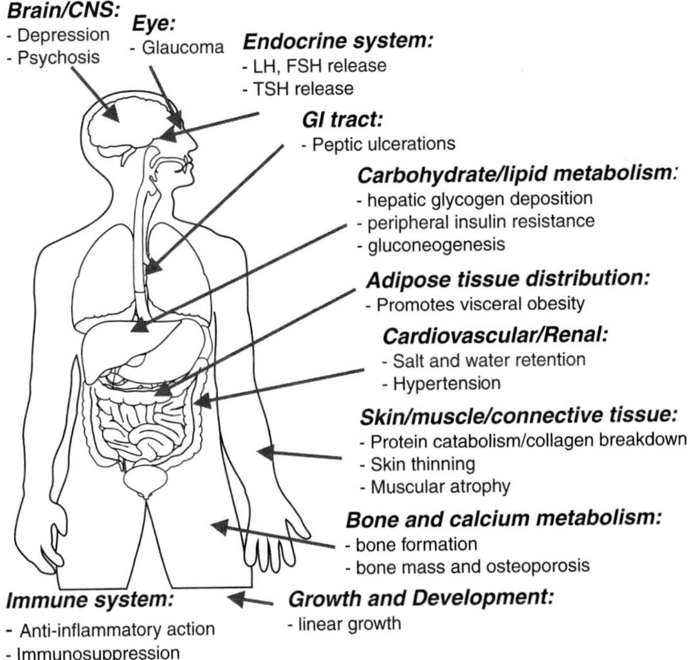

Fig. 4. The principal sites of action of glucocorticoids in people highlighting some of the diverse effects of cortisol upon many tissues.

cortisol stimulates glycogen deposition by increasing glycogen synthase and inhibiting the glycogen mobilizing enzyme, glycogen phosphorylase. Hepatic glucose output increases through the activation of key enzymes involved in gluconeogenesis, principally glucose-6-phosphatase and phosphoenolpyruvate kinase (PEPCK) [67]. In peripheral tissues (muscle and fat), cortisol inhibits glucose uptake and use. In adipose tissue, lipolysis is activated, resulting in the release of free fatty acids into the circulation. An increase in total circulating cholesterol and triglycerides is observed, but HDL cholesterol levels fall. Glucocorticoids also have a permissive effect upon other hormones including catecholamines and glucagon. The resultant effect is to cause insulin resistance and an increase in blood glucose concentrations, at the expense of protein and lipid catabolism. In Cushing's syndrome, glucose intolerance frequently occurs, and overt diabetes mellitus is present in up to one-third of patients in some series. Hepatic lipoprotein synthesis is stimulated, and increases in circulating cholesterol and triglycerides may be found.

Glucocorticoids stimulate adipocyte differentiation, promoting adipogenesis through the transcriptional activation of key differentiation genes including lipoprotein lipase, glycerol-3-phosphate dehydrogenase, and leptin [68]. Chronically, the effects of glucocorticoid excess upon adipose tissue is more complex, at least in people, where the deposition of visceral or central adipose tissue is stimulated, providing a useful discriminatory sign for diagnosing Cushing's syndrome. The explanation for the predilection for visceral obesity may relate to the increased expression of both the GR and type 1 isozyme of 11β-HSD (generating cortisol from cortisone) in omental compared with subcutaneous adipose tissue [63].

Weight gain and obesity are the most common signs in patients who have Cushing's syndrome, and, at least in adults, this is invariably centripetal in nature [69]. Indeed, generalized obesity is more common in the general population than it is in patients who have Cushing's syndrome. One exception to this is childhood, where glucocorticoid excess may result in generalized obesity. In addition to centripetal obesity, patients develop fat depots over the thoraco–cervical spine (buffalo hump), in the supraclavicular region and over the cheeks and temporal regions giving rise to the rounded moon-like facies. The epidural space is another site of abnormal fat deposition, and this may lead to neurologic deficits.

Skin, muscle, and connective tissue

In addition to inducing insulin resistance in muscle tissue, glucocorticoids also cause catabolic changes in muscle, skin, and connective tissue. In the skin and connective tissue, glucocorticoids inhibit epidermal cell division and DNA synthesis and reduce collagen synthesis and production. In muscle, glucocorticoids cause atrophy (but not necrosis), and this seems to be specific for type II or phasic muscle fibers. Muscle protein synthesis is reduced. As a result, patients who have Cushing's syndrome present with muscle weakness and atrophy, characteristically affecting the gluteal and femoral proximal muscles.

Bone and calcium metabolism

The effects of glucocorticoids upon osteoclast function are debated, but osteoblast function is inhibited by glucocorticoids, and this is thought to explain the osteopenia and osteoporosis that characterize glucocorticoid excess [70]. With 0.5% to 1% of Western populations taking chronic glucocorticoid therapy, glucocorticoid-induced osteoporosis is becoming a prevalent health concern. Glucocorticoids also induce negative calcium balance by inhibiting intestinal calcium absorption and increasing renal calcium excretion. As a consequence, parathyroid hormone secretion usually is increased.

In childhood, the most common presentation of Cushing's syndrome is with poor linear growth and weight gain. Many patients who have long-standing Cushing's syndrome have lost height because of osteoporotic vertebral collapse. This can be assessed by measuring the patient's height and comparing it with his or her span; in normal subjects, these measurements should be equal. Pathologic fractures, either spontaneous or after minor trauma, are not uncommon. Rib fractures, in contrast to those of the vertebrae, are often painless. The radiograph appearances are typical, with exuberant callus formation at the site of the healing fracture. In addition, aseptic necrosis of the femoral and humeral heads, a recognized feature of high-dose exogenous corticosteroid therapy, can occur in endogenous Cushing's syndrome. Hypercalciuria may lead to renal calculi, but hypercalcemia is not a feature, because glucocorticoid excess prevents gastrointestinal (GI) calcium absorption.

Salt and water homeostasis and blood pressure control

Glucocorticoids increase blood pressure by several mechanisms involving actions on the kidney and vasculature [71]. In vascular smooth muscle, they increase sensitivity to pressor agents such as catecholamines and angiotensin II while reducing nitric oxide-mediated endothelial dilatation. Angiotensinogen synthesis is increased by glucocorticoids. In the kidney, depending upon the activity of the type 2 isozyme of 11β-HSD, cortisol can act on the distal nephron to cause sodium retention and potassium loss (mediated by means of the MR). Elsewhere across the nephron, glucocorticoids increase glomerular filtration rate, proximal tubular epithelial sodium transport, and free water clearance [72]. This latter effect involves antagonism of the action of vasopressin and explains the dilutional hyponatremia seen in patients who have glucocorticoid deficiency [73].

Hypokalemic alkalosis is found in 10% to 15% of patients who have Cushing's disease but over 95% of patients who have ectopic ACTH syndrome. Several factors may contribute to this mineralocorticoid excess state, including corticosterone and deoxycorticosterone excess, but the principal culprit is thought to be cortisol itself. Depending upon the prevailing cortisol production rate, cortisol swamps the protective 11β-HSD2 in the kidney to act as a mineralocorticoid. Hypokalemic alkalosis is more common in ectopic ACTH syndrome, because cortisol production rates are higher than in patients who have Cushing's disease [74,75]. This can be diagnosed by documenting an increase in the ratio of urinary cortisol/cortisone metabolites. In addition, hepatic 5α-reductase activity is inhibited, resulting in a greater excretion of 5β-cortisol metabolites.

Hypertension is another prominent feature in Cushing's syndrome, occurring in up to 75% of cases. Even though epidemiologic data show a strong association between blood pressure and obesity, hypertension is much more common in patients who have Cushing's syndrome than in those who have simple obesity [76]. This, together with the established metabolic consequences of the disease (diabetes, hyperlipidemia), is thought to explain the increased cardiovascular mortality in untreated cases. In addition, thromboembolic events may be more common in Cushing's disease patients.

Anti-inflammatory actions and the immune system

Glucocorticoids suppress immunologic responses, and this has been the stimulus to develop a series of highly potent pharmacologic glucocorticoids to treat several autoimmune and inflammatory conditions. The inhibitory effects are mediated at many levels. In peripheral blood, glucocorticoids reduce lymphocyte counts acutely (T lymphocytes > B lymphocytes) by redistributing lymphocytes from the intravascular compartment to the spleen, lymph nodes, and bone marrow [77]. Conversely, neutrophil counts increase following glucocorticoid administration. Eosinophil counts rapidly fall, an effect, which historically was used as a bioassay for glucocorticoids. The immunologic actions of glucocorticoids involve direct actions on both T and B lymphocytes, and these include inhibition of immunoglobulin synthesis and stimulation of lymphocyte apoptosis [78]. Inhibition of cytokine production from lymphocytes is mediated through inhibition of the action of nuclear factor kappa B (NF-κB). NF-κB plays a crucial and generalized role in inducing cytokine gene transcription; glucocorticoids can bind directly to NF-κB to prevent nuclear translocation, and, in addition induce NF-κB inhibitors, which sequester NF-κB in the cytoplasm, thereby inactivating its effect [79].

Additional anti-inflammatory effects involve inhibition of monocyte differentiation into macrophages and macrophage phagocytosis and cytotoxic activity. Glucocorticoids reduce the local inflammatory response by preventing the action of histamine and plasminogen activators.

Prostaglandin synthesis is impaired through the induction of lipocortins that inhibit phospholipase A2 activity.

Infections are more common in patients who have Cushing's disease [79,80]. In many instances, these are asymptomatic and occur because the normal inflammatory response is suppressed. Reactivation of tuberculosis has been reported and has even been the presenting feature in some cases. Fungal infections of the skin (notably tinea versicolor) and nails may occur, as may opportunistic fungal infections. Bowel perforation is more common in patients who have extreme hypercortisolism, and in turn, the hypercortisolism may mask the usual symptoms and signs of the condition. Wound infections are common and contribute to poor wound healing.

Central nervous system and mood

Clinical observations on patients who have glucocorticoid excess and deficiency reveal that the brain is an important target tissue for glucocorticoids, with depression, euphoria, psychosis, apathy, and lethargy being important manifestations. Both glucocorticoid and mineralocorticoid receptors are expressed in discrete regions of the rodent, brain including hippocampus, hypothalamus, cerebellum, and cortex [81]. Glucocorticoids cause neuronal death, notably in the hippocampus, and this may underlie the recent interest in glucocorticoids and cognitive function, memory, and neurodegenerative diseases such as Alzheimer's disease. Of note, DHEA has been shown to have neuroprotective effects in the hippocampus region [82,83]. CYP7B, an enzyme metabolizing DHEA to its 7α-hydroxylated metabolite, was shown to be highly expressed in brain, with increased expression in the hippocampus. Moreover, it has been shown that in the brain of Alzheimer's disease patients CYP7B expression in dentate neurons is decreased significantly [84]. In Cushing's syndrome, a characteristic shrinkage of the hippocampus region has been observed, caused by glucocorticoid excess, and it may be worthwhile to speculate whether the suppression of DHEA in adrenal Cushing's syndrome may result in a more pronounced effect because of the loss of a putative hippocampus protective factor.

Psychiatric abnormalities occur in approximately 50% of patients who have Cushing's syndrome regardless of cause [85]. Agitated depression and lethargy are among the most common problems [86], but paranoia and overt psychosis also are recognized. Memory and cognitive function also may be affected, and increased irritability may be an early feature. Insomnia is common, and both rapid eye movement and delta wave sleep patterns are reduced. Lowering of plasma cortisol by medical or surgical therapy usually results in a rapid improvement in the psychiatric state. Psychosis occurs most frequently in patients who have ACTH-dependent disease, and once this is cured, psychosis usually cannot be provoked by exogenous glucocorticoid treatment.

In the eye, glucocorticoids act to raise intraocular pressure through an increase in aqueous humor production and deposition of matrix within the trabecular meshwork that inhibits aqueous drainage. 11β-HSD1 is expressed in the ciliary epithelium, and this may augment corticosteroid-induced aqueous humor production [61]. Steroid-induced glaucoma appears to have a genetic predisposition, but the underlying mechanisms are unknown [87]. Ocular effects in Cushing's syndrome include raised intraocular pressure and exophthalmos (in up to one third of patients in Cushing's original series), the latter occurring because of increased retro-orbital fat deposition. Cataracts, a well-recognized complication of corticosteroid therapy, seem to be uncommon [88], except as a complication of diabetes. In the authors' experience, chemosis is a sensitive and under-reported feature of Cushing's syndrome.

Gut

Chronic, but not acute administration of glucocorticoids increases the risk of developing peptic ulcer disease [89]. Pancreatitis with fat necrosis is reported in patients who have glucocorticoid excess. The GR is expressed throughout the GI tract and the MR in the distal colon, and these mediate the corticosteroid control of epithelial ion transport.

Endocrine effects

Glucocorticoids suppress the thyroid axis, probably through a direct action on thyrotropin secretion. In addition, they inhibit 5′ deiodinase activity, mediating the conversion of thyroxine to active triiodothyronine. Growth hormone secretion is reduced, possibly mediated through an increase in somatostatinergic tone. Glucocorticoids also act centrally to inhibit GnRH pulsatility and luteinizing hormone and follicle-stimulating hormone release [90]. These physiologic effects of glucocorticoids explain the functional suppression of the pituitary–thyroid axis and pituitary–gonadal axis in patients who have Cushing's syndrome. Cortisol causes a reversible form of hypogonadotrophic hypogonadism but also directly inhibits Leydig cell function.

In Cushing's syndrome, gonadal dysfunction is very common, with menstrual irregularity in females and loss of libido in both sexes. Hirsutism frequently is found in female patients, as is acne. The most common form of hirsutism is vellous hypertrichosis on the face, and this should be distinguished from darker terminal differentiated hirsutism that may occur, but usually signifies concomitant androgen excess (as may occur secondary to ACTH-mediated adrenal androgen secretion).

Summary

Insights into the physiology and pathophysiology of adrenal steroids help to explain how the clinical sequelae of Cushing's syndrome evolve.

Endogenous glucocorticoid excess does not impact only on glucocorticoid action, but it also affects adrenal steroidogenesis and steroid metabolism, thereby contributing to the manifestations of the disease. Further understanding of the underlying pathophysiology will enable clinicians to improve diagnostic assessment and therapeutic management of patients suffering from Cushing's syndrome.

References

[1] Gwynne JT, Strauss JF III. The role of lipoprotein in steroidogenesis and cholesterol metabolism in steroidogenic glands. Endocr Rev 1982;3:299–329.

[2] Borkowski AJ, Levin S, Delcroix C, et al. Blood cholesterol and hydrocortisone production in man: quantitative aspects of the utilization of circulating cholesterol by the adrenals at rest and under adrenocorticotropin stimulation. J Clin Invest 1967;46:797–811.

[3] Acton S, Rigotti A, Landschulz KT, et al. Identification of scavenger receptor SR-BI as a high-density lipoprotein receptor. Science 1996;27:518–20.

[4] Stocco DM, Clark BJ. Regulation of the acute production of steroids in steroidogenic cells. Endocr Rev 1996;17:221–44.

[5] Bernhardt R. The role of adrenodoxin in adrenal steroidogenesis. Current Opinion in Endocrinology & Diabetes 2000;7:109–15.

[6] Onoda M, Hall PF. Cytochrome b_5 stimulates purified testicular microsomal cytochrome P450 (C_{21} side-chain cleavage). Biochem Biophys Res Commun 1982;108:454–60.

[7] Lee TC, Miller WL, Auchus RJ. Cytochrome b5 augments the 17,20-lyase activity of human P450c17 without direct electron transfer. J Biol Chem 1998;273:3158–65.

[8] Miller WL. Molecular biology of steroid hormone synthesis. Endocr Rev 1988;9:295–318.

[9] White PC, Mune T, Agarwal AK. 11β-Hydroxysteroid dehydrogenase and the syndrome of apparent mineralocorticoid excess. Endocr Rev 1997;18:135–56.

[10] Rheaume E, Simard J, Morel Y, et al. Congenital adrenal hyperplasia due to point mutations in the type II 3 beta-hydroxysteroid dehydrogenase gene. Nat Genet 1992;1:239–45.

[11] Geller DH, Auchus RJ, Mendonca BB, et al. The genetic and functional basis of isolated 17,20-lyase deficiency. Nat Genet 1997;17:201–5.

[12] Tajima T, Fujieda K, Kouda N, et al. Heterozygous mutation in the cholesterol side chain cleavage enzyme (p450scc) gene in a patient with 46,XY sex reversal and adrenal insufficiency. J Clin Endocrinol Metab 2001;86:3820–5.

[13] Arlt W, Walker EA, Draper N, et al. Congenital adrenal hyperplasia caused by mutant P450 oxidoreductase and human androgen synthesis: analytical study. Lancet 2004;363:2128–35.

[14] John ME, John MC, Ashley P, MacDonald RJ, et al. Identification and characterization of cDNA clones specific for cholesterol side-chain cleavage cytochrome P-450. Proc Natl Acad Sci U S A 1984;81:5628–32.

[15] Lorence MC, Murray BA, Trant JM, et al. Human 3β-hydroxysteroid dehydrogenase/Δ^5-Δ^4 isomerase from placenta: expression in nonsteroidogenic cells of a protein that catalyses the dehydrogenation/isomerization of C21 and C19 steroids. Endocrinology 1990;126:2493–8.

[16] Bradshaw KD, Waterman MR, Couch RT, et al. Characterization of complementary deoxyribonucleic acid for human adrenocortical 17α-hydroxylase: a probe for analysis of 17α-hydroxylase deficiency. Mol Endocrinol 1987;1:348–54.

[17] White PC, New MI, Dupont B. Cloning and expression of cDNA encoding a bovine adrenal cytochrome P450 specific for steroid 21-hydroxylation. Proc Natl Acad Sci U S A 1984;81: 1986–90.

[18] Chua SC, Szabo P, Vitek A, et al. Cloning of cDNA encoding steroid 11β-hydroxylase (P450c11). Proc Natl Acad Sci U S A 1987;84:7193–7.

[19] Mornet E, Dupont J, Vitek A, et al. Characterization of two genes encoding human steroid 11β-hydroxylase (P-450(11)β). J Biol Chem 1989;264:20961–7.

[20] Curnow KM, Tusie-Luna MT, Pascoe L, et al. The product of the CYP11B2 gene is required for aldosterone biosynthesis in the human adrenal cortex. Mol Endocrinol 1991;5:1513–22.
[21] Suzuki T, Sasano H, Takeyama J, et al. Developmental changes in steroidogenic enzymes in human postnatal adrenal cortex: immunohistochemical studies. Clin Endocrinol (Oxf) 2000; 53:739–47.
[22] Strott CA. Sulfonation and molecular action. Endocr Rev 2002;23:703–32.
[23] Siiteri PK, MacDonald PC. The utilization of dehydroisoandrosterone sulphate for estrogen synthesis during human pregnancy. Steroids 1963;2:713–30.
[24] Rainey WE, White PC. Functional adrenal zonation and regulation of aldosterone biosynthesis. Current Opinion in Endocrinology & Diabetes 1998;5:175–82.
[25] Quinn SJ, Williams GH. Regulation of aldosterone secretion. Annu Rev Physiol 1988;50: 409–26.
[26] Dluhy RG, Axelrod L, Underwood RH, et al. Studies of the control of plasma aldosterone concentration in normal man: effect of dietary potassium and acute potassium infusion. J Clin Invest 1972;51:1950–7.
[27] Labrie F, Belanger A, Simard J, et al. DHEA and peripheral androgen and oestrogen formation: intracrinology. Ann N Y Acad Sci 1995;774:16–28.
[28] Longcope C. Adrenal and gonadal secretion in normal females. Clin Endocrinol Metab 1986;15:213–28.
[29] Orentreich N, Brind JL, Rizer RL, Vogelman JH. Age changes and sex differences in serum dehydroepiandrosterone sulfate concentrations throughout adulthood. J Clin Endocrinol Metab 1984;59:551–5.
[30] Reiter EO, Fuldauer VG, Root AW. Secretion of the adrenal androgen, dehydroepiandrosterone sulfate, during normal infancy, childhood, and adolescence, in sick infants, and in children with endocrinologic abnormalities. J Pediatr 1977;90:766–70.
[31] Sklar CA, Kaplan SL, Grumbach MM. Evidence for dissociation between adrenarche and gonadarche: studies in patients with idiopathic precocious puberty, gonadal dysgenesis, isolated gonadotropin deficiency, and constitutionally delayed growth and adolescence. J Clin Endocrinol Metab 1980;51:548–56.
[32] Orentreich N, Brind JL, Vogelman JH, et al. Long-term longitudinal measurements of plasma dehydroepiandrosterone sulfate in normal men. J Clin Endocrinol Metab 1992;75: 1002–4.
[33] Laughlin GA, Barrett-Connor E. Sexual dimorphism in the influence of advanced aging on adrenal hormone levels: the Rancho Bernardo Study. J Clin Endocrinol Metab 2000;85: 3561–8.
[34] Parker CR, Mixon RL, Brissie RM, et al. Aging alters zonation in the adrenal cortex of men. J Clin Endocrinol Metab 1997;82:3898–901.
[35] Liu CH, Laughlin GA, Fischer UG, et al. Marked attenuation of ultradian and circadian rhythms of dehydroepiandrosterone in postmenopausal women: evidence for a reduced 17,20-desmolase enzymatic activity. J Clin Endocrinol Metab 1990;71:900–6.
[36] Parker CR, Slayden SM, Azziz R, et al. Effects of aging on adrenal function in the human: responsiveness and sensitivity of adrenal androgens and cortisol to adrenocorticotropin in premenopausal and postmenopausal women. J Clin Endocrinol Metab 2000;85:48–54.
[37] Weinberger C, Hollenberg SM, Rosenfeld MG, et al. Domain structure of the human glucocorticoid receptor and its relationship to the v-erb-A oncogene product. Nature 1985; 318:670–2.
[38] Arriza JL, Weinberger C, Cerelli G, et al. Cloning of human mineralocorticoid receptor complementary DNA: structural and functional kinship with the glucocorticoid receptor. Science 1987;237:268–75.
[39] Gustafsson JA, Carlstedt-Duke J, Poellinger L, et al. Biochemistry, molecular biology, and physiology of the glucocorticoid receptor. Endocr Rev 1987;8:185–234.
[40] Lu NZ, Cidlowski JA. The origin and function of multiple human glucocorticoid receptor isoforms. Ann N Y Acad Sci 2004;1024:102–23.

[41] Zennaro MC, Farman N, Bonvalet JP, et al. Tissue-specific expression of α and β mRNA isoforms of the human mineralocorticoid receptor in normal and pathological states. J Clin Endocrinol Metab 1997;82:1345–52.

[42] Pratt WB. The role of heat shock protein in regulating the function, folding and trafficking of the glucocorticoid receptor. J Biol Chem 1993;268:21455–8.

[43] Beato M, Sanchez-Pacheco A. Interaction of steroid hormone receptors with the transcription initiation complex. Endocr Rev 1996;17:587–609.

[44] Hollenberg SM, Giguere V, Segui P, et al. Colocalization of DNA-binding and transcriptional activation functions in the human glucocorticoid receptor. Cell 1987;49: 39–46.

[45] Rusconi S, Yamamoto KR. Functional dissection of the hormone and DNA binding activities of the glucocorticoid receptor. EMBO J 1987;6:1309–15.

[46] McKenna NJ, Lanz RB, O'Malley BW. Nuclear receptor coregulators: cellular and molecular biology. Endocr Rev 1999;20:321–44.

[47] Krozowski ZS, Funder JW. Renal mineralocorticoid receptors and hippocampal corticosterone-binding species have identical intrinsic steroid specificity. Proc Natl Acad Sci U S A 1983;80:6056–60.

[48] Edwards CR, Stewart PM, Burt D, et al. Localisation of 11β-hydroxysteroid dehydrogenase—tissue-specific protector of the mineralocorticoid receptor. Lancet 1988;ii:836–41.

[49] Funder JW, Pearce PT, Smith R, et al. Mineralocorticoid action: target tissue specificity is enzyme, not receptor, mediated. Science 1988;242:583–5.

[50] Verrey F, Kraehenbuhl JP, Rossier BC. Aldosterone induces a rapid increase in the rate of Na, K-ATPase gene transcription in cultured kidney cells. Mol Endocrinol 1989;3:1369–76.

[51] Chen SY, Bhargava A, Mastroberardino L, et al. Epithelial sodium channel regulated by aldosterone-induced protein sgk. Proc Natl Acad Sci U S A 1999;93:6025–30.

[52] Rocha R, Funder JW. The pathophysiology of aldosterone in the cardiovascular system. Ann N Y Acad Sci 2002;970:89–100.

[53] Pitt B, Remme W, Zannad F, et al. Eplerenone Post-Acute Myocardial Infarction Heart Failure Efficacy and Survival Study investigators. Eplerenone, a selective aldosterone blocker, in patients with left ventricular dysfunction after myocardial infarction. N Engl J Med 2003;348:1309–21.

[54] Christ M, Haseroth K, Falkenstein E, et al. Nongenomic steroid actions: fact or fancy? Vitam Horm 1999;57:325–73.

[55] Hammond GL. Molecular properties of corticosteroid binding globulin and the sex-steroid binding proteins. Endocr Rev 1990;11:65–79.

[56] Zumoff B, Bradlow HL, Levin J, et al. Influence of thyroid function on the in vivo cortisol–cortisone equilibrium in man. J Steroid Biochem 1983;18:437–40.

[57] Moore JS, Monson JP, Kaltsas G, et al. Modulation of 11β-hydroxysteroid dehydrogenase isozymes by growth hormone and insulin-like growth factor: in vivo and in vitro studies. J Clin Endocrinol Metab 1999;84:4172–7.

[58] Yamada S, Iwai K. Induction of hepatic cortisol-6-hydroxylase by rifampicin. Lancet 1976; 2:366–7.

[59] Morris DJ, Brem AS. Metabolic derivatives of aldosterone. Am J Physiol 1987;252:F365–73.

[60] White PC, Mune T, Agarwal AK. 11β-hydroxysteroid dehydrogenase and the syndrome of apparent mineralocorticoid excess. Endocr Rev 1997;18:135–6.

[61] Tomlinson JW, Walker EA, Bujalska IJ, et al. 11β-Hydroxysteroid dehydrogenase type 1: a tissue-specific regulator of glucocorticoid response. Endocr Rev 2004;25:831–66.

[62] Quinkler M, Stewart PM. Hypertension and the cortisol–cortisone shuttle. J Clin Endocrinol Metab 2003;88:2384–92.

[63] Bujalska IJ, Kumar S, Stewart PM. Does central obesity reflect Cushing's disease of the omentum? Lancet 1997;349:1210–3.

[64] Kotelevtsev Y, Holmes MC, Burchell A, et al. 11β-hydroxysteroid dehydrogenase type 1 knockout mice show attenuated glucocorticoid-inducible responses and resist hyperglycemia on obesity or stress. Proc Natl Acad Sci U S A 1997;94:14924–9.
[65] Draper N, Walker EA, Bujalska IJ, et al. Mutations in the genes encoding 11β-hydroxysteroid dehydrogenase type 1 and hexose-6-phosphate dehydrogenase interact to cause cortisone reductase deficiency. Nat Genet 2003;34:434–9.
[66] Cooper MS, Blumsohn A, Goddard PE, et al. 11β-Hydroxysteroid dehydrogenase type 1 activity predicts the effects of glucocorticoids on bone. J Clin Endocrinol Metab 2003;88: 3874–7.
[67] Exton JH. Regulation of gluconeogenesis by glucocorticoids. In: Baxter JD, Rousseau GG, editors. Glucocorticoid hormone action. New York: Springer-Verlag; 1979. p. 535–46.
[68] Hauner H, Entenmann G, Wabitsch M, et al. Promoting effects of glucocorticoids on the differentiation of human adipocyte precursor cells cultured in a chemically defined medium. J Clin Invest 1989;84:1663–70.
[69] Rebuffe-Scrive M, Krotkiewski M, Elfverson J, et al. Muscle and adipose morphology and metabolism in Cushing's syndrome. J Clin Endocr Metab 1988;67:1122–8.
[70] Canalis E. Clinical review 83. Mechanisms of glucocorticoid action in bone: implications to glucocorticoid-induced osteoporosis. J Clin Endocrinol Metab 1996;81:3441–7.
[71] Fraser R, Davies DL, Connell JMC. Hormones and hypertension. Clin Endocrinol (Oxf) 1989;31:701–46.
[72] Marver D. Evidence of corticosteroid action along the nephron. Am J Physiol 1984;246: F111–23.
[73] Raff H. Glucocorticoid inhibition of neurohypophysial vasopressin secretion. Am J Physiol 1987;252:R635–44.
[74] Ulick S, Wang JZ, Blumenfeld JD, et al. Cortisol inactivation overload: a mechanism of mineralocorticoid hypertension in the ectopic adrenocorticotropin syndrome. J Clin Endocrinol Metab 1992;74:963–7.
[75] Stewart PM, Walker BR, Holder G, et al. 11β-Hydroxysteroid dehydrogenase activity in Cushing's syndrome: explaining the mineralocorticoid excess state of the ectopic ACTH syndrome. J Clin Endocrinol Metab 1995;80:3617–20.
[76] Saruta T, Suzuki H, Handa M, et al. Multiple factors contribute to the pathogenesis of hypertension in Cushing's syndrome. J Clin Endocrinol Metab 1986;62:275–9.
[77] Yu DT, Clements PJ, Paulus HE, et al. Human lymphocyte subpopulations: effect of corticosteroids. J Clin Invest 1974;53:565–71.
[78] McKay LI, Cidlowski JA. Molecular control of immune/inflammatory responses: interactions between nuclear factor-kB and steroid receptor-signalling pathways. Endocr Rev 1999;20:435–59.
[79] Dale DC, Petersdorf RG. Corticosteroids and infectious diseases. Med Clin North Am 1973; 57:1277–87.
[80] Graham BS, Tucker WS Jr. Opportunistic infections in endogenous Cushing's syndrome. Ann Intern Med 1984;101:334–8.
[81] McEwen BS, deKloet ER, Rostene W. Adrenal steroid receptors and action in the central nervous system. Physiol Rev 1986;66:1121–88.
[82] MacLusky NJ, Hajszan T, Leranth C. Effects of dehydroepiandrosterone and flutamide on hippocampal CA1 spine synapse density in male and female rats: implications for the role of androgens in maintenance of hippocampal structure. Endocrinology 2004;145:4154–61.
[83] Hajszan T, MacLusky NJ, Leranth C. Dehydroepiandrosterone increases hippocampal spine synapse density in ovariectomized female rats. Endocrinology 2004;145:1042–5.
[84] Yau JL, Rasmuson S, Andrew R, et al. Dehydroepiandrosterone 7-hydroxylase CYP7B: predominant expression in primate hippocampus and reduced expression in Alzheimer's disease. Neuroscience 2003;121:307–14.
[85] Jeffcoate WJ, Silverstone JT, Edwards CRW, et al. Psychiatric manifestations of Cushing's syndrome: response to lowering of plasma cortisol. Q J Med 1979;48:465–72.

[86] Dorn LD, Burgess ES, Dubbert B, et al. Psychopathology in patients with endogenous Cushing's syndrome: atypical or melancholic features. Clin Endocrinol (Oxf) 1995;43: 433–42.
[87] Clark AF. Steroids, ocular hypertension, and glaucoma. J Glaucoma 1995;4:354–69.
[88] Bouzas EA, Mastorakos G, Friedman G, et al. Posterior subcapsular catarct in endogenous Cushing's syndrome: an uncommon manifestation. Invest Ophthalmol Vis Sci 1993;34: 3497–500.
[89] Messer J, Reitman D, Sacks HS, et al. Association of adrenocorticosteroid therapy and peptic ulcer disease. N Engl J Med 1983;309:21–4.
[90] Saketos M, Sharma N, Santoro NF. Suppression of the hypothalmo-pituitary-ovarian axis in normal women by glucocorticoids. Biol Reprod 1993;49:1270–6.

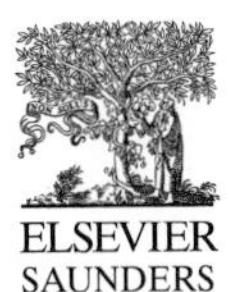
ELSEVIER
SAUNDERS

Endocrinol Metab Clin N Am
34 (2005) 315–326

ENDOCRINOLOGY
AND METABOLISM
CLINICS
OF NORTH AMERICA

Glucocorticoid Resistance and Hypersensitivity

Carl D. Malchoff, MD, PhD*,
Diana M. Malchoff, PhD

Division of Endocrinology, University of Connecticut Health Center, 263 Farmington Avenue, Farmington, CT 06030, USA

Cortisol, a critical mediator of energy and blood pressure homeostasis, is produced in the adrenal cortex in response to corticotropin (ACTH) stimulation and circulates within a tightly controlled concentration range with diurnal variation. Syndromes of glucocorticoid (GC) resistance and hypersensitivity to cortisol are rare and present a diagnostic and therapeutic challenge to the clinician. Clinically, these syndromes can be categorized according to the tissue location of resistance and hypersensitivity. Altered sensitivity may be present in all tissues, present in peripheral tissues only with the hypothalamus and pituitary being unaffected, or limited to specific tissues (Box 1). In most instances, careful clinical and biochemical observations have stimulated detailed and successful mechanistic studies. This article emphasizes the disorders caused by mutations and polymorphisms of the alpha form of the GC receptor (GRα). These disorders usually present with increased circulating cortisol concentrations and must be distinguished from Cushing's syndrome, because the therapies are markedly different. The other disorders present with clinical features limited to a specific organ system. Although they illustrate important physiologic and pathophysiologic principles, they usually are not confused with Cushing's syndrome.

Generalized glucocorticoid resistance

Generalized GC resistance (GGR), also known as primary cortisol resistance, is a familial GC receptor-mediated disorder that first was

* Corresponding author.
E-mail address: malchoff@nso2.uchc.edu (C.D. Malchoff).

0889-8529/05/$ - see front matter
doi:10.1016/j.ecl.2005.02.002 *endo.theclinics.com*

Box 1. Syndromes of glucocorticoid resistance and hypersensitivity

Resistance

Generalized

- Generalized GC resistance
- GRα polymorphism with mild resistance
- Apparent resistance: corticosteroid-binding globulin (CBG) excess

Peripheral

- Cushing's disease without central obesity

Localized

- Cortisone reductase deficiency
- Neoplasms: pituitary and hematologic
- Asthma?

Hypersensitivity

Generalized

- GRα polymorphisms
- GRα polymorphism with mild hypersensitivity
- Apparent hypersensitivity: CBG deficiency

Peripheral

- Cushing's syndrome with normal hypothalamic–pituitary–adrenal (HPA) axis

Localized

- Apparent mineralocorticoid excess
- Metabolic syndrome?

described by Vingerhoeds et al in 1976 [1]. Biochemical features include increased circulating concentrations of all three classes of adrenal steroids: GCs (cortisol), androgens (dehydroepiandrosterone, dehydroepiandrosterone sulfate, and androstenedione), and mineralocorticoids (deoxycorticosterone). In contrast the clinical features include only evidence of excess androgens and mineralocorticoids. The Cushingoid features usually associated with cortisol excess are absent.

The endocrine pathophysiology of this disorder is described in Fig. 1 and contrasted with the normal endocrine physiology of the HPA axis. Resistance to GCs is partial and generalized to all tissues. Hence the pituitary and hypothalamus are partially resistant to the negative feedback of cortisol. As expected, the production of ACTH and the ACTH-dependent adrenal steroids is reset at higher concentrations than normal. Because the peripheral tissues are relatively insensitive to cortisol, the Cushingoid features do not develop. In contrast, the peripheral tissues remain sensitive to androgens and mineralocorticoids. Therefore, the clinical

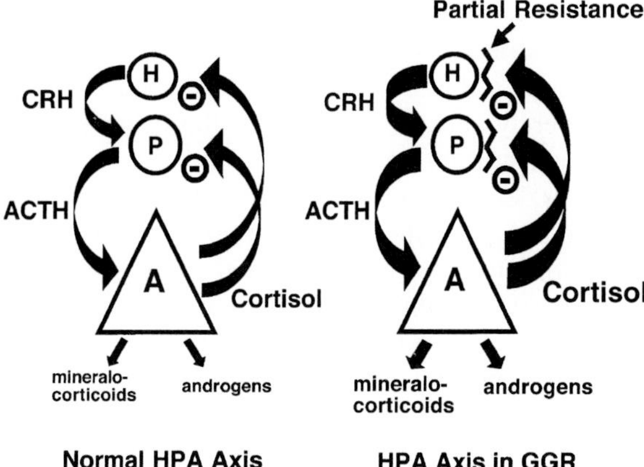

Fig. 1. Regulation of the HPA axis. Normal compared with GGR. The normal HPA axis is shown diagrammatically and compared with HPA axis in GGR. The primary lesion within the HPA axis is the resistance at the level of the pituitary and hypothalamus to the normal negative feedback effects of cortisol on secretion of corticotropin-releasing hormone (CRH) and ACTH. The net result is an increase in production of CRH, ACTH, cortisol, mineralocorticoids, and adrenal androgens. Therefore in GGR, the HPA axis is reset at higher cortisol and ACTH concentrations than normal. Like the hypothalamus and pituitary, the peripheral tissues are relatively resistant to cortisol, so that the expected features of excess GCs do not develop. In contrast, the peripheral tissues remain normally sensitive to mineralocorticoids and androgens. Therefore the clinical presentations include volume-dependent hypertension with hypokalemia, hirsutism and acne in women, isosexual precocious pseudopuberty in boys, and heterosexual precocious pseudopuberty and pseudohermaphroditism in girls. (*Adapted from* Malchoff DM, Malchoff CM. Generalized glucocorticoid resistance. In: DeGroot LJ, Jameson JL, editors. Endocrinology. vol. 2. 4th edition. Philadelphia: W.B. Saunders; 2001. p. 1716.)

features are secondary to increased production of these hormones. Other features of the HPA axis are left intact. In particular, the diurnal variation in cortisol production and responses to stress persists. These features and the inheritance pattern have important diagnostic and therapeutic implications.

The most common feature of GGR is hypercortisolism without Cushingoid features. Because most patients who do not have Cushingoid features are not tested for hypercortisolism, this initial finding is often serendipitous. The excess adrenal androgens cause hirsutism, acne, and altered menstruation in women, and this may be the most common presentation of this disorder [2,3]. Isosexual precocious pseudopuberty in a boy [4] and pseudohermaphroditism in a female neonate [5] have been described. Features of excess mineralocorticoids include volume-dependent hypertension with low plasma renin activity and sometimes hypokalemia [1,2,6,7]. The clinical features are quite variable and generally reflect the biochemical abnormalities and the degree of resistance. Resistance is usually relatively mild, but it can be severe. Presumably, complete resistance is incompatible with life.

Both hypercortisolism and decreased responsiveness to dexamethasone occur in almost all patients, although there have been a small number of patients described with only mild resistance to dexamethasone suppression [2]. In the most severely affected individuals, the urinary cortisol excretion may exceed the upper normal limit by 200-fold [1,2]. The diurnal variation of serum cortisol is left intact, but reset at higher concentrations than normal. This finding distinguishes GGR from Cushing's syndrome. Plasma ACTH concentrations may be in the normal range or elevated, but they are always inappropriately high for the degree of hypercortisolism. In women and children, the serum adrenal androgen concentrations usually are elevated above the normal range [1,2,4–9]. Because the normal ranges of these hormones are higher in adult men, adult male subjects may not demonstrate any apparent biochemical abnormalities of these hormones. The adrenal androgens produce the clinical features of precious pseudopuberty in children [4] and the features of hirsutism and acne in women [2,3].

The hypertension of GGR is volume-dependent and associated with a low plasma renin activity and sometimes with a low serum potassium concentration [1,2,6,7]. It likely is caused by high circulating concentrations of deoxycorticosterone (DOC) and cortisol. DOC may be elevated two- to fourfold above the upper normal limit [4,6–8]. At high circulating concentrations, these hormones can activate the mineralocorticoid receptor in the renal distal tubule. Corticosterone production also is increased, but this likely contributes little to the clinical features, because it is not a potent GC or mineralocorticoid in people. Aldosterone production is not increased, because renin stimulation of angiotensin II production is necessary to permit conversion of corticosterone to aldosterone.

The inheritance patterns are variable. Both autosomal dominant and recessive inheritance have been described. In addition, a gene dose effect or codominant inheritance occurs in some kindreds, and homozygotes are affected to a greater degree than the heterozygotes [8,10]. In the dominant syndromes, the mutant GRα interferes with the function of the normal receptor. This is a dominant negative effect [11]. In the recessive syndromes, one might expect the normal receptor to rescue the mutant receptor so that the heterozygotes would be clinically normal. This has not been demonstrated in laboratory assays, however [12].

The differential diagnosis of GGR includes Cushing's syndrome, interference with the urinary cortisol assay, increased cortisol-binding globulin, and depression. Two characteristics help to distinguish GGR from Cushing's syndrome: the diurnal variation of cortisol production and the cortisol response to insulin-induced hypoglycemia [4,13]. Because the HPA axis is reset at an abnormally high circulating hormone concentration, there is a diurnal change in serum cortisol concentration, and cortisol production increases following hypoglycemic stress. In Cushing's syndrome, the cortisol response to a hypoglycemic stress is diminished, and the diurnal variation of serum cortisol is absent. In addition, a familial association of hypercortisolism and an evaluation of linear growth in children may help to distinguish GC resistance from Cushing's syndrome. Although there are probably rare exceptions, familial ACTH-dependent hypercortisolism is caused by GC resistance and not Cushing's syndrome. The absence of a familial association of hypercortisolism does not exclude GC resistance. Some etiologic GC receptor mutations are new, and the disorder is recessive in some kindreds. In children, the growth curve is useful in distinguishing GGR from Cushing's syndrome. Hypercortisolism reduces the rate of linear growth, while androgens stimulate it [4]. Accelerated growth with advanced bone age suggests GGR, while growth delay suggests Cushing's syndrome. Both carbamazepine and fenofibrate or their metabolites interfere with the assays for urinary cortisol excretion and produce false elevations [14,15]. Therefore, ingestion of these pharmaceutical agents may give the false impression of hypercortisolism and suggest GGR.

Mutations in the alpha form of the GC receptor are the most common cause of this disorder. In some patients, however, the GRα complementary DNA sequence is normal, and the molecular etiology remains unknown [16,17]. Deletions of the *GRα* gene reduce GR number and cause dominantly inherited GC resistance [18]. Fig. 2 summarizes the point mutations causing GGR that have been identified in the DNA-binding [3] and ligand-binding domains of the GRα [3,5,18–20]. These point mutations interfere with several GRα activities, including GRα binding to cortisol and other GCs, GRα transport into the nucleus, and GRα interaction with coactivators [12]. Increased expression of the beta form of the GC receptor (GRβ) combined

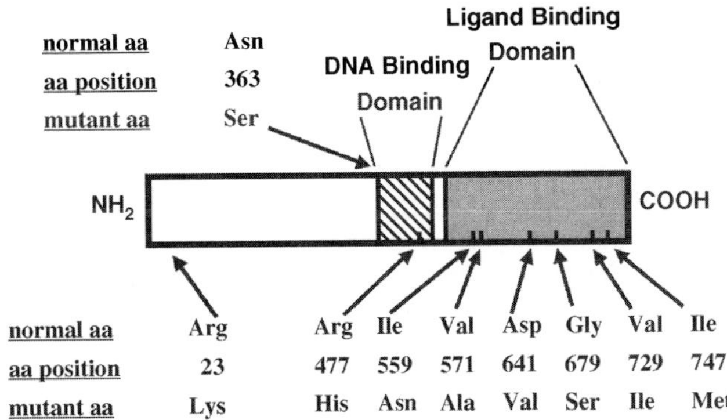

Fig. 2. Mutations and polymorphisms of the alpha GC receptor (GRα). The primary sequence of the GRα is shown with the DNA binding domain and ligand binding domains indicated. The single polymorphism shown above the GRα is associated with obesity and possible GC hypersensitivity, while the GRα mutations and polymorphisms shown below the GRα diagram are associated with GC resistance. (*Adapted from* Malchoff DM, Malchoff CM. Generalized glucocorticoid resistance. In: DeGroot LJ, Jameson JL, editors. Endocrinology. vol. 2. 4th edition. Philadelphia: W.B. Saunders; 2001. p. 1718.)

with decreased expression of the GRα caused GC resistance in one subject [21]. The GRβ interferes with the activity of GRα. Analysis of the *GRα* gene is not available on a commercial basis. Therefore, biochemical and clinical features are used most commonly to make the diagnosis of GC resistance, and DNA sequencing is performed in research laboratories.

Treatment of generalized GC resistance depends upon the clinical situation. If the subjects are asymptomatic, then no treatment is indicated. Dexamethasone will lower ACTH production and serum concentrations of both adrenal androgens and mineralocorticoids will decrease along with the circulating cortisol concentration. For individuals who have features caused by excess adrenal androgens or mineralocorticoids, this therapy is appropriate. The authors' approach has been to titrate the morning cortisol concentration into the usual normal range so that the subjects do not develop exogenous Cushing's syndrome [19]. Alternatively, mineralocorticoid antagonists or androgen antagonists could be used.

Mild glucocorticoid resistance associated with a GRα *receptor polymorphism*

Lamberts' group has investigated a large cohort in which 8% of subjects carry a *GRα* polymorphism that changes codon 23 from arginine to lysine [22,23]. There is evidence of mild central GC resistance in vivo, since the heterozygotes responded slightly less vigorously to a 1 mg dexamethasone test than normal subjects. Serum cortisol concentrations, however, are not different in the two groups, suggesting that central sensitivity to cortisol is similar. Heterozygotes who have this polymorphism have lower cholesterol levels, and heterozygote males with this polymorphism are taller, stronger, and have greater lean body mass and greater longevity than males that who not carry the polymorphism. This seems to confer a greater beneficial effect in men than women.

Apparent glucocorticoid resistance

Cortisol circulates bound to CBG. High concentrations of CBG, which occur during pregnancy and estrogen therapy, are associated with increased total cortisol concentrations [24,25]. The clinical features and measurements of CBG and free cortisol help to distinguish the increased circulating cortisol of pregnancy from Cushing's syndrome.

Localized glucocorticoid resistance

Glucocorticoid resistance caused by cortisone reductase deficiency

The role of cortisone reductase activity in human disease is being investigated. The interconversion of cortisol and cortisone is summarized in Fig. 3. The enzyme 11β-hydroxysteroid dehydrogenase type 1 (11β-HSD1)

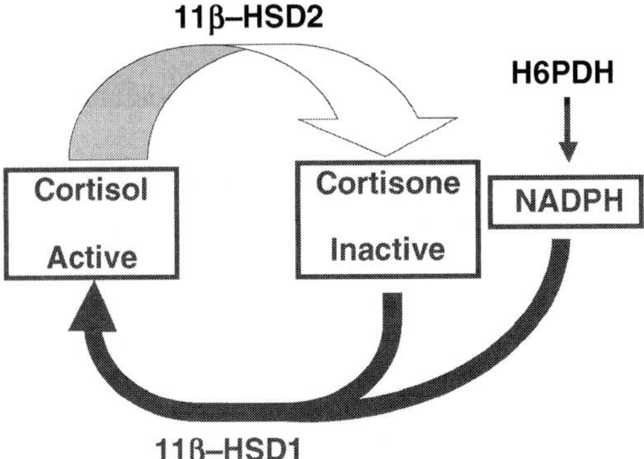

Fig. 3. Local tissue concentrations of cortisol are regulated by the interconversion of cortisol and cortisone. Changes in local cortisol concentrations cause hypersensitivity and resistance to cortisol. An example of local cortisol hypersensitivity is the syndrome of apparent mineralocorticoid excess. In this disorder, the kidney distal tubule fails to inactivate cortisol by conversion to cortisone. It is caused by mutations and deletions of the *11β-HSD2* gene. Local cortisol concentrations in other tissues may be diminished by a cortisone reductase deficiency that may be caused not only by a deficiency in 11β-HSD1, but also by a deficiency of H6PDH that generates the NADPH for cortisone reduction to cortisol. Hence, a cortisol resistance syndrome develops. Increased cortisone reductase activity in adipose tissue may contribute to the development of the metabolic syndrome. If this hypothesis is correct, then the metabolic syndrome could be viewed as a cortisol hypersensitivity state.

reduces cortisone to cortisol in liver and other tissues. Hexose-6-phosphate dehydrogenase (H6PDH) generates the nicotinamide adenosine dinucleotide phosphate (NADPH) substrate necessary for cortisone reductase activity [26]. It has been suggested that some of the effects of GCs are not caused by circulating cortisol, but by higher cortisol concentrations produced in the target tissues by the conversion of cortisone to cortisol. Several subjects have been described with a cortisone reductase activity deficiency [26]. In the most marked example, a subject who had proven pituitary Cushing's disease did not develop Cushingoid features [27]. Other subjects who have this disorder tend to be women presenting with increased adrenal androgens. The genetic mechanism causing cortisone reductase activity is polygenic. There are intronic polymorphisms of the *11β-HSD1* gene and polymorphisms in the *H6PDH* gene. Therefore decreased 11β-HSD and decreased available NADPH combine to cause cortisone reductase deficiency [26].

Glucocorticoid resistance localized to neoplasms

Resistance of ACTH secretion to the effects of GCs characterizes Cushing's disease caused by ACTH secreting pituitary adenomas. This is the basis of the 1 mg dexamethasone suppression test. There are probably multiple mechanisms that contribute to this resistance. In one study, about a third of ACTH-secreting pituitary tumors demonstrated loss of heterozygosity at the *GRα* locus, although no point mutations of the *GRα* were found [28]. Because investigations of generalized GC resistance demonstrate that a haploinsufficiency of the GRα causes GC resistance, then pituitary resistance to GCs contributes to the development of Cushing's disease. The resistance to GCs in most ACTH-secreting pituitary tumors and the loss of diurnal variation, however, likely are caused by other mechanisms. Some hematologic malignancies have altered *GRα* that may contribute to GC resistance [29,30].

Glucocorticoid resistance localized to bronchial smooth muscle in asthma

Recent studies by Roth et al provide evidence that asthma in some subjects may be caused by decreased expression of the CCAAT/enhancer binding protein α (C/EBPα) in bronchial smooth muscle cells [31]. The C/EBPα protein is necessary for the antiproliferative effect of GCs in bronchial smooth muscle cells. Therefore, those individuals who do not express this cofactor in their bronchial smooth muscle cells are at risk for developing asthma, and presumably the rest of the body's cells express C/EBPα, so that GC resistance is localized.

Glucocorticoid hypersensitivity syndrome

Generalized glucocorticoid hypersensitivity

Lamberts' group identified a *GRα* polymorphism that is associated with increased body mass index (BMI), but not with increased blood pressure. Individuals who have this polymorphism are more sensitive to a 0.25-mg dexamethasone challenge than normal subjects [32]. Circulating cortisol concentrations were normal. Therefore, this *GRα* polymorphism may confer a slight increase in GC sensitivity and subsequent increase in BMI as compared with controls. Another large population study identified a three-marker haplotype in *GRα* intron B associated with increased responsiveness to 0.25 mg dexamethasone [33]. Therefore, polymorphisms in the GRα DNA coding region and within *GRα* introns have modest influences on GC sensitivity.

Apparent generalized glucocorticoid hypersensitivity

An apparent generalized GC hypersensitivity syndrome can occur in individuals with low CBG caused by inherited mutations of the *CBG* gene [34–36]. Total circulating cortisol concentration is low, but the subjects do not have adrenal insufficiency, because the circulating concentrations of unbound (free) cortisol are normal. Some of these individuals have somewhat low blood pressure and depression, but it is not clear if this represents a selection bias or a true cause-and-effect relationship. Severe illness is a more common cause of low CBG, and many of these subjects have low ACTH-stimulated serum cortisol concentrations, but normal

ACTH-stimulated free cortisol concentrations. There is controversy as to whether these individuals require GC supplementation [37,38].

Peripheral glucocorticoid hypersensitivity

Two patients have been described with increased peripheral sensitivity to GCs. One was a young girl with significant Cushingoid features, but normal diurnal variation of serum cortisol and normal urinary cortisol excretion [39]. The cause of this increased sensitivity was felt to be an increase in the GC receptor number, because her circulating mononuclear leukocytes demonstrated this abnormality. The patient's Cushingoid features resolved later in life coincident with a fall in GC receptor number [39]. The mechanism of this transient GC receptor abnormality is unknown. Because the patient's circulating cortisol concentration was normal, and because cortisol production suppressed normally with dexamethasone, the GC sensitivity was limited to the periphery and did not involve the pituitary gland. Presumably a syndrome with generalized GC sensitivity would be clinically normal with biochemical evidence of hypocortisolism. The second subject with peripheral hypersensitivity [39] did have hypocortisolism with Cushingoid features, suggesting that the hypersensitivity in the peripheral tissues was greater than that in the hypothalamus and pituitary. Although the hypersensitivity could be reproduced in vitro by measuring the aromatase response of fibroblasts to dexamethasone, the mechanism for hypersensitivity remains unexplained [40].

Localized glucocorticoid hypersensitivity

Apparent mineralocorticoid excess

An apparent localized hypersensitivity to cortisol occurs in the kidney and is known as the syndrome of apparent mineralocorticoid excess [41]. This rare autosomal recessive disorder presents with hypertension and hypokalemia and is caused by mutations of 11β-HSD2, which converts cortisol to cortisone in the renal tubule. Cortisol binds the mineralocorticoid receptor with the same affinity as aldosterone. Cortisone is not a potent activator of this receptor, however. Individuals unable to convert cortisol to cortisone have excess cortisol in the renal tubule. Subsequently, the mineralocorticoid receptor is activated by cortisol, and the patient develops hypertension and hypokalemia. Dexamethasone suppresses cortisol production and can be used to treat this disorder.

Hypersensitivity in adipose tissue and the metabolic syndrome

It is attractive to speculate that components of the metabolic syndrome (obesity, insulin resistance, type 2 diabetes, and hypertension) may be caused by an apparent localized hypersensitivity to cortisol. Transgenic mice that overexpress 11β-HSD1 in adipose tissue develop the metabolic syndrome [42]. There is increased conversion of 11-dehydrocorticosterone to corticosterone (the active GC in mice) in the adipose tissue. This causes central obesity and insulin resistance. The validity of this model in the metabolic syndrome of humans is being investigated. Even if this is not a cause of the metabolic syndrome, it has been suggested that inhibition of the 11β-HSD1 in humans may reverse the metabolic syndrome [26]. A discussion of the potential for this mechanism to cause cortisol hypersensitivity in other tissues is discussed elsewhere [26].

Summary

GC resistance and hypersensitivity syndromes may be generalized or localized to specific tissues. Mechanisms of altered GC sensitivity include mutations or deletions of the *GRα* gene, decreased GRα cofactors, alterations in cortisol binding globulin, and perturbations of local cortisol concentrations. *GRα* gene mutations and deletions produce GGR. Polymorphisms of the *GRα* may contribute to mild syndromes of GGR and hypersensitivity. *GRα* gene deletions localized to ACTH-secreting pituitary tumors may contribute to pituitary GC resistance of some patients with Cushing's disease. Similarly, *GRα* gene abnormalities may contribute to GC resistance of a small number of hematologic malignancies. Decreased expression of the C/EBPα GRα cofactor in bronchial smooth muscle has been implicated in the development of asthma. Altered tissue concentrations of cortisol by increased or decreased interconversion of cortisol and cortisone cause apparent GC resistance and hypersensitivity syndromes. Best described is the syndrome of apparent mineralocorticoid excess that is caused by decreased 11β-HSD2 activity in the kidney. Cortisone reductase converts cortisone to active cortisol in local tissues. Decreased cortisone reductase activity may cause local resistance, while increased cortisone reductase activity may cause a local cortisol hypersensitivity syndrome. Finally, apparent GGR and sensitivity may be caused by increases and decreases in circulating CBG concentrations.

References

[1] Vingerhoeds A, Thijssen J, Shwarz F. Spontaneous hypercortisolism without Cushing's syndrome. J Clin Endocrinol Metab 1976;43:1128–33.

[2] Lamberts SWJ, Koper JW, Biemond P, et al. Cortisol receptor resistance: the variability of its clinical presentation and response to treatment. J Clin Endocrinol Metab 1992;74(2): 313–21.

[3] Ruiz M, Lind U, Gafvels M, Eggertsen G, et al. Characterization of two novel mutations in the glucocorticoid receptor gene in patients with primary cortisol resistance. Clin Endocrinol 2001;55:363–71.

[4] Malchoff C, Javier E, Malchoff D, et al. Primary cortisol resistance presenting as isosexual precocity. J Clin Endocrinol Metab 1990;70:503–7.
[5] Mendonca B, Leite M, de Castro M, et al. Female pseudohermaphroditism caused by a novel homozygous missense mutation of the GR gene. J Clin Endocrinol Metab 2002;87: 1805–9.
[6] Iida S, Gomi M, Moriwaki K, et al. Primary cortisol resistance accompanied by a reduction in glucocorticoid receptors in two members of the same family. J Clin Endocrinol Metab 1985;60:967–71.
[7] Nawata H, Sekiya K, Higuchi K, et al. Decreased deoxyribonucleic acid binding of glucocorticoid-receptor complex in cultured skin fibroblasts from a patient with glucocorticoid resistance syndrome. J Clin Endocrinol Metab 1987;65:219–26.
[8] Chrousos GP, Vingerhoeds ACM, Brandon D, et al. Primary cortisol resistance in man: a glucocorticoid receptor-mediated disease. J Clin Invest 1982;69:1261–9.
[9] Lamberts SWJ, Poldermans D, Zweens M, et al. Familial cortisol resistance: differential diagnostic and therapeutic aspects. J Clin Endocrinol Metab 1986;63:1328–33.
[10] Chrousos G, Vingerhoeds A, Loriaux D, et al. Primary cortisol resistance: a family study. J Clin Endocrinol Metab 1983;56:1243–5.
[11] Kino T, Stauber RH, Resau JH, et al. Pathologic human GR mutant has a transdominant negative effect on the wild-type GR by inhibiting its translocation into the nucleus: Importance of the ligand-binding domain for intracellular GR trafficking. J Clin Endocrinol Metab 2001;86:5600–8.
[12] Charmandari E, Kino T, Souvatzoglou E, et al. Natural glucocorticoid receptor mutants causing generalized glucocorticoid resistance: molecular genotype, genetic transmission, and clinical phenotype. J Clin Endocrinol Metab 2004;89:1939–49.
[13] Besser G, Edwards C. Cushing's syndrome. Clin Endocrinol Metab 1972;1:451–90.
[14] Findling JW, Shaker J, Raff H, et al. Pseudohypercortisoluria: spurious elevation of urinary cortisol due to carbamazepine. Endocrinologist 1998;8:51–4.
[15] Meikle A, Findling J, Kushnir M, et al. Pseudo-Cushing's syndrome caused by fenofibrate interference with urinary cortisol assayed by high-performance liquid chromatography. J Clin Endocrinol Metab 2003;88:3521–4.
[16] New M, Nimkarn S, Brandon D, et al. Resistance to multiple steroids in two sisters. J Clin Endocrinol Metab 2001;76:161–6.
[17] Huizenga N, de Lange P, Koper J, et al. Five patients with biochemical and/or clinical generalized glucocorticoid resistance without alterations in the glucocorticoid receptor gene. J Clin Endocrinol Metab 2000;85:2076–81.
[18] Karl M, Lamberts SWJ, Detera-Wadleigh SD, et al. Familial glucocorticoid resistance caused by a splice site deletion in the human glucocorticoid receptor gene. J Clin Endocrinol Metab 1993;76:683–9.
[19] Malchoff DM, Brufsky A, Reardon G, et al. A point mutation of the human glucocorticoid receptor in primary cortisol resistance. J Clin Invest 1993;91:1918–25.
[20] Hurley D, Accili D, Stratakis C, et al. Point mutation causing a single amino acid substitution in the hormone binding domain of the glucocorticoid receptor in familial glucocorticoid resistance. J Clin Invest 1991;87:680–6.
[21] Shahadi H, Vottero A, Stratakis C, et al. Imbalanced expression of the glucocorticoid receptor isoforms in cultured lymphocytes from a patient with systemic glucocorticoid resistance and chronic lymphocytic leukemia. Biochem Biophys Res Commun 1999;254: 559–65.
[22] van Rossum E, Voorhoeve P, te Velde S, et al. The ER2/23EK polymorphism in the glucocorticoid receptor gene is associated with a beneficial body composition and muscle strength in young adults. J Clin Endocrinol Metab 2004;89:4004–9.
[23] van Rossum E, Koper J, Huizenga N, et al. A polymorphism in the glucocorticoid receptor gene, which decreases sensitivity to glucocorticoids in vivo, is associated with low insulin and cholesterol levels. Diabetes 2002;51:3128–34.

[24] Dorr H, Heller A, Versmold H, et al. Longitudinal study of progestins, mineralocorticoids, and glucocorticoids throughout pregnancy. J Clin Endocrinol Metab 1989;68:683–8.
[25] Demey-Ponsart E, Foidart J, Sulon J, et al. free and total cortisol and circadian patterns of adrenal function in normal pregnancy. J Steroid Biochem 1982;16:165–9.
[26] Tomlinson J, Walker E, Bujalska I, et al. 11β-hydroxysteroid dehydrogenase type 1: a tissue-specific regulator of glucocorticoid response. Endocr Rev 2004;25:831–66.
[27] Tomlinson J, Mackie D, Johnson A, et al. Absence of Cushingoid phenotype in a patient with Cushing's disease due to defective cortisone to cortisol conversion. J Clin Endocrinol Metab 2002;87:57–62.
[28] Huizenga NA, de Lange P, Koper JW, et al. Human adrenocorticotropin-secreting pituitary adenomas show frequent loss of heterozygosity at the glucocorticoid receptor gene locus. J Clin Endocrinol Metab 1998;83(3):917–21.
[29] Hala M, Hartmann BL, Bock G, et al. Glucocorticoid-receptor-gene defects and resistance to glucocorticoid-induced apoptosis in human leukemic cell lines. Int J Cancer 1996;68: 663–8.
[30] Strasser-Wozak EM, Hattmannstorfer R, Hala M, et al. Splice site mutation in the glucocorticoid receptor gene causes resistance to glucocorticoid-induced apoptosis in a human acute leukemic cell line. Cancer Res 1995;55:348–53.
[31] Roth M, Johnson P, Borger P, et al. Dysfunctional interaction of C/EBPα and the glucocorticoid receptor in asthmatic bronchial smooth muscle cells. N Engl J Med 2004;351: 560–74.
[32] Huizenga NA, Koper JW, de Lange P, et al. A polymorphism in the glucocorticoid receptor gene may be associated with an increased sensitivity to glucocorticoids in vivo. J Clin Endocrinol Metab 1998;83:144–51.
[33] Stevens A, Ray D, Zeggini E, et al. Glucocorticoid sensitivity is determined by a specific glucocorticoid receptor haplotype. J Clin Endocrinol Metab 2004;89:892–7.
[34] Emptoz-Bonneton A, Cousin P, Segichi K, et al. A novel human corticosteroid-binding globulin variant with low cortisol-binding affinity. J Clin Endocrinol Metab 2000;85:361–7.
[35] Roitman A, Bruchis S, Bauman B, et al. Total deficiency of corticosteroid-binding globulin. Clin Endocrinol 1984;21:541–8.
[36] Torpy D, Bachmann A, Grice J, et al. Familial corticosteroid-binding globulin deficiency due to a novel null mutation: association with fatigue and relative hypotension. J Clin Endocrinol Metab 2001;86:3692–700.
[37] Annane D, Sebille V, Charpentier C, et al. Effect of treatment with low doses of hydrocortisone and fludrocortisone on mortality in patients with septic shock. JAMA 2002; 288:862–71.
[38] Hamrahian A, Oseni T, Arafah B. Measurements of serum free cortisol in critically ill patients. N Engl J Med 2004;350:1629–38.
[39] Newfield R, Kalaitzoglou G, Licholai T, et al. Normocortisolemic Cushing's syndrome initially presenting with increased glucocorticoid receptor numbers. J Clin Endocrinol Metab 2000;85:14–21.
[40] Iida S, Nakamura Y, Fujii H, et al. A patient with hypocortisolism and Cushing's syndrome-like manifestations: cortisol hyper-reactive syndrome. J Clin Endocrinol Metab 1990;70: 729–37.
[41] White P, Mune T, Agarwal A. 11β-hydroxysteroid dehydrogenase and the syndrome of apparent mineralocorticoid excess. Endocr Rev 1997;18:135–56.
[42] Masuzaki H, Paterson J, Shinyama H, et al. A transgenic model of visceral obesity and the metabolic syndrome. Science 2001;294:2166–70.

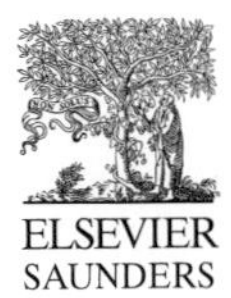
ELSEVIER
SAUNDERS

Endocrinol Metab Clin N Am
34 (2005) 327–339

ENDOCRINOLOGY
AND METABOLISM
CLINICS
OF NORTH AMERICA

The Metabolic Syndrome and Cardiovascular Risk in Cushing's Syndrome

Rosario Pivonello, MD, PhD, Dr*,
Antongiulio Faggiano, MD, Dr,
Gaetano Lombardi, MD, Dr Prof,
Annamaria Colao, MD, PhD, Dr Prof

Department of Molecular and Clinical Endocrinology and Oncology, "Federico II" University, Via Sergio Pansini 5, Naples, 80131, Italy

Cushing's syndrome (CS) is characterized by a series of systemic complications, including abdominal obesity, systemic arterial hypertension, impairment of glucose tolerance, dyslipidemia, and thrombotic diatesis, which increase cardiovascular risk [1,2]. Cardiovascular complications associated with CS include coronary artery disease, congestive heart failure, and cardiac stroke, which significantly increase the mortality rate of CS patients compared with normal population [3]. The remission or cure of CS usually reduces but does not eliminate these systemic complications completely. Therefore, a history of CS is associated with persistent increased cardiovascular risk, despite the normalization of cortisol secretion [4]. Most studies on cardiovascular risk associated with CS have been performed in patients who have Cushing's disease (CD), the most common form of CS, caused by an adrenocorticotropin (ACTH)–secreting pituitary tumor. The results of these studies, however, are extended to patients who have adrenal CS caused by a cortisol-secreting adrenal tumor or ectopic CS caused by an ACTH-secreting nonpituitary tumor.

Metabolic syndrome in Cushing's syndrome

Metabolic syndrome is a severe clinical condition associated with an increased cardiovascular risk affecting approximately 20% of the general

* Corresponding author.
E-mail address: rpivone@tin.it (R. Pivonello).

doi:10.1016/j.ecl.2005.01.010 ***endo.theclinics.com***

population [5,6]. It is characterized by abdominal obesity, systemic arterial hypertension, insulin resistance, dyslipidemia, and thrombotic diatesis. The etiopathogenesis of metabolic syndrome is unclear, and the differential diagnostic criteria have been proposed [7]. The World Health Organization criteria are focused on abdominal obesity ad insulin resistance [8]. Indeed, either abdominal obesity or insulin resistance has been indicated as the main candidate in the development of metabolic syndrome [9]. On the other hand, cortisol secretion was found to be higher in patients who have metabolic syndrome than in the general population [10] and allelic variants of the glucocorticoid receptor are associated with the progression of metabolic syndrome [11]. In addition, abdominal obesity and insulin resistance also have been suggested to be the starting points of the peculiar metabolic syndrome associated with CS [2].

Abdominal obesity, systemic arterial hypertension, insulin resistance with consequent impaired glucose tolerance or diabetes mellitus, dyslipidemia, and thrombotic diathesis are common features of patients who have CS [12–15]. The authors recently demonstrated that overweight/obesity occurred in approximately 75%, systemic arterial hypertension in 70%, impaired glucose tolerance in 60%, diabetes mellitus in 20%, increased total cholesterol levels in 50%, increased total/high-density lipoprotein (HDL) cholesterol ratio in 55%, and increased triglycerides levels in approximately 20% of patients who have active CD (Fig. 1) [2]. These metabolic abnormalities were more severe in CD patients characterized by abdominal obesity than in age-, sex-, and BMI-matched controls characterized by general obesity [2]. This suggests that abdominal obesity is associated more than general obesity with metabolic syndrome, although other factors, including insulin resistance and the possible direct effect of glucocorticoid excess, may participate to induce and maintain metabolic syndrome in patients who have CD.

Insulin resistance associated with CS was found to be characterized by decreased insulin responsiveness and insulin clearance distinct from that

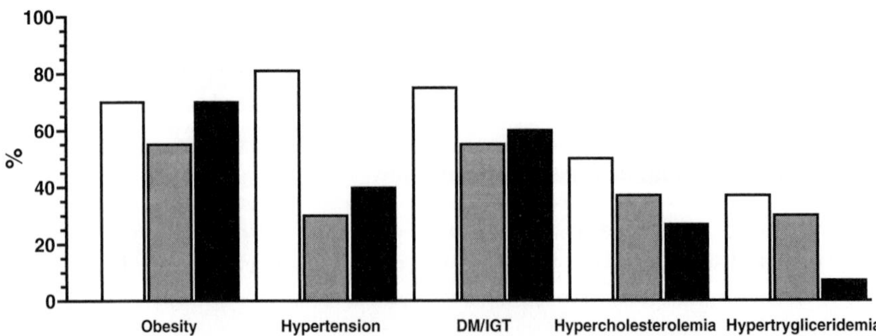

Fig. 1. Prevalence of metabolic syndrome abnormalities in patients who have active CD (*white bars*), patients in short-term remission (*gray bars*), and patients in long-term remission (*black bars*) from CD. DM, diabetes mellitus; IGT, impaired glucose tolerance.

occurring and to be in obesity. A defect at or distal to the glucose transport was shown to be responsible for insulin resistance of CS by insulin euglycemic clamp techniques [12]. This evidence partially contradicts the findings of the authors' studies in which insulin responsiveness, at least at the oral glucose load, increased compared with obese and normal control subjects [2].

Nonetheless, the main metabolic abnormalities were corrected with the waist-to-hip ratio, a relevant index of abdominal obesity and, indirectly, of insulin resistance [2]. Indeed, these two factors interact reciprocally. Abdominal obesity, but not peripheral obesity, is associated with low peripheral insulin sensitivity and hepatic insulin extraction [16], and hyperinsulinemia is predictive of the accumulation of visceral adipose tissue in the abdomen in nondiabetic subjects [17]. Insulin resistance is a prerequisite for the development of metabolic syndrome [18]. In patients who have hypercortisolism, insulin resistance and abdominal obesity induce gluconeogenesis [19] and promote a cascade of metabolic abnormalities that results in an overt metabolic syndrome.

Two important enzymes involved in the glucocorticoid metabolism also have been indicated as potential factors for the development of metabolic syndrome in CS. The 11β-hydroxysteroid dehydrogenase type 2 is a peripheral regulator of the glucocorticoid activity by converting cortisol to cortisone and protecting the mineralocorticoid receptor from high levels of cortisol. Insufficient activity of this enzyme is associated with CS because the cortisol/cortisone ratio was found to be higher in patients who have CS than in normal subjects [20]. This effect may contribute to the occurrence of systemic arterial hypertension in patients who have CS. On the other hand, the 11β-hydroxysteroid dehydrogenase type 1, which converts inactive cortisone to active cortisol, has been reported to be hyperactivated in the adipocytes of idiopathic obese subjects, thus producing a local hypercortisolism in adipose tissue despite normal circulating cortisol levels [21]. Several studies on animals and humans confirmed a causal role of this enzyme activity in the development of visceral obesity and glucose intolerance [22,23]. In summary, hypercortisolism plays a prominent role in the development of metabolic syndrome in patients who have CS, characterized by increased serum cortisol concentrations, and in non-CS patients who have increased intracellular cortisol concentration [24].

Changes of metabolic syndrome after remission of Cushing's syndrome

Metabolic syndrome associated with CS after the disease remission has had limited evaluation, probably because it was assumed that the normalization of cortisol secretion induced a recovery of the complications of the disease, including metabolic syndrome. No study has evaluated the persistence of metabolic syndrome in patients subjected to long-term treatments with corticosteroids for different nonendocrine diseases who have stopped treatment.

However, the presence of a metabolic syndrome also has been demonstrated in patients in remission or cured from CS. Indeed, 1 year after a stable remission from hypercortisolism, metabolic syndrome did not follow the normalization of cortisol levels in a cohort of patients who had CD [2]. In these patients, most metabolic parameters were still significantly higher than those observed in obese control subjects and in the general population, despite a partial decrease compared with the active phase of the disease. By comparing CD patients before and 1 year after remission from hypercortisolism, body mass index (BMI) did not change, whereas waist-to-hip ratio and blood pressure decreased but remained significantly higher than normal subjects. Moreover, overweight/obesity persisted in 55%, systemic arterial hypertension in 30%, impaired glucose tolerance or diabetes mellitus in 55%, dyslipidemia in 30%, and increased total/HDL cholesterol ratio in 20% of patients who have cured CD (see Fig. 1).

These results were similar to those reported in a transversal study evaluating patients cured from CD for at least 5 years. The authors also found the presence of a metabolic syndrome in this cohort of cured CD patients [4]. These patients maintained several clinical and biochemical abnormalities typical of the active phase of CD, such as overweight or obesity in 73%, arterial hypertension in 40%, impairment of glucose tolerance or diabetes mellitus in 60%, and dyslipidemia in 30% of patients (see Fig. 1). Insulin levels were increased compared with normal subjects at fasting and after glucose load, suggesting a state of insulin resistance with hyperinsulinemia (Fig. 2). Fasting insulinemia was the best predictor of waist-to-hip ratio and vice versa, confirming the strong relationship between these two parameters in patients cured of CD. Finally, the significant correlation between waist-to-hip ratio or fasting insulin levels with most metabolic abnormalities confirmed the role of abdominal obesity and insulin resistance in the development of metabolic syndrome of patients cured of CD.

These data indicate that either short- or long-term normalization of cortisol levels are characterized by persistence of a metabolic syndrome similar to that observed in active CS. Abdominal/visceral obesity and insulin resistance represent the pathogenic mechanism of metabolic syndrome in patients who have active CS and those who have a history of CS. This is in line with a previous study evaluating patients cured of adrenal CS, after removal of cortisol-secreting adrenal tumors, which described a postoperative persistence of hypertension correlated to hypertension severity and duration during the active phase of hypercortisolism [25].

Cardiovascular risk in Cushing's syndrome

Cardiovascular risk associated with CS is caused not only by clinical and metabolic complications, such as metabolic syndrome, but also by the vascular alterations resulting from chronic glucocorticoid excess. An

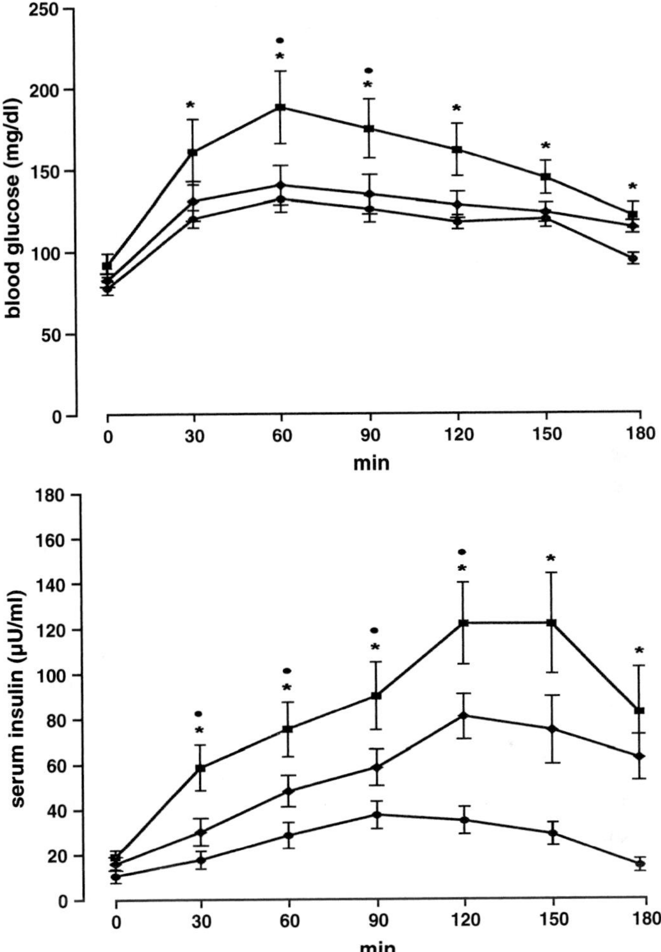

Fig. 2. Blood glucose and serum insulin response to oral glucose tolerance test in patients cured from CD (*squares*), sex- and age-matched controls (*circles*), and BMI-matched controls (*diamonds*). Asterisk indicates $P < .05$ compared with sex- and age-matched controls; solid circle above data points indicates $P < .05$ compared with BMI-matched controls. (*From* Colao A, Pivonello R, Spiezia S, et al. J Clin Endocrinol Metab 1999;84:2664–72; with permission.)

increased cardiovascular risk and increased occurrence of cardiovascular events recently has been associated with exogenous [26,27] as well as endogenous [2,3] glucocorticoid excess.

The main vascular alteration in CS is atherosclerosis. The link between cortisol and atherosclerosis first was suggested by indications that prolonged corticosteroid therapy accelerates the development of atherosclerosis. In animal experiments, ACTH and cortisone produced vascular injury [28] and enhanced experimentally induced atherosclerosis [29]. In humans, the use of glucocorticoids caused significant changes in vascular connective tissue [30]. Furthermore, a significant association between coronary artery disease and serum cortisol concentrations has been found in patients subjected to coronary angiography for heart angina or stroke [31]. In addition, a cause/effect relationship between corticosteroid treatment and premature atherosclerosis was hypothesized in patients who have rheumatoid arthritis or systemic lupus erythematosus chronically treated with corticosteroids [32–34]. The occurrence of atherosclerosis and coronary artery disease has been confirmed recently in patients who have systemic lupus erythematosus treated with corticosteroids, although a direct effect of the primary disease or its systemic complications on the cardiovascular system has to be considered [35,36].

Atherosclerosis also is associated with CS. The authors recently demonstrated that patients who have active CD, have an increased intima-media thickness (IMT) and a decreased distensibility coefficient (DC), which are considered preatherosclerotic lesions, or an increased prevalence of well-defined carotid plaques compared with controls. Carotid wall plaques were detected in 32% of patients, 0% of control subjects matched with patients for sex and age, and 6% of control subjects matched with patients for sex, age, and BMI (Fig. 3). Carotid plaques were found bilaterally in 16% of patients who had active CD. In these patients, waist-to-hip ratio as well as fasting and post–glucose load insulin levels were correlated to common carotid IMT and DC, whereas duration of hypercortisolism was correlated significantly only to common carotid IMT and DC. At the multiple regression analysis, waist-to-hip ratio was the best predictor of carotid IMT and DC beyond insulin resistance [2].

The results of the study suggested that beyond a direct effect of glucocorticoid excess on the vascular system, metabolic syndrome may play a pivotal role in determining the premature carotid atherosclerosis associated

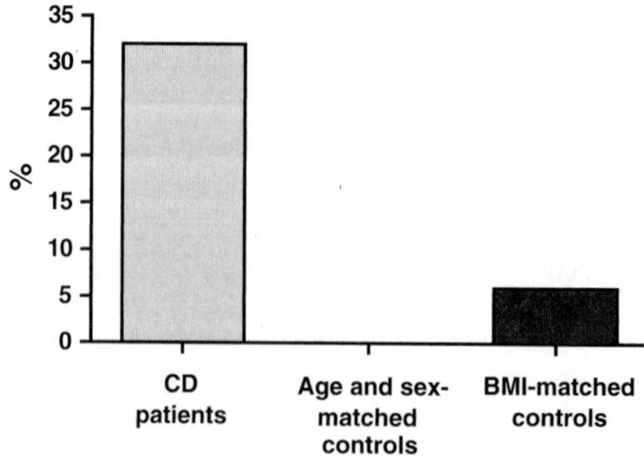

Fig. 3. Prevalence of atherosclerotic plaques in patients who have active CD and in controls.

with CS. In particular, among the multiple factors influencing metabolic syndrome, abdominal obesity and insulin resistance seem to have the major role in initiating and maintaining atherosclerosis. Excessive accumulation of central adiposity is related to increased mortality and cardiovascular risk for disorders such as systemic arterial hypertension, diabetes mellitus, dyslipidemia, and atherosclerosis [37]. Therefore, abdominal obesity is a likely explanation for the increased vascular risk in patients who have chronic hypercortisolism.

Insulin resistance is recognized as a basic prerequisite to metabolic syndrome [18], and when associated with abdominal obesity, as in patients who have hypercortisolism, it increases cardiovascular risk [12]. The vascular damage of patients who have metabolic syndrome starts with endothelial dysfunction [38]. Impaired vasodilation after acetylcholine or hyperemia [39], enhanced large artery stiffness [40], and increased thrombotic diatesis [41] have been demonstrated in all states associated with metabolic syndrome/insulin resistance development, such as obesity [42], impairment of glucose tolerance [43], diabetes mellitus [44], and gestational diabetes mellitus [45]. Summarizing, the sequence of events leading to atherosclerotic plaque formation in patients who have CD seems to begin with visceral adiposity excess and reduced insulin sensitivity, followed by gradual development of an overt metabolic syndrome with endothelial damage and atherosclerotic plaque formation.

Increased homocysteine and decreased taurine levels have been reported recently as new atherogenic factors associated with cardiovascular risk. Increased levels of homocysteine and decreased levels of taurine have been identified in patients who have renal failure, a pathologic condition sharing with CS clinical features such as hypercatabolism, systemic arterial hypertension, glucose and lipid abnormalities, and increased cardiovascular risk [46]. Increased homocysteine levels also have been documented recently in patients who have CS [47]. Moreover, the authors observed an increased prevalence of hyperhomocysteinemia and hypotaurinemia in patients who have CD without renal failure (Antongiulio Faggiano, MD, Dr, and Rosario Pivonello, MD, PhD, Dr, unpublished data, 2005). These elements complicate the spectrum of clinical and biochemical alterations induced by hypercortisolism and associated with cardiovascular risk, and help explain why the cardiovascular consequences of patients who have CS are more precocious and severe than those who have obesity.

Change of cardiovascular risk after remission of Cushing's syndrome

The cardiovascular risk associated with CS after disease remission has had limited evaluation, probably because it was assumed that normalization of cortisol secretion induced a recovery of the complications of the disease, including cardiovascular risk. No study has evaluated the persistence of cardiovascular risk in patients subjected to long-term treatments with corticosteroids for various nonendocrine diseases who have stopped this treatment. A recent study found that the mortality of patients cured of CS was not different than that expected in normal population [3]. This evidence should be confirmed, however, by studies involving large populations and different reference centers considering homogeneous criteria for the remission or cure of CS.

The authors recently found that the cardiovascular risk of patients who have CD, although reduced after 1 year of disease remission, remained higher than in the normal population [2]. Common carotid artery IMT decreased, whereas DC increased compared with the active disease, but remained abnormal compared with controls (Fig. 4). Well-defined carotid wall plaques were detected in 32% of patients, with no change compared with the active disease. After remission, waist-to-hip ratio as well as fasting and post–glucose load insulin levels were correlated significantly to common carotid IMT and DC. Therefore, 1 year after remission from hypercortisolism, despite a moderate improvement of clinical, biochemical, and vascular parameters, reduced caliber and increased stiffness of the carotid

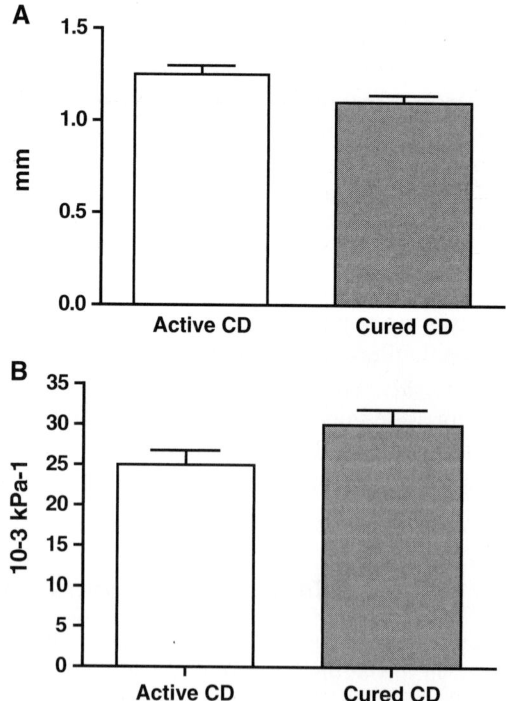

Fig. 4. IMT (*A*) and DC (*B*) in CD patients during active disease and 1 year after disease remission. $P < 0.05$.

arteries wall and atherosclerotic plaques persisted. Disease remission, defined by endocrine and radiologic parameters, is not followed by decreased cardiovascular risk.

This evidence is similar to that found in a transversal study on subjects cured of CD for at least 5 years. In this cohort, common carotid arteries' IMT was significantly higher, whereas DC was significantly lower compared with sex-, age-, and BMI-matched control groups. Moreover, well-defined carotid wall plaques were detected in approximately 30% of subjects. Fig. 5 shows an example of IMT in a subject long-term cured of CD and in a control. Waist-to-hip ratio and insulin levels were correlated significantly to common carotid IMT and DC. These results and the finding of a persistent metabolic syndrome in this cohort suggest that cardiovascular risk persists after long-term remission from CD.

The atherogenic consequences of metabolic syndrome seem to be worse in patients in long-term remission from hypercortisolism compared with those in short-term remission [2,4], although a longitudinal long-term study is necessary to draw final conclusions. This finding may be related to a persistent

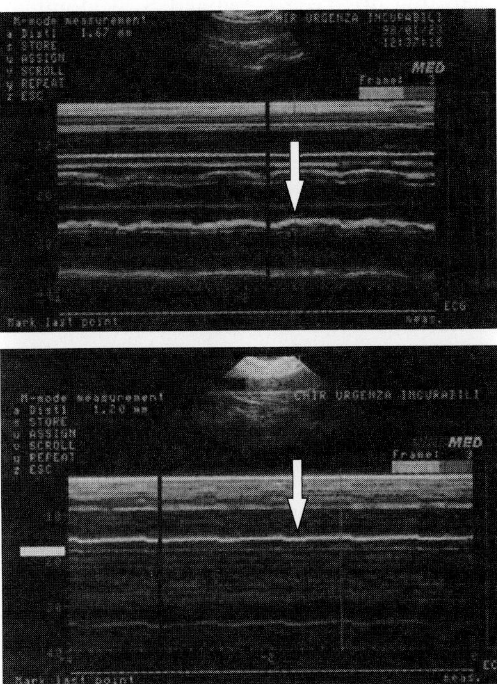

Fig. 5. M-mode ultrasonography showing a measurement of IMT at the level of common carotid wall in a patient in long-term remission from CD (*top*), and in a control (*bottom*). Arrow indicates the site of IMT measurement. (*From* Colao A, Pivonello R, Spiezia S, et al. J Clin Endocrinol Metab 1999;84:2664–72; with permission.)

but not marked presence of abdominal obesity or insulin resistance with associated metabolic syndrome, representing a low but continuous stimulus for the atherogenesis. In addition, an immune system rebound following the shift from chronic hypercortisolism to normal cortisol levels may play a role. Indeed, the removal of cortisol-induced suppression of the immune system has been suggested as an explanation for the increased prevalence of autoimmune diseases in patients cured from CS [48]. Therefore, the aggravation of metabolic syndrome and especially atherosclerosis over time in subjects cured from CS may be sustained partially by inflammatory processes damaging the regulative mechanisms of glucose and lipid homeostasis and the vasculature.

No abnormality of homocysteine and taurine metabolism seems to persist after remission from hypercortisolism (Antongiulio Faggiano, MD, Dr, and Rosario Pivonello, MD, PhD, Dr, unpublished data, 2005), suggesting that hyperhomocysteinemia and hypotaurinemia are reversible metabolic complications of CS that do not contribute to the persistent and progressively worsening cardiovascular risk of patients cured from the disease.

To conclude, these data indicate that either short- or long-term normalization of cortisol levels are characterized by persistent cardiovascular risk similar to that observed in active CS. Abdominal/visceral obesity and insulin resistance, together with the consequent metabolic syndrome, represent the pathogenic mechanisms of the increased cardiovascular risk in patients who have active CS and in those who have a history of CS. The severity of glucocorticoid excess and the disease duration also influence the severity of atherosclerosis and cardiovascular risk, especially in patients with cured CS.

Summary

CS is associated with severe atherosclerotic damage, indicated by reduced caliber and increased stiffness of the carotid artery wall and increased prevalence of atherosclerotic plaques. Vascular damage develops in concert with an acquired metabolic syndrome. Metabolic and vascular alterations correlate markedly to visceral obesity and insulin resistance, and seem to interact with each other. Short-term remission from hypercortisolism is followed by improvement, but not normalization, of metabolic and vascular damage. Moreover, long-term remission from CS seems to be associated with similar or worse metabolic and vascular damage, probably as a result of persistent abdominal obesity or insulin resistance syndrome years after normalization of cortisol secretion. The results of this study suggest that increased cardiovascular risk also may persist in patients who undergo treatment with exogenous glucocorticoids after therapy withdrawal. Considering the many patients subjected to corticosteroid treatment, this finding could be of great clinical relevance and should be investigated thoroughly.

References

[1] Etxabe J, Vazquez JA. Morbidity and mortality in Cushing's disease: an epidemiological approach. Clin Endocrinol (Oxf) 1994;40:479–84.

[2] Faggiano A, Pivonello R, Spiezia S, et al. Cardiovascular risk factors and common carotid artery caliber and stiffness in patients with Cushing's disease during active disease and 1 year after disease remission. J Clin Endocrinol Metab 2003;88:2527–33.

[3] Lindholm J, Juul S, Jorgensen JO, et al. Incidence and late prognosis of Cushing's syndrome: a population-based study. J Clin Endocrinol Metab 2001;86:117–23.

[4] Colao A, Pivonello R, Spiezia S, et al. Persistence of increased cardiovascular risk in patients with Cushing's disease after five years of successful cure. J Clin Endocrinol Metab 1999;84: 2664–72.

[5] Cameron AJ, Shaw JE, Zimmet PZ. The metabolic syndrome: prevalence in worldwide populations. Endocrinol Metab Clin North Am 2004;33:351–75.

[6] Scheen AJ, Luyckx FH. Metabolic syndrome: definitions and epidemiological data. Rev Med Liege 2003;58:479–84.

[7] Davidson MB. Metabolic syndrome/insulin resistance syndrome/pre-diabetes: new section in diabetes care. Diabetes Care 2003;26:3179.

[8] Aguilar-Salinas CA, Rojas R, Gomez-Perez FJ, et al. Analysis of the agreement between the World Health Organization criteria and the National Cholesterol Education Program-III definition of the metabolic syndrome: results from a population-based survey. Diabetes Care 2003;26:1635.

[9] Garber AJ. The metabolic syndrome. Med Clin North Am 2004;88:837–46.

[10] Andrew R, Gale CR, Walker BR, et al. Glucocorticoid metabolism and the metabolic syndrome: associations in an elderly cohort. Exp Clin Endocrinol Diabetes 2002;110:284–90.

[11] Rosmond R. The glucocorticoid receptor gene and its association to metabolic syndrome. Obes Res 2002;10:1078–86.

[12] Karnieli E, Cohen P, Barzilai N, et al. Insulin resistance in Cushing's syndrome. Horm Metab Res 1985;17:518–21.

[13] Bowes SB, Benn JJ, Scobie IN, et al. Glucose metabolism in patients with Cushing's syndrome. Clin Endocrinol (Oxf) 1991;34:311–6.

[14] Friedman TC, Mastorakos G, Newman TD, et al. Carbohydrate and lipid metabolism in endogenous hypercortisolism: shared features with metabolic syndrome X and NIDDM. Endocr J 1996;43:645–55.

[15] Fatti LM, Bottasso B, Invitti C, et al. Markers of activation of coagulation and fibrinolysis in patients with Cushing's syndrome. J Endocrinol Invest 2000;23:145–50.

[16] Peiris AN, Mueller RA, Smith GA, et al. Splanchnic insulin metabolism in obesity. Influence of body fat distribution. J Clin Invest 1986;78:1648–57.

[17] Boyko EJ, Leonetti DL, Bergstrom RW, et al. Low insulin secretion and high fasting insulin and C-peptide levels predict increased visceral adiposity. 5-year follow-up among initially nondiabetic Japanese-American men. Diabetes 1996;45:1010–5.

[18] Reaven GM. Banting lecture 1988. Role of insulin resistance in human disease. Diabetes 1988;37:1595–607.

[19] Khani S, Tayek JA. Cortisol increases gluconeogenesis in humans: its role in the metabolic syndrome. Clin Sci (Lond) 2001;101:739–47.

[20] Dotsch J, Dorr HG, Stalla GK, et al. Effect of glucocorticoid excess on the cortisol/cortisone ratio. Steroids 2001;66:817–20.

[21] Wake DJ, Walker BR. 11 beta-hydroxysteroid dehydrogenase type 1 in obesity and the metabolic syndrome. Mol Cell Endocrinol 2004;215:45–54.

[22] Stulnig TM, Waldhausl W. 11beta-Hydroxysteroid dehydrogenase type 1 in obesity and type 2 diabetes. Diabetologia 2004;47:1–11.

[23] Engeli S, Bohnke J, Feldpausch M, et al. Regulation of 11beta-HSD genes in human adipose tissue: influence of central obesity and weight loss. Obes Res 2004;12:9–17.

[24] Bahr V, Pfeiffer AF, Diederich S. The metabolic syndrome X and peripheral cortisol synthesis. Exp Clin Endocrinol Diabetes 2002;110:313–8.
[25] Suzuki T, Shibata H, Ando T, et al. Risk factors associated with persistent postoperative hypertension in Cushing's syndrome. Endocr Res 2000;26:791–5.
[26] Souverein PC, Berard A, Van Staa TP, et al. Use of oral glucocorticoids and risk of cardiovascular and cerebrovascular disease in a population based case-control study. Heart 2004;90:859–65.
[27] Wei L, MacDonald TM, Walker BR. Taking glucocorticoids by prescription is associated with subsequent cardiovascular disease. Ann Intern Med 2004;141:764–70.
[28] Stamler J, Pick R, Katz LN. Effects of cortisone, hydrocortisone and corticotropin on lipemia, glycemia and atherogenesis in cholesterol-fed chicks. Circulation 1954;10:237–46.
[29] Rosenfeld S, Marmorston J, Sobel H, et al. Enhancement of experimental atherosclerosis by ACTH in the dog. Proc Soc Exp Biol Med 1960;103:83–6.
[30] Lorenzen I, Hansen LK. Effect of glucocorticoids on human vascular connective tissue. Biochemical and microscopic studies of vein biopsies. Vasc Dis 1967;4:335–41.
[31] Troxler RG, Sprague EA, Albanese RA, et al. The association of elevated plasma cortisol and early atherosclerosis as demonstrated by coronary angiography. Atherosclerosis 1977; 26:151–62.
[32] Tsakraklides VG, Blieden LC, Edwards JE. Coronary atherosclerosis and myocardial infarction associated with systemic lupus erythematosus. Am Heart J 1974;87:637–41.
[33] Kalbak K. Incidence of arteriosclerosis in patients with rheumatoid arthritis receiving long-term corticosteroid therapy. Ann Rheum Dis 1972;31:196–200.
[34] Nashel DJ. Is atherosclerosis a complication of long-term corticosteroid treatment? Am J Med 1986;80:925–9.
[35] Doria A, Shoenfeld Y, Wu R, et al. Risk factors for subclinical atherosclerosis in a prospective cohort of patients with systemic lupus erythematosus. Ann Rheum Dis 2003; 62:1071–7.
[36] Sella EM, Sato EI, Leite WA, et al. Myocardial perfusion scintigraphy and coronary disease risk factors in systemic lupus erythematosus. Ann Rheum Dis 2003;62:1066–70.
[37] Wajchenberg BL. Subcutaneous and visceral adipose tissue: their relation to the metabolic syndrome. Endocr Rev 2000;21:697–738.
[38] Calles-Escandon J, Cipolla M. Diabetes and endothelial dysfunction: a clinical perspective. Endocr Rev 2001;22:36–52.
[39] Cosentino F, Luscher TF. Endothelial dysfunction in diabetes mellitus. J Cardiovasc Pharmacol 1998;32(Suppl 3):S54–61.
[40] Westerbacka J, Vehkavaara S, Bergholm R, et al. Marked resistance of the ability of insulin to decrease arterial stiffness characterizes human obesity. Diabetes 1999;48:821–7.
[41] Kario K, Matsuo T, Kobayashi H, et al. Activation of tissue factor-induced coagulation and endothelial cell dysfunction in non-insulin-dependent diabetic patients with microalbuminuria. Arterioscler Thromb Vasc Biol 1995;15:1114–20.
[42] Steinberg HO, Chaker H, Leaming R, et al. Obesity/insulin resistance is associated with endothelial dysfunction. Implications for the syndrome of insulin resistance. J Clin Invest 1996;97:2601–10.
[43] Ferri C, Desideri G, Baldoncini R, et al. Early activation of vascular endothelium in nonobese, nondiabetic essential hypertensive patients with multiple metabolic abnormalities. Diabetes 1998;47:660–7.
[44] Hogikyan RV, Galecki AT, Pitt B, et al. Specific impairment of endothelium-dependent vasodilation in subjects with type 2 diabetes independent of obesity. J Clin Endocrinol Metab 1998;83:1946–52.
[45] Anastasiou E, Lekakis JP, Alevizaki M, et al. Impaired endothelium-dependent vasodilatation in women with previous gestational diabetes. Diabetes Care 1998;21:2111–5.

[46] Suliman ME, Qureshi AR, Barany P, et al. Hyperhomocysteinemia, nutritional status, and cardiovascular disease in hemodialysis patients. Kidney Int 2000;57:1727–35.
[47] Terzolo M, Allasino B, Bosio S, et al. Hyperhomocysteinemia in patients with Cushing's syndrome. J Clin Endocrinol Metab 2004;89:3745–51.
[48] Colao A, Pivonello R, Faggiano A, et al. Increased prevalence of thyroid autoimmunity in patients successfully treated for Cushing's disease. Clin Endocrinol (Oxf) 2000;53:13–9.

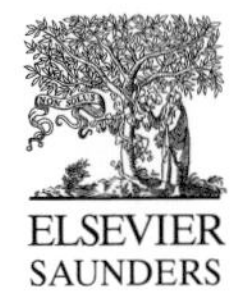

ELSEVIER
SAUNDERS

Endocrinol Metab Clin N Am
34 (2005) 341–356

ENDOCRINOLOGY
AND METABOLISM
CLINICS
OF NORTH AMERICA

Osteoporosis Associated with Excess Glucocorticoids

Joseph L. Shaker, MD[a,*], Barbara P. Lukert, MD[b]

[a] *Endocrine–Diabetes Center, St. Luke's Medical Center, University of Wisconsin School of Medicine, 2801 West KK River Parkway, Suite 245, Milwaukee, WI 53215, USA*

[b] *Division of Metabolism, Endocrinology and Genetics, University of Kansas School of Medicine, 3901 Rainbow Boulevard, Kansas City, KS 66160, USA*

In his original description of basophil adenomas of the pituitary in 1932, Cushing noted the presence of bone disease [1]. It subsequently has become clear that excess corticosteroids, whether endogenous or exogenous, are associated with decreased bone mass and fractures. This article addresses the effects of endogenous and exogenous corticosteroids on the skeleton, the pathogenesis of bone loss caused by corticosteroids, the effect of cure of endogenous hypercortisolism on the skeleton, and the management of glucocorticoid-induced osteoporosis.

Endogenous hypercortisolism

In Cushing's original series of 12 patients published in 1932, one was reported to have radiographic osteoporosis; six were reported to have kyphosis, and two were reported to have spontaneous fractures [1]. In 1971, Welbourne et al [2] reported radiographic osteoporosis in 28 of 60 patients who had Cushing's syndrome and reported many had rib fractures, some of which were found at the time of adrenalectomy. Nine of the 60 patients were reported to have vertebral fractures. Decreased bone mass on radiographs has been reported in 40% to 60% of patients, and pathologic fractures have been reported in 16% to 67% of patients who have endogenous hypercortisolism [3]. In a study of 10 patients who had childhood-onset and 18 patients who had adult-onset Cushing's disease, the mean lumbar spine dual

Dr. Lukert has received research grants from Procter & Gamble and Lilly.

* Corresponding author.
E-mail address: joseph.shaker@aurora.org (J.L. Shaker).

doi:10.1016/j.ecl.2005.01.014

radiograph absorptiometry (DXA) Z-score was −2.6 in the children and −2.1 in the adults [4]. The authors reported biochemical evidence of decreased osteoblastic function (decreased osteocalcin) and increased osteoclastic function (increased urinary N-telopeptide) [4]. In a study of 18 eugonadal women who had Cushing's syndrome (12 pituitary, 6 adrenal), Chiodini et al [5] found significantly reduced spinal trabecular bone mass by quantitative CT (QCT), decreased spinal bone density by DXA, decreased forearm trabecular bone density by QCT, and decreased femoral bone density when compared with controls. Forearm cortical bone was not decreased. Osteocalcin was decreased, and markers of bone resorption were increased [5]. Vestergaarde et al [6] compared the fracture rate in 104 patients who had Cushing's syndrome with controls and found an increased incidence rate ratio of 6.0 (confidence interval of 2.1 to 17.2) in patients who had Cushing's syndrome in the 2 years before diagnosis. Indeed, osteoporosis and fractures may be the presenting features of Cushing's syndrome [7]. The prevalence of osteoporosis and fragility fractures may be higher in adrenal Cushing's syndrome than in pituitary Cushing's disease, perhaps because the higher adrenal androgens in corticotropin (ACTH)-dependent Cushing's syndrome have a protective effect on the skeleton [8,9].

Adrenal incidentalomas

In recent years, it has become clear that adrenal incidentalomas are not uncommon on abdominal CT scanning, occurring in 0.3% to 5% of scans [10]. Some of these patients have evidence of mild glucocorticoid excess or subclinical Cushing's syndrome [10]. Some studies have found biochemical evidence of decreased bone formation and increased bone resorption in patients who have adrenal incidentalomas and subclinical Cushing's syndrome [10–12]. Reductions in bone mass have been reported in men and women who have adrenal incidentalomas and subclinical hypercortisolism compared with patients who have adrenal incidentalomas without subclinical hypercortisolism [11–13]. These studies suggest that the mild hypercortisolism seen in some patients who have adrenal incidentalomas may have adverse skeletal effects.

Exogenous corticosteroids

Exogenous glucocorticoids are used in approximately 0.5% of the population for several inflammatory conditions, and fractures may occur in 30% to 50% of patients on chronic glucocorticoid therapy [14]. Bone loss appears to be fastest in the first 6 months of therapy, but bone loss persists at a slower rate thereafter [14]. Trabecular bone [15,16] and the cortical rim of vertebral bodies [16] appear to be more susceptible to the effects of glucocorticoids. In a randomized clinical trial of rheumatoid arthritis patients, there was an 8.2% decrease in lumbar spine bone density by QCT at 20 weeks in patients treated with approximately 50 mg/wk of prednisone [17]. The bone density improved rapidly 24 weeks after stopping prednisone [17].

Although the effects of glucocorticoid treatment on fractures are complicated by the effects of the underlying disorders on bone, fracture risk appears to increase with glucocorticoid therapy. Adinoff and Hollister [18] found increased rib and vertebral fractures in asthma patients on long-term glucocorticoids as compared with matched asthma patients not on glucocorticoids. Van Staa et al conducted a retrospective cohort study of 244,235 adult using oral glucocorticoids compared with controls and found an increase in nonvertebral (risk ratio [RR], 1.33), hip (RR, 1.61), forearm (RR, 1.09), and vertebral fractures (RR, 2.60) [19]. The increase in risk was dose-related and occurred with doses as low as 2.5 mg/d of prednisolone [19]. The fracture risk may decrease rapidly after glucocorticoids are stopped [19]. A meta-analysis of 42,500 men and women from seven prospective cohorts also found that prior or current glucocorticoid use was associated with increased fracture risk [20]. Oral glucocorticoid use also appears to increase fracture risk in children [21]. In the placebo group of a randomized clinical trial of risedronate, 17% of the control patients (mean prednisone dose of 11 mg/d) had vertebral fractures within 1 year of initiating prednisone [22]. In that study, the mean decrease in lumbar spine, femoral neck, and greater trochanter bone density after 1 year in the placebo group was approximately 3% [22].

There are conflicting data about whether glucocorticoid-treated patients fracture at higher or similar bone densities compared with patients not treated with glucocorticoids [23–25]. This issue needs further study. Despite the high risk of fracture in patients on glucocorticoids, evaluation of such patients is inadequate. In a recent study of 6517 adults on glucocorticoids, only 33% had bone density measured, and only 37% had some form of osteoporosis treatment [26].

Inhaled corticosteroids

Inhaled glucocorticoids frequently are used for managing chronic asthma. Studies on the effects of inhaled glucocorticoids on bone have yielded conflicting results. Osteocalcin (a marker of bone formation) may decrease after use of inhaled beclomethasone [27,28]. Lau et al [29] compared patients on inhaled glucocorticoids with matched controls and found that inhaled glucocorticoid use was associated with decreased hip but not spine bone mineral density (BMD) in men (but not women). In a study of 196 asthmatics aged 20 to 40 years, there was a negative relationship between cumulative dose of inhaled glucocorticoids and BMD of spine and hip [30]. Fujita et al [31] found reduced lumbar spine BMD and reduced serum osteocalcin in early postmenopausal women but not premenopausal women treated with inhaled beclomethasone. Another study found that inhaled triamcinolone was associated with a dose-dependent decrease in hip

BMD in premenopausal women [32]. A 2-year randomized trial of inhaled fluticasone propionate (88 and 440 μg twice daily) found no adverse effects on BMD [33]. A retrospective cohort study of 170,818 inhaled glucocorticosteroid users compared with bronchodilator users and controls found increased fractures in inhaled glucocorticoid users as compared with controls but no increase in fractures compared with bronchodilator users, suggesting the increased fracture risk may be related to the pulmonary disease [34]. The studies on effects of inhaled glucocorticoids on bone have yielded mixed results, possibly because of effects of underlying lung disease on skeleton, differences in potencies and doses of the drugs, and other confounding variables. Measurement of bone density is indicated in patients on chronic, high doses of inhaled glucocorticoids, particularly if other risk factors are present.

Pathogenesis of bone loss caused by corticosteroids

The mechanisms of bone loss caused by exogenous and endogenous glucocorticoids are complicated (Fig. 1). Glucocorticoids appear to have

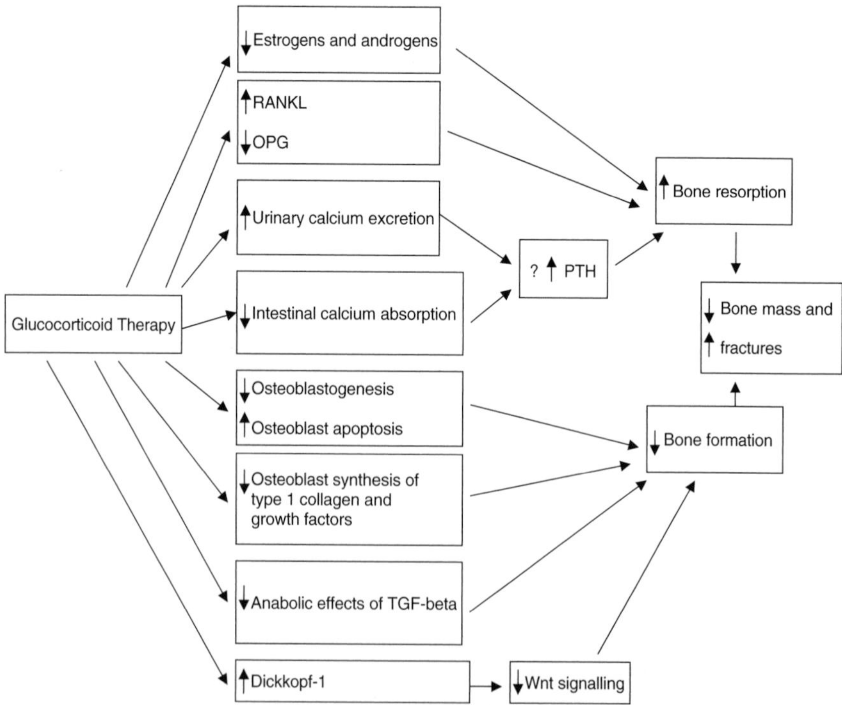

Fig. 1. Mechanisms that have been implicated in the pathogenesis of bone loss caused by glucocorticoid excess.

multiple adverse effects on bone remodeling that result in decreased bone formation and increased bone resorption. Glucocorticoids decrease levels of the gonadal steroids estrogen and testosterone [35,36]. The reduction in gonadal hormones likely is related to direct gonadal effects and hypothalamic-pituitary effects [14,35]. In addition, exogenous glucocorticoids are associated with suppression of adrenal androgen production [36]. Sex hormone deficiency is associated with increased bone resorption and therefore bone loss. Glucocorticoids also appear to increase production of receptor activator of NF-kappa beta ligand (RANKL), which is formed by osteoblasts and increases osteoclastogenesis [37]. Additionally, glucocorticoids decrease osteoprotegerin (OPG) [37], a decoy receptor for RANKL that acts to decrease osteoclast differentiation. The combination of increased RANKL and decreased OPG results in increased osteoclastic bone resorption.

Glucocorticoids may decrease intestinal calcium absorption [38] and decrease renal tubular reabsorption of calcium [39] resulting in hypercalciuria. Both of these could contribute to secondary hyperparathyroidism and increased bone resorption. A recent review, however, suggested secondary hyperparathyroidism is not an important factor in glucocorticoid-induced bone loss [40].

Inhibitory effects on osteoblastic function and number resulting in decreased bone formation are probably the most important skeletal effects of glucocorticoids. Glucocorticoids reduce osteoblastogenesis and increase apoptosis of osteoblasts and osteocytes [41]. A recent study [42] found that high-dose glucocorticoids (methylprednisolone 15 mg/kg intravenously for 10 days) promptly decreased biochemical markers of bone formation, decreased insulin-like growth factor 1 (IGF-1), and transiently increased biochemical markers of bone resorption. Glucocorticoids decrease osteoblastic synthesis of type 1 collagen and IGF-1 [43]. Glucocorticoids alter the binding of transforming growth factor β (TGF-β) and decrease its anabolic effects on bone [44]. Glucocorticoids also may enhance the expression of dickkopf-1 in osteoblasts, which inhibits Wnt signaling (a stimulus for osteoblastic function) [45].

Local conversion between cortisol and cortisone may mediate some of the effects of glucocorticoids on bone. 11β-hydroxysteroid dehydrogenase type 1 (11β-HSD1) converts cortisone to cortisol and prednisone to prednisolone. 11β-HSD type 2 (11β-HSD2) converts cortisol to cortisone [46]. Inflammatory cytokines may decrease 11β-HSD2 and increase 11β-HSD1, thus increasing local production of active steroids [47]. Furthermore, glucocorticoids may induce 11β-HSD1, increasing local production of the active steroids [46].

Effect of cure of endogenous hypercortisolism on bone

In 1971, Welbourn et al [2] reported remineralization of the skeleton and healing of fractures after treatment of Cushing's syndrome. BMD appears to improve substantially after cure of endogenous hypercortisolism [48,49]. In a study of 17 adults cured of Cushing's syndrome 8.6 plus or minus 1.6 years earlier, BMD was normal, and there was a positive relationship between bone density and time since cure of Cushing's syndrome [50]. Hermus et al [51] studied bone density and bone turnover after cure of Cushing's syndrome in 18 patients. Significant improvement in bone density was found by 1 year. There was an early increase in markers of bone formation and bone resorption at 3 months, followed by gradual decline. Dobnig et al [52] reported a patient who had Cushing's syndrome caused by ectopic ACTH production who experienced spontaneous rib fractures and whose lumbar spine bone density increased 79% over 3 years after cure of the Cushing's syndrome. In a study of six childhood- and nine adult-onset Cushing's disease patients, 2 years of cortisol normalization were associated with significantly improved lumbar spine BMD Z-scores (although still below controls) [53]. These studies suggest that bone density improves significantly after cure of endogenous hypercortisolism.

Avascular necrosis

Avascular necrosis (AVN) or osteonecrosis is a known complication of glucocorticoid therapy. The most commonly involved site is the proximal femur [54]; however, the proximal humerus and distal femur are other frequent locations [55]. Patients typically present with pain that worsens with joint use [55]. The risk of AVN is greater with higher doses of glucocorticoids [56], but AVN may occur with low doses of glucocorticoids for long periods and after intra-articular glucocorticoids [57].

Mechanisms for AVN that have been proposed include fat cell hypertrophy causing venous obstruction, vascular occlusion, compression of small veins causing increased intraosseous pressure, and intravascular fat embolization [54]. Apoptosis of osteocytes also has been reported in patients who have osteonecrosis of the femoral head [58]. The use of statin drugs may be associated with a decreased risk of AVN in glucocorticoid-treated patients [59].

Health care providers should consider AVN in a patient on glucocorticoids (or who has endogenous hypercortisolism) who develops hip, shoulder, or knee pain. This condition may be unilateral or bilateral. Radiographs should be done, and if the symptoms are not explained, MRI should be obtained, as AVN has a characteristic appearance on MRI [54]. Therapy includes avoidance of weight-bearing activities and use of crutches or a cane [57]. Several surgical approaches such as core decompression, bone grafting, and osteotomies have been used; however, many patients will require total joint replacement [55,60].

Evaluation of patients on glucocorticoid therapy

Patients on chronic glucocorticoid therapy and those initiating glucocorticoid therapy should have their skeletal health assessed. This evaluation should include a complete history and physical with specific attention to the presence of prior fragility fractures (prior fragility fractures increase the risk of subsequent fractures), signs or symptoms of hypogonadism, history of nephrolithiasis, tobacco use, and excess alcohol use. Dietary and supplemental calcium intake should be assessed. The patient should be evaluated for myopathy, which could increase the risk of falls and fracture.

Appropriate laboratory studies include a chemistry panel and a 24-hour urine collection for calcium, sodium, and creatinine (to evaluate for hypercalciuria). A measurement of serum 25-hydroxyvitamin D to assess vitamin D status is prudent. In men, measurement of serum testosterone is appropriate to evaluate gonadal status. In women who have uncertain gonadal status, measurement of follicle-stimulating hormone (FSH) and estradiol may be useful. A baseline BMD of the spine and hip by DXA should be performed. Peripheral measurements are less useful in detecting glucocorticoid-associated bone loss, because trabecular bone may be lost preferentially.

Management of patients on glucocorticoid therapy

The American College of Rheumatology has published its recommendations for preventing and treating glucocorticoid-induced osteoporosis [61]. Conservative management includes lifestyle changes such as tobacco cessation and reduction of excess alcohol consumption. Physical therapy and an exercise program may be useful, especially in patients who have or are at risk for myopathy. Calcium and vitamin D are important for managing osteoporosis; however, calcium therapy alone is probably not adequate to prevent bone loss associated with glucocorticoid therapy [62]. Calcium 1000 mg/d with vitamin D3 500 IU/d together prevented bone loss of the spine in patients with rheumatoid arthritis on a mean of 5.6 mg/d of prednisone [63]. A 3-year study of calcium 1000 mg/d and vitamin D 50,000 U/wk, however, did not show a benefit in patients on approximately 20 mg/d of prednisone [64]. Studies using meta-analysis suggest that vitamin D is useful for preventing bone loss associated with glucocorticoid therapy [62,65]. Activated forms of vitamin D such as calcitriol [66,67] and alfacalcidiol [68] appear to help prevent bone loss but may be associated with increased risk of hypercalciuria and hypercalcemia [66]. A study of 195 patients on glucocorticoid therapy suggested that calcitriol was no better than plain vitamin D for managing glucocorticoid-induced bone loss [69].

If hypercalciuria is present, sodium restriction may be useful to decrease urinary calcium excretion. If hypercalciuria persists, thiazide diuretic therapy should be considered to decrease urinary calcium excretion. Furthermore, there are some data that thiazide use is associated with beneficial effects on bone density in older adults [70] and perhaps decreased fracture risk [71].

Sex hormone deficiency is common in glucocorticoid-treated patients. In a study of asthmatic men on chronic glucocorticoid therapy, 12 months of testosterone therapy were associated with a 5% increase in lumbar spine bone density [72]. A more recent trial studied the effect of testosterone and nandrolone in men on a mean of 12.6 mg/d of prednisone [73]. At 12 months, both drugs improved muscle mass and muscle strength. Testosterone increased lumbar spine bone density 4.7%. There was no benefit on bone density of the hip or total body. There are no fracture data with the use of testosterone in glucocorticoid-associated osteoporosis.

In a study of 15 postmenopausal or amenorrheic women on glucocorticoid therapy (prednisone 5 to 15 mg/d), hormone therapy (conjugated equine estrogen plus medroxyprogesterone) was associated with an increase in bone density of the spine at 1 year [74]. A 2-year, randomized trial of transdermal estradiol (plus norethisterone in patients who have an intact uterus) in women on glucocorticoid therapy for rheumatoid arthritis demonstrated a 3.75% increase in lumbar spine bone density [75]. There are no data to suggest that hormone therapy has a benefit for the hip, and no trials are available to suggest fracture efficacy. In view of the findings of the women's health initiative [76], hormone therapy may be less than ideal preventing bone loss associated with corticosteroid therapy. Raloxifene, a selective estrogen receptor modulator, increases lumbar spine bone density and decreases vertebral fractures in patients who have postmenopausal osteoporosis [77], and raloxifene is approved by the Food and Drug Administration (FDA) for preventing and treating postmenopausal osteoporosis. There are no data available on the use of raloxifene for glucocorticoid-induced osteoporosis.

Salmon calcitonin, 100 IU subcutaneously every other day, was studied for 6 months in 36 patients who had steroid-dependent chronic obstructive pulmonary disease (COPD), and a benefit on bone density was suggested at the radius [78]. Another study of subcutaneous salmon calcitonin 100 IU three times weekly in patients who have temporal arteritis or polymyalgia rheumatica showed that calcitonin, calcium, and vitamin D therapy was no better than calcium and vitamin D alone [79]. In a study of intranasal calcitonin 100 IU/d in patients on low-dose glucocorticoids for rheumatoid arthritis, there was a benefit with calcitonin on proximal femur bone density at 1 year [80]. A meta-analysis suggested calcitonin was more effective than no treatment or calcium alone in protecting against glucocorticoid-induced osteoporosis [65].

Bisphosphonates are the best-studied drugs for preventing and treating glucocorticoid-induced osteoporosis, and they are important tools for managing these patients. Adachi et al found intermittent cyclic etidronate prevented vertebral bone loss in patients on chronic glucocorticoid treatment [81]. Another study found that intermittent cyclic etidronate increased bone density at the spine and total hip in patients on chronic glucocorticoid therapy (more than 10 mg/d of prednisone) and with established osteoporosis [82]. In a randomized controlled trial of 141 patients who recently began corticosteroid treatment (mean dose 21 to 23 mg/d prednisone or equivalent) intermittent cyclic etidronate prevented bone loss at the lumbar spine and greater trochanter [83]. Other studies also have suggested intermittent cyclic etidronate has a BMD benefit in patients on chronic corticosteroids or initiating glucocorticoids [84–86]. A pooled data analysis suggested the use of intermittent cyclic etidronate in corticosteroid-treated patients has a vertebral fracture benefit in postmenopausal women initiating glucocorticoid therapy [87].

In a randomized control trial lasting 48 weeks, 477 men and women on glucocorticoid therapy were randomized to alendronate with calcium and vitamin D or calcium and vitamin D alone. The group taking alendronate demonstrated BMD benefits at the spine and hip when compared with the group taking calcium and vitamin D alone [88]. In this study, there was a borderline significant decrease in the number of patients who had new vertebral fractures in the subgroup of postmenopausal women ($P = 0.05$). No fractures occurred in the premenopausal women. A 12-month extension of this trial (62 men and 142 women) demonstrated a significant decrease in the number of patients who had morphometric vertebral fractures (0.7% in the alendronate-treated group versus 6.8% in placebo-treated patients) [89]. Bone biopsies in glucocorticoid-treated patients taking alendronate revealed decreased turnover but no adverse effects on bone structure or mineralization [90].

A 1-year study of patients initiating glucocorticoid therapy demonstrated that risedronate prevented bone loss at the spine and proximal femur [22]. In this study, risedronate therapy was associated with a trend toward a decrease in the percentage of patients who have new vertebral fractures. In another study of risedronate in glucocorticoid-treated patients, 5 mg/d resulted in an increase in spine and hip bone density and a 70% reduction in the number of patients who have new vertebral fractures at 1 year (no fractures occurred in the premenopausal women) [91]. An additional study with risedronate in patients on high-dose, oral glucocorticoid therapy found an increase in spine and hip bone density and a 70% reduction in the number of patients who have new vertebral fractures [92].

Intravenous pamidronate also has been studied for prevention of bone loss caused by glucocorticoid therapy. Intravenous pamidronate 90 mg at baseline followed by 30 mg every 3 months or a single 90-mg infusion has been shown to prevent bone loss in glucocorticoid-treated patients [93,94]. In a study of patients who had established glucocorticoid therapy, intravenous ibandronate 2 mg every 3 months was compared with oral alfacalcidol. Ibandronate had significantly greater bone density benefits at the femoral neck and lumbar spine, and there was a significant reduction in the number of patients who had vertebral fractures in the ibandronate group at 36 months (8.6% versus 22.8%) [95].

A review of the studies of pharmacotherapy for management of glucocorticoid-associated osteoporosis found bisphosphonates to be the most effective treatment, especially when combined with vitamin D [65]. Currently, alendronate (treatment) and risedronate (prevention and treatment) are approved by the FDA for managing glucocorticoid-induced osteoporosis. Intermittent cyclic etidronate and the intravenous bisphosphonates pamidronate and zoledronic acid are not FDA-approved for this indication. Oral ibandronate is approved by the FDA for postmenopausal osteoporosis, but it is not available in the United States.

Anabolic therapy with parathyroid hormone (PTH) 1-34 for 12 months was studied in postmenopausal women on glucocorticoids who already had low bone density. The women were also taking estrogen. PTH therapy was associated with a dramatic increase in BMD at the lumbar spine with an increase of 9.8% by DXA and 33.5% by QCT [96]. There was no significant difference in hip or forearm BMD between the groups [96]. In a follow-up study (1 year off the PTH), the spine bone density increase was maintained in the PTH group, but there was an approximately 5% increase in BMD at the hip with PTH compared with 1.3% to 2.6% in the hormone replacement therapy group alone [97]. PTH also may increase vertebral cross-sectional area in patients on glucocorticoids [98], an effect that theoretically could decrease the risk of fractures. There are no studies on parathyroid hormone in glucocorticoid-associated osteoporosis powered to assess fracture risk, and PTH 1-34 is not approved by the FDA for glucocorticoid-induced osteoporosis.

Sodium fluoride has been studied in glucocorticoid-induced osteoporosis [99,100]. BMD of the spine but not hip increased on sodium fluoride therapy. Studies in women who had postmenopausal osteoporosis suggest that sodium fluoride increases bone density but may not reduce fractures [101]. Fluoride is not currently used for glucocorticoid-induced osteoporosis.

Strontium ranelate, which has anabolic and antiresorptive effects and recently has been shown to increase bone density and decrease vertebral fractures in postmenopausal women [102], has not been studied in glucocorticoid-induced osteoporosis. It not approved by the FDA.

Summary

Excess glucocorticoid, whether endogenous or exogenous, can cause osteoporosis and fractures. Even low doses of oral glucocorticoids and possibly inhaled glucocorticoids may have adverse skeletal effects. Mild endogenous hypercortisolism as is present in some patients who have adrenal incidentalomas may be associated with bone loss. Patients treated with glucocorticoids, however, often are not evaluated and treated for this problem. Patients on chronic glucocorticoids or initiating these drugs should have their bone density measured and undergo appropriate laboratory studies. They should be treated with adequate calcium and vitamin D.

Box 1. Summary of prevention and treatment of glucocorticoid-induced osteoporosis

- Use the lowest dose of glucocorticoids with the shortest half-life possible
- Use topical glucocorticoids when possible
- Maintain physical activity; arrange physical therapy if necessary.
- Restrict dietary sodium intake
- Thiazide diuretics can be considered if hypercalciuria persists despite sodium restriction
- Provide a total calcium intake from diet and supplements totaling ~1500 mg/d
- Provide adequate vitamin D and try to keep the 25-hydroxyvitamin D level > 30 ng/mL
- Gonadal hormone replacement is a consideration in postmenopausal women who develop glucocorticoid-induced amenorrhea and men who have low testosterone levels if the benefits are believed to outweigh the risks
- Measure bone mineral density at baseline, 6–12 months, and yearly thereafter
- Pharmacologic therapy should be considered in patients initiating glucocorticoids or those on chronic glucocorticoid therapy, particularly if the bone density is low. The oral bisphosphonates, alendronate and risedronate, are FDA-approved for the management of glucocorticoid-induced osteoporosis. Intermittent cyclic etidronate and the intravenous bisphosphonates are off-label alternatives. Calcitonin is considered if the patient is unable to take bisphosphonates. Teriparatide (PTH 1–34) is a consideration in patients who have steroid-associated osteoporosis at very high risk for fracture.

Antiresorptive therapy (preferably bisphosphonates) should be considered in patients initiating or on chronic corticosteroid therapy, particularly if their bone mass is low. Box 1 summarizes the management of glucocorticoid-induced osteoporosis.

Acknowledgments

The authors appreciate the help of Virginia Wiatrowski in the preparation of this manuscript.

References

[1] Cushing H. The basophil adenomas of the pituitary body and their clinical manifestations (pituitary basophilism). Bull Johns Hopkins Hosp 1932;1(3):137–95.
[2] Welbourn RB, Montgomery DAD, Kennedy TL. The natural history of treated Cushing's syndrome. Br J Surg 1971;58(1):1–16.
[3] Hodgson SF. Corticosteroid-induced osteoporosis. Endocrinol Metab Clin North Am 1990;19(1):95–111.
[4] Di Somma C, Pivonello R, Loche S, et al. Severe impairment of bone mass and turnover in Cushing's disease: comparison between childhood-onset and adulthood-onset disease. Clin Endocrinol 2002;56:153–8.
[5] Chiodini I, Carnevale V, Torlontano M, et al. Alterations of bone turnover and bone mass at different skeletal sites due to pure glucocorticoid excess: study in eumenorrheic patients with Cushing's syndrome. J Clin Endocrinol Metab 1998;83:1863–7.
[6] Vestergaard P, Lindholm J, Jorgensen JOL, et al. Increased risk of osteoporotic fractures in patients with Cushing's syndrome. Eur J Endocrinol 2002;146:51–6.
[7] Kleerekoper M, Rao SD, Frame B, et al. Occult Cushing's syndrome presenting with osteoporosis. Henry Ford Hosp Med J 1980;28:132–6.
[8] Ohmori N, Nomura K, Ohmori K, et al. Osteoporosis is more prevalent in adrenal than in pituitary Cushing's syndrome. Endocr J 2003;50:1–7.
[9] Minetto M, Reimondo G, Osella G, et al. Bone loss is more severe in primary adrenal than in pituitary-dependent Cushing's syndrome. Osteoporos Int 2004;15:855–61.
[10] Osella G, Terzolo M, Reimondo G, et al. Serum markers of bone and collagen turnover in patients with Cushing's syndrome and in subjects with adrenal incidentalomas. J Clin Endocrinol Metab 1997;82:3303–7.
[11] Torlontano M, Chiodini I, Pileri M, et al. Altered bone mass and turnover in female patients with adrenal incidentaloma: the effect of subclinical hypercortisolism. J Clin Endocrinol Metab 1999;84:2381–5.
[12] Hadjidakis D, Tsagarakis S, Roboti C, et al. Does subclinical hypercortisolism adversely affect the bone mineral density of patients with adrenal incidentalomas? Clin Endocrinol 2003;58:72–7.
[13] Chiodini I, Tauchmanova L, Torlontano M, et al. Bone involvement in eugonadal male patients with adrenal incidentaloma and subclinical hypercortisolism. J Clin Endocrinol Metab 2002;87:5491–4.
[14] Graves L, Lukert BP. Glucocorticoid-induced osteoporosis. Clinical Reviews in Bone and Mineral Metabolism 2004;2(2):79–90.
[15] Carbonare LD, Arlot ME, Chavassieux APM, et al. Comparison of trabecular bone microarchitecture and remodeling in glucocorticoid-induced and postmenopausal osteoporosis. J Bone Miner Res 2001;16:97–103.
[16] Laan RF, Buijs WC, van Erning LJ, et al. Differential effects of glucocorticoids on cortical appendicular and cortical vertebral bone mineral content. Calcif Tissue Int 1993; 52:5–9.
[17] Laan RFJM, van Riel PLCM, van de Putte LBA, et al. Low-dose prednisone induces rapid reversible axial bone loss in patients with rheumatoid arthritis. Ann Intern Med 1993;119: 963–8.
[18] Adinoff AD, Hollister JR. Steroid-induced fractures and bone loss in patients with asthma. N Engl J Med 1983;309:265–8.
[19] Van Staa TP, Leufkens HGM, Abenhaim L, et al. Use of oral corticosteroids and risk of fractures. J Bone Miner Res 2000;15:993–1000.
[20] Kanis JA, Johansson H, Oden A, et al. A meta-analysis of prior corticosteroid use and fracture risk. J Bone Miner Res 2004;19:893–9.
[21] Van Staa TP, Cooper C, Leufkens HGM, et al. Children and the risk of fractures caused by oral corticosteroids. J Bone Miner Res 2003;18:913–8.

[22] Cohen S, Levy RM, Keller M, et al. Risedronate therapy prevents corticosteroid-induced bone loss. Arthritis Rheum 1999;42(11):2309–18.

[23] Luengo M, Picado C, Del Rio L, et al. Vertebral fractures in steroid-dependent asthma and involutional osteoporosis: a comparative study. Thorax 1991;46:803–6.

[24] Selby PL, Halsey JP, Adams KRH, et al. Corticosteroids do not alter the threshold for vertebral fracture. J Bone Miner Res 2000;15:952–6.

[25] Van Staa TP, Laan RF, Barton IP, et al. Bone density threshold and other predictors of vertebral fracture in patients receiving oral glucocorticoid therapy. Arthritis Rheum 2003; 48:3224–9.

[26] Curtis JR, Allison J, Becker A, et al. Screening and treatment of glucocorticoid induced osteoporosis among 6517 adults [abstract]. J Bone Miner Res 2004;19(Suppl 1):1114.

[27] Pouw EM, Prummel MF, Oosting H, et al. Beclomethasone inhalation decreases serum osteocalcin concentrations. BMJ 1991;302:627–8.

[28] Poulijoki H, Liippo K, Herrala J, et al. Inhaled beclomethasone decreases serum osteocalcin in postmenopausal asthmatic women. Bone 1992;13:285–8.

[29] Lau EMC, Li M, Woo J, et al. Bone mineral density and body composition in patients with airflow obstruction–the role of inhaled steroid therapy, disease and lifestyle. Clin Exp Allergy 1998;28:1066–71.

[30] Wong CA, Walsh LJ, Smith CJP, et al. Inhaled corticosteroid use and bone mineral density in patients with asthma. Lancet 2000;355:1399–403.

[31] Fujita K, Kasayama S, Hashimoto J, et al. Inhaled corticosteroids reduce bone mineral density in early postmenopausal but not premenopausal asthmatic women. J Bone Miner Res 2001;16:782–7.

[32] Israel E, Banerjee TR, Fitzmaurice GM, et al. Effects of inhaled glucocorticoids on bone density in premenopausal women. N Engl J Med 2001;345:941–7.

[33] Kemp JP, Osur S, Shrewsbury SB, et al. Potential effects of fluticasone propionate on bone mineral density in patients with asthma: a 2-year randomized, double-blind, placebo-controlled trial. Mayo Clin Proc 2004;79:458–66.

[34] Van Staa TP, Leufkens HGM, Cooper C. Use of inhaled corticosteroids and risk of fractures. J Bone Miner Res 2001;16:581–8.

[35] MacAdams MR, White RH, Chipps BE. Reduction of serum testosterone levels during chronic glucocorticoid therapy. Ann Intern Med 1986;104:648–51.

[36] Hampson G, Bhargava N, Cheung J, et al. Low circulating estradiol and adrenal androgens concentrations in men on glucocorticoids. a potential contributory factor in steroid-induced osteoporosis. Metabolism 2002;51:1458–62.

[37] Hofbauer LC, Gori F, Riggs L, et al. Stimulation of osteoprotegerin ligand and inhibition of osteoprotegerin production by glucocorticoids in human osteoblastic lineage cells: potential paracrine mechanisms of glucocorticoid-induced osteoporosis. Endocrinology 1999;140:4382–9.

[38] Morris HA, Need AG, O'Loughlin PD, et al. Malabsorption of calcium in corticosteroid-induced osteoporosis. Calcif Tissue Int 1990;46:305–8.

[39] Reid IR, Ibbertson HK. Evidence for decreased tubular reabsorption of calcium in glucocorticoid-treated asthmatics. Horm Res 1987;27:200–4.

[40] Rubin ME, Bilezikian JP. The role of parathyroid hormone in the pathogenesis of glucocorticoid-induced osteoporosis: a re-examination of the evidence. J Clin Endocrinol Metab 2002;87(9):4033–41.

[41] Weinstein RS, Jilka RL, Parfitt AM, et al. Inhibition of osteoblastogenesis and promotion of apoptosis of osteoblasts and osteocytes by glucocorticoids: potential mechanisms of their deleterious effects on bone. J Clin Invest 1998;102(2):274–82.

[42] Dovio A, Perazzolo L, Osella G, et al. Immediate fall of bone formation and transient increase in bone resorption in the course of high-dose, short-term glucocorticoid therapy in young patients with multiple sclerosis. J Clin Endocrinol Metab 2004;89: 4923–8.

[43] Canalis E, Delany AM. Mechanisms of glucocorticoid action in bone. Ann N Y Acad Sci 2002;966:73–81.
[44] Centrella M, McCarthy TL, Canalis E. Glucocorticoid regulation of transforming growth factor β1 activity and binding in osteoblast-enriched cultures from fetal rat bone. Mol Cell Biol 1991;11:4490–6.
[45] Ohnaka K, Taniguchi H, Kawate H, et al. Glucocorticoid enhances the expression of dickkopf-1 in human osteoblasts: novel mechanism of glucocorticoid-induced osteoporosis. Biochem Biophys Res Com 2004;318:259–64.
[46] Cooper MS, Rabbitt EH, Goddard PE, et al. Osteoblastic 11β-hydroxysteroid dehydrogenase type 1 activity increases with age and glucocorticoid exposure. J Bone Miner Res 2002;17(6):979–86.
[47] Cooper MS, Bujalska I, Rabbit EH, et al. Modulation of 11 beta-hydroxysteroid dehydrogenase isoenzymes by proinflammatory cytokines in osteoblasts: an autocrine switch from glucocorticoid inactivation to activation. J Bone Miner Res 2001;17: 1037–44.
[48] Pocock NA, Eisman JA, Dunstan CR, et al. Recovery from steroid-induced osteoporosis. Ann Intern Med 1987;107:319–23.
[49] Lufkin EG, Wahner HW, Bergstralh EJ. Reversibility of steroid-induced osteoporosis. Am J Med 1988;85:887–8.
[50] Manning PJ, Evans MC, Reid IR. Normal bone mineral density following cure of Cushing's syndrome. Clin Endocrinol 1992;36:229–34.
[51] Hermus AR, Smals AG, Swinkels LM, et al. Bone mineral density and bone turnover before and after surgical cure of Cushing's syndrome. J Clin Endocrinol Metab 1995;80: 2859–65.
[52] Dobnig H, Stepan V, Leb G, et al. Recovery from severe osteoporosis following cure from ectopic ACTH syndrome caused by an appendix carcinoid. J Intern Med 1996;239:365–9.
[53] Di Somma C, Pivonello R, Loche S, et al. Effect of 2 years of cortisol normalization on the impaired bone mass and turnover in adolescent and adult patients with Cushing's disease: a prospective study. Clin Endocrinol 2003;58:302–8.
[54] Gebhard KL, Mailbach HI. Relationship between systemic corticosteroids and osteonecrosis. American Journal of Clinical Dermatology 2001;2(6):377–88.
[55] Lane NE, Lukert B. The science and therapy of glucocorticoid-induced bone loss. Endocrinol Metab Clin North Am 1998;27(2):465–83.
[56] Felson DT, Anderson JJ. A cross-study evaluation of association between steroid dose and bolus steroids and avascular necrosis of bone. Lancet 1987;1(8538):902–6.
[57] Mankin HJ. Nontraumatic necrosis of bone (osteonecrosis). N Engl J Med 1992;326(22): 1473–9.
[58] Weinstein RS, Nicholas RW, Manolagas S. Apoptosis of osteocytes in glucocorticoid-induced osteonecrosis of the hip. J Clin Endocrinol Metab 2000;85:2907–12.
[59] Pritchett JW. Statin therapy decreases the risk of osteonecrosis in patients receiving steroids. Clinical Orthopedics and Related Research 2001;1(386):173–8.
[60] Lieberman JR, Berry DJ, Mont MA, et al. Osteonecrosis of the hip: management in the twenty-first century. J Bone Joint Surg 2002;84-A(5):834–53.
[61] American College of Rheumatology Ad Hoc Committee on Glucocorticoid-Induced Osteoporosis. Recommendations for the prevention and treatment of glucocorticoid-induced osteoporosis. Arthritis Rheum 2001;44:1496–503.
[62] Amin S, LaValley P, Simms R, et al. The role of vitamin D in corticosteroid-induced osteoporosis: a meta-analytic approach. Arthritis Rheum 1999;42(8):1740–51.
[63] Buckley LM, Leib ES, Cartularo KS, et al. Calcium and vitamin D3 supplementation prevents bone loss in the spine secondary to low-dose corticosteroids in patients with rheumatoid arthritis. Ann Intern Med 1996;125:961–8.
[64] Adachi JD, Bensen WG, Bianchi F, et al. Vitamin D and calcium in the prevention of corticosteroid induced osteoporosis: a 3-year follow-up. J Rheumatol 1996;23:995–1000.

[65] Amin S, Lavalley MP, Simms RW, et al. The comparative efficacy of drug therapies used for the management of corticosteroid-induced osteoporosis: a meta-regression. J Bone Miner Res 2002;17(8):1512–26.
[66] Sambrook P, Birmingham J, Kelly P, et al. Prevention of corticosteroid osteoporosis: a comparison of calcium, calcitriol, and calcitonin. N Engl J Med 1993;328:1747–52.
[67] Gram J, Junker P, Nielsen HK, et al. Effects of short-term treatment with prednisolone and calcitriol on bone and mineral metabolism in normal men. Bone 1998;23:297–302.
[68] Reginster JY, Kuntz D, Verdickt W, et al. Prophylactic use of alfacalcidiol in corticosteroid-induced osteoporosis. Osteoporos Int 1999;9:75–81.
[69] Sambrook PN, Kotowicz M, Nash P, et al. Prevention and treatment of glucocorticoid-induced osteoporosis: a comparison of calcitriol, vitamin D plus calcium, and alendronate plus calcium. J Bone Miner Res 2003;18:919–24.
[70] LaCroix AZ, Ott SM, Ichikawa L, et al. Low-dose hydrochlorothiazide and preservation of bone mineral density in older adults; a randomized, double-blind, placebo-controlled trial. Ann Intern Med 2000;133:516–26.
[71] Jones G, Nguyen T, Sambrook PN, et al. Thiazide diuretics and fractures: can meta-analysis help? J Bone Miner Res 1995;10:106–11.
[72] Reid IR, Wattie DJ, Evans MC, et al. Testosterone therapy in glucocorticoid-treated men. Arch Intern Med 1996;156:1173–7.
[73] Crawford BAL, Liu PY, Kean MT, et al. Randomized placebo-controlled trial of androgen effects on muscle and bone in men requiring long-term systemic glucocorticoid treatment. J Clin Endocrinol Metab 2003;88:3167–76.
[74] Lukert BP, Johnson BE, Robinson RG. Estrogen and progesterone replacement therapy reduces glucocorticoid-induced bone loss. J Bone Min Res 1992;7(9):1063–9.
[75] Hall GM, Daniels M, Dolye DV, et al. Effect of hormone replacement therapy on bone mass in rheumatoid arthritis with and without steroids. Arthritis Rheum 1994;37: 1499–505.
[76] Writing Group for the Womens Health Initiative Investigators. Risks and benefits of estrogen plus progestin in healthy postmenopausal women. JAMA 2002;282:321–33.
[77] Ettinger B, Black DM, Mitlak BH, et al. Reduction in vertebral fracture risk in postmenopausal women with osteoporosis treated with raloxifene: results from a 3-year, randomized clinical trial. Multiple outcome of Raloxifene (MORE) Investigators. JAMA 1999;282:637–45.
[78] Ringe JD, Welzel D. Salmon calcitonin in the therapy of corticoid-induced osteoporosis. Eur J Clin Pharmacol 1987;33:35–9.
[79] Healey JH, Paget SA, Williams-Russo P, et al. A randomized controlled trial of salmon calcitonin to prevent bone loss in corticosteroid-treated temporal arteritis and polymyalgia rheumatica. Calcif Tissue Int 1996;58:73–80.
[80] Kotaniemi A, Piirainen H, Paimela L, et al. Is continuous intranasal salmon calcitonin effective in treating axial bone loss in patients with active rheumatoid arthritis receiving low dose glucocorticoid therapy? J Rheumatol 1996;23:1875–9.
[81] Adachi JD, Cranney A, Goldsmith CH, et al. Intermittent cyclic therapy with etidronate in the prevention of corticosteroid-induced bone loss. J Rheumatol 1994;21:1922–6.
[82] Struys A, Snelder AA, Mulder H. Cyclical etidronate reverses bone loss of the spine and proximal femur in patients with established corticosteroid-induced osteoporosis. Am J Med 1995;99:235–42.
[83] Adachi JD, Bensen WG, Brown J, et al. Intermittent etidronate therapy to prevent corticosteroid-induced osteoporosis. N Engl J Med 1997;337:382–7.
[84] Geusens P, Dequeker J, Vanhoof J, et al. Cyclical etidronate increases bone density in the spine and hip of postmenopausal women receiving long term corticosteroid treatment. A double-blind, randomized placebo-controlled study. Ann Rheum Dis 1998;57:724–7.
[85] Jenkins EA, Walker-Bone KE, Wood A, et al. The prevention of corticosteroid-induced bone loss with intermittent cyclical etidronate. Scand J Rheumatol 1999;28:152–6.

[86] Roux C, Oriente P, Laan R, et al. Randomized trial of effect of cyclical etidronate in the prevention of corticosteroid-induced bone loss. J Clin Endocrinol Metab 1998;83:1128–33.
[87] Adachi JD, Roux C, Pitt PI, et al. A pooled data analysis on the use of intermittent cyclical etidronate therapy for the prevention and treatment of corticosteroid induced bone loss. J Rheumatol 2000;27:2424–31.
[88] Saag KG, Emkey R, Schnitzer TJ, et al. Alendronate for the prevention and treatment of glucocorticoid-induced osteoporosis. N Engl J Med 1998;339(5):292–9.
[89] Adachi JD, Saag KG, Delmas PD, et al. Two-year effects of alendronate on bone mineral density and vertebral fracture in patients receiving glucocorticoids. Arthritis Rheum 2001; 44(1):202–11.
[90] Chavassieux PM, Arlot ME, Roux JP, et al. Effects of alendronate on bone quality and remodeling in glucocorticoid-induced osteoporosis: a histomorphometric analysis of transiliac biopsies. J Bone Miner Res 2000;15(4):754–62.
[91] Wallach S, Cohen S, Reid DM, et al. Effects of risedronate treatment on bone density and vertebral fracture in patients on corticosteroid therapy. Calcif Tissue Int 2000;67:277–85.
[92] Reid DM, Hughes RA, Laan RF, et al. Efficacy and safety of daily risedronate in the treatment of corticosteroid-induced osteoporosis in men and women: a randomized trial. J Bone Miner Res 2000;15:1006–13.
[93] Boutsen Y, Jamart J, Esselinckx W, et al. Primary prevention of glucocorticoid-induced osteoporosis with intravenous pamidronate and calcium: a prospective controlled 1-year study comparing a single infusion, an infusion given once every 3 months, and calcium alone. J Bone Miner Res 2001;16:104–12.
[94] Boutsen Y, Jamart J, Esselinckx W, et al. Primary prevention of glucocorticoid-induced osteoporosis with intermittent intravenous pamidronate: a randomized trial. Calcif Tissue Int 1997;61:266–71.
[95] Ringe JD, Dorst A, Faber H, et al. Intermittent intravenous ibandronate injections reduce vertebral fracture risk in corticosteroid-induced osteoporosis: results from a long-term comparative study. Osteoporos Int 2003;14:801–7.
[96] Lane NE, Sanchez S, Modin GW, et al. Parathyroid hormone treatment can reverse corticosteroid-induced osteoporosis. J Clin Invest 1998;102:1627–33.
[97] Lane NE, Sanchez S, Modin GW, et al. Bone mass continues to increase at the hip after parathyroid hormone treatment is discontinued in glucocorticoid-induced osteoporosis: results of a randomized controlled clinical trial. J Bone Miner Res 2000;15:944–51.
[98] Rehman Q, Lang TF, Arnaud CD, et al. Daily treatment with parathyroid hormone is associated with an increase in vertebral cross-sectional area in postmenopausal women with glucocorticoid-induced osteoporosis. Osteoporos Int 2003;14:77–81.
[99] Lems WF, Jacobs WG, Bijlsma JWJ, et al. Effect of sodium fluoride in the prevention of corticosteroid-induced osteoporosis. Osteoporos Int 1997;7:575–82.
[100] Lems WF, Jacobs JWG, Bijlsma JWJ, et al. Is addition of fluoride to cyclical etidronate beneficial in the treatment of corticosteroid induced osteoporosis? Ann Rheum Dis 1997;56: 357–63.
[101] Riggs BL, Hodgson SF, O'Fallon WM, et al. Effect of fluoride treatment on the fracture rate in postmenopausal women with osteoporosis. N Engl J Med 1990;322:802–9.
[102] Meunier PJ, Roux C, Seeman E, et al. The effects of strontium ranelate on the risk of vertebral fractures in women with postmenopausal osteoporosis. N Engl J Med 2004;350: 459–68.

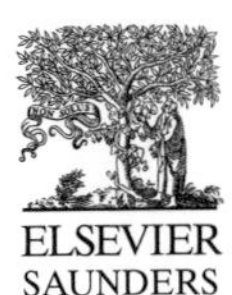

ELSEVIER
SAUNDERS

Endocrinol Metab Clin N Am
34 (2005) 357–369

ENDOCRINOLOGY
AND METABOLISM
CLINICS
OF NORTH AMERICA

Cognitive Function and Cerebral Assessment in Patients Who Have Cushing's Syndrome

Isabelle Bourdeau, MD[a,*], Céline Bard, MD[b], Hélène Forget, PhD[c], Yvan Boulanger, PhD[d], Henri Cohen, PhD[e], André Lacroix, MD[a]

[a]*Division of Endocrinology, Department of Medicine, Hôtel-Dieu du Centre Hospitalier de l'Université de Montréal, 3840 Saint-Urbain Street, Montreal, QC H2W 1T8, Canada*

[b]*Department of Radiology, Hôtel-Dieu du Centre Hospitalier de l'Université de Montréal, 3840 Saint-Urbain Street, Montreal, QC H2W 1T8, Canada*

[c]*Department of Psychology, Université du Québec en Outaouais, 283 Alexandre Taché, CP 1250, suc. Hull, Gatineau, QC J8X 3X7, Canada*

[d]*Department of Radiology, Hôpital Saint-Luc du Central Hospitalier de l'Université de Montréal, 1058 St-Denis, Montreal, QC H2X 3J4, Canada*

[e]*Cognitive Neuroscience Center, Université du Québec à Montréal, P.O. Box 8888, Succ. Centre-Ville, Montreal, QC H3C 3P8, Canada*

Corticosteroids play an important role in the function and homeostasis of the central nervous system (CNS). Chronic exposure to supraphysiologic levels of glucocorticoids (GCs) in Cushing's syndrome (CS) is associated with an increased prevalence of sleep disturbances, mood alterations, psychiatric diseases, cognitive impairment, and anatomical brain changes. Thus, patients who have CS provide a natural model to demonstrate the interactions between hypercortisolism and brain function in people. This article presents data on alterations of brain anatomy and metabolism and cognitive and neuropsychologic impairments for patients who have CS.

Loss of brain volume in endogenous Cushing's syndrome

Previous pathologic and imaging studies suggested that some morphologic anatomic modifications did occur in the brain of patients who have CS. The authors first wish to point out that the terminology cerebral atrophy has been

* Corresponding author.
E-mail address: isabelle.bourdeau@umontreal.ca (I. Bourdeau).

0889-8529/05/$ - see front matter
doi:10.1016/j.ecl.2005.01.016

used widely in the literature for the description of morphologic changes observed in the brain of patients who have CS. Considering the facts that cell atrophy or cell loss has not been demonstrated pathologically and that the observed changes are potentially reversible, the authors now prefer to use the terminology of loss of brain volume until the precise pathophysiology is determined more accurately.

Although limited in number, some autopsy studies revealed modifications of brain anatomy in CS. Momose et al found a mild loss of brain volume and ventricular enlargement at autopsy in four of eight patients suffering from CS [1]. Other reports described a lower brain weight associated with enlarged ventricles in a subgroup of patients who have CS [2,3].

In 1971, a high incidence of cortical atrophy of the cerebral (90%) and cerebellar (74%) hemispheres was described in 31 patients who had Cushing's disease (CD) using pneumoencephalography [1]. Similar findings were reported in 1992 by Starkman et al [4], with decreases in hippocampal formation volume in 27% of patients who had CS, in whom the values being below the 95% confidence interval were compared with a normal population taken from the literature. An association was found in affected patients between reduced hippocampal formation, memory dysfunction, and elevated cortisol levels, suggesting a possible link between anatomic structure and neuropsychologic function [4]. More recently, Simmons et al [5] also described significant subjective loss of brain volume in 63 patients who had CD, compared with an age- and sex-matched control group studied using CT and MRI scans.

The authors' group also confirmed the presence of loss of brain volume in patients affected with CS. They retrospectively studied 38 patients, including 21 who had CD and 17 who had adrenal CS, to assess the presence and distribution of loss of brain volume. Both objective (third ventricle diameter and bicaudate diameter) and subjective measures were obtained from CT or MRI examinations. These objective measures were used as indirect signs of volume loss in correlation with the subjective assessment. The authors found subjective loss of brain volume in 86% of patients who had CD and 100% of patients who had adrenal CS [6]. The values for third ventricle diameter, bicaudate diameter, and subjective evaluation were increased significantly in CS groups compared with the control group comprising 20 normal individuals and 18 patients who had non-ACTH secreting pituitary tumors. The authors' data suggested that loss of brain volume is highly prevalent in patients who had CS. Additionally, it is not limited to hippocampal volume formation but also with increased subarachnoid space and ventricles in agreement with other previous reports (Fig. 1).

Reversibility of loss of brain volume after correction of hypercortisolism

Data on the anatomic outcome of apparent cerebral atrophy following correction of hypercortisolism are limited. The authors re-evaluated

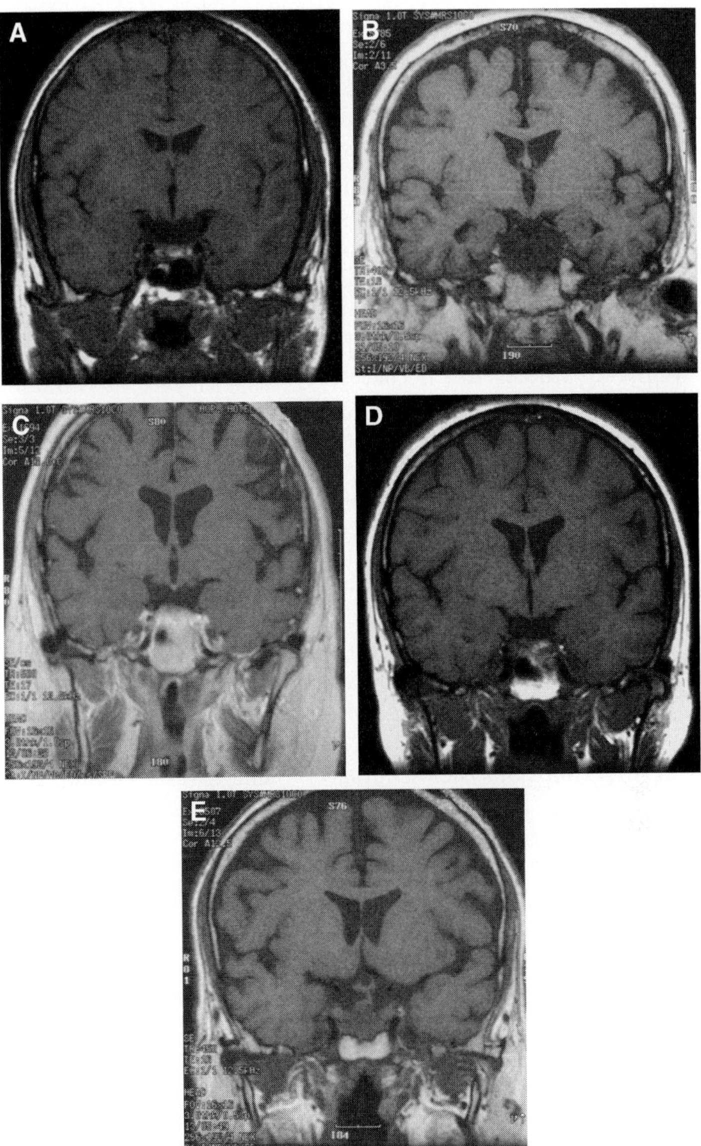

Fig. 1. (*A*) Coronal T_1-weighted MRI image of a 40-year-old normal control woman. (*B*) A 45-year-old woman who has CS from a surgically proven adrenal adenoma presenting brain volume loss characterized by increased sulci and ventricle enlargement. (*C, D*) A 22-year-old woman who has adrenal CS presenting an apparent complete anatomical regression of brain volume loss on a control MRI 7 years after correction of hypercortisolism (*D*) compared with the her initial MRI when CS was diagnosed (*C*). (*E*) A 46-year-old man who has a delayed diagnosis of CS, 4 years after surgery for an ACTH-secreting pituitary adenoma still showing signs of brain volume loss for his age.

22 patients who had CS at 39.7 ± 34.1 months after achieving eucortisolism. The subjective score of apparent brain volume loss, the third ventricle diameter, and the bicaudate diameter improved (see Fig. 1) [6] but did not reach the normal control group values (see Fig. 1). The objective parameters of brain volumes progressively improved but did not reach a plateau after 45 months of normalization of cortisol levels in one patient. Starkman et al [7] reported that the volume of hippocampal formation increased by 3% following treatment in 22 patients who had CS with a mean follow-up of 16 ± 9.3 months. This increase was found to correlate significantly with the reduction in urinary free cortisol levels. Interestingly, they also observed a trend toward an increased volume in the head of the caudate nucleus. These studies suggested that loss of brain volume is at least partially reversible, but longer follow-up studies will be necessary to determine whether complete correction can be achieved.

Loss of brain volume in exogenous Cushing's syndrome

Synthetic GCs are used widely, and their systemic adverse effects are well known. Their impact on brain volume, however, largely remains unrecognized. A few reports underlined the association of supraphysiologic administration of exogenous GCs with apparent brain atrophy. Bentson et al [8] studied a population less than 40 years old that had a diagnosis of cerebral atrophy and found that approximately 10% of them were on chronic GC therapy. Pharmacologic doses of GCs also were related to apparent cerebral atrophy in two groups of systemic lupus erythematosus or nonlupus patients compared with age- and sex-matched normal subjects [9]. Other studies demonstrated a possible link between conditions associated with the increased activity of the pituitary-adrenal axis such as alcoholism [10], depression [11–13], and stress [14] and apparent cerebral atrophy.

Cerebral magnetic resonance spectroscopy in Cushing's syndrome

Patients affected by endogenous and exogenous CS were studied by proton magnetic resonance spectroscopy (MRS) of the brain. Thirteen untreated patients who had endogenous CS, including seven who had pituitary corticotroph adenomas and six who had primary adrenal disease, were examined in the frontal, thalamic, and temporal areas, and compared with 40 normal control subjects. A statistically significant decrease in the choline to creatine ratio (Cho/Cr) was measured in the frontal (−24%) and thalamic (−17%) areas of CS patients (Fig. 2), while no significant variation was found in the temporal area [15]. The Cho/Cr ratio is a membrane marker reflecting mostly the phosphatidylcholine metabolism. When comparing patients who had CD and patients who had CS secondary to an adrenal disease, the Cho/Cr change was larger for the second group in the thalamic

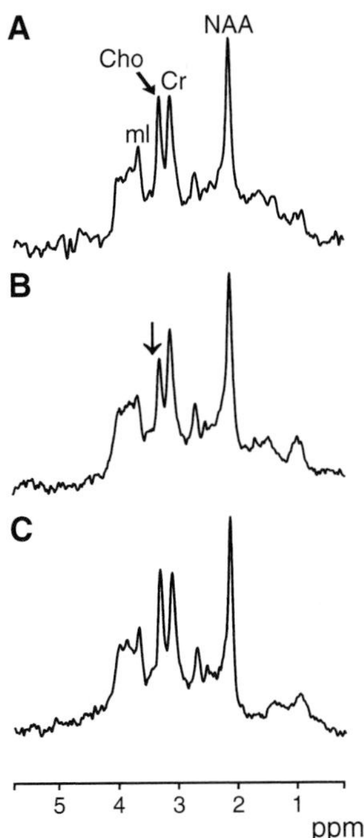

Fig. 2. Proton magnetic resonance spectra from the thalamic area of the brain for (*A*) a normal subject and a patient who has pituitary CD (*B*) before and (*C*) after correction of hypercortisolism. The intensity of the choline (Cho) signal is reduced for the CD patient relative to the normal subject but recovers after correction of hypercortisolism. (*Reprinted from* Khiat A, Bard C, Lacroix A, et al. Recovery of the brain choline level in treated Cushing's patients as monitored by proton magnetic resonance spectroscopy. Brain Res 2000;862:304; with permission.)

area, but not in the frontal area. The authors noted that Cho decreases also were observed in diseases with similar symptoms such as depression, ischemia, neuronal necrosis, hepatic encephalopathy, and schizophrenia. The other metabolite ratios (ie, *N*-acetylaspartate [NAA/Cr], a neuron marker, and myoinositol [mI/Cr], a glial marker) were unaffected by CS. In a follow-up study, MRS data were obtained for 10 CS patients whose hypercortisolism had been corrected for at least 6 months [16]. A statistically significant recovery of the choline levels was found in the frontal and thalamic areas. The results were interpreted as an inhibition by GCs of the action of phospholipases that degrade phosphatidylcholine in the presence of CS. After correction of hypercortisolism, this inhibition disappears.

The effects of exogenous CS on brain metabolism were also investigated in 13 patients who were treated with 5 to 50 mg of prednisone per day for periods varying between 2 to 22 years for various pathologic conditions without specific effects on brain volume [17]. When compared with normal subjects, none of the MRS metabolites showed any significant variation. A refined analysis, however, revealed a significant decrease of the Cho/H_2O ratio as a function of the treatment period at a rate of −1.3% per year. This decrease was not found to be dose- or age-dependent.

Pathophysiology of glucocorticoids on brain

Corticosteroid hormones enter the brain compartment and bind to intracellular receptors. Two receptor subtypes mediate GC actions: GC receptors (GRs) and mineralocorticoid receptors (MRs). GRs are distributed widely in cerebral neurons and glial cells, whereas MRs are expressed highly in limbic brain areas such as the hippocampus. MRs bind corticosterone with an affinity 10-fold higher than GRs. Thus, low basal corticosterone levels predominantly occupy high-affinity MRs, whereas GRs can be activated concomitantly to MRs when GC concentrations are elevated during the active period of the circadian cycle, during stress, and in CS [18].

In addition to the amount of circulating steroids available to activate the receptors, prereceptor metabolism of GCs occurs intracellularly [19] and is mediated by the enzyme 11β-hydroxysteroid dehydrogenase (11β-HSD). Two distinct isoforms of 11β-HSDs exist. 11β-HSD type 1 elevates intracellular GC levels, and 11β-HSD type 2 inactivates GCs by converting cortisol into the inactive cortisone molecule. Two mechanisms lead to GC effects in hippocampal cells: (1) only 11β-HSD type 1 is expressed, leading to conversion of inert into active GCs [20], and (2) 11β-HSD type 2 is not expressed in hippocampus or other limbic structures, allowing MR activation by GCs in these brain areas.

What are the mechanisms underlying loss of brain volume in Cushing's syndrome?

The pathogenesis of loss in brain volume induced by chronic GC excess is probably multi-factorial [18]. Previous animal and in vitro studies examined the effects of GCs on the morphology and survival of neurons on the brain; it must be mentioned that this work has been conducted mainly on hippocampus cells. Woolley et al [21] reported that treatment of young adult rats with exogenous corticosterone for 3 weeks induced atrophy of the apical dendrites of CA3 pyramidal neurons, whereas a longer exposure of 3 months to corticosterone injections resulted in loss of CA3 pyramidal neurons [22]. Atrophy of dendritic processes seemed to be GC-dependent and reversible and correlated with impaired explicit memory [23]. Similarly, Watanabe et al demonstrated that daily stress for 21 days in rats leads to significant decreases in the total dendritic length and the number of branch points of apical dendrites of CA3 pyramidal neurons [24–26]. In contrast, removal of adrenal glands resulted in apoptotic-like degeneration of mature, granule cells in the rat dentate gyrus, but not in other hippocampal fields [18,27,28]. In addition to the induction of reversible atrophy of dendritic processes, GCs act also by inhibiting neurogenesis. Recently, Tag et al reported that dexamethasone has an inhibitory effect on proliferation, but not on differentiation in rat fetal hippocampal progenitor cells [29]. In contrast, in aged rats, the neurogenesis can be restored by removing the elevated GC levels associated with aging [30].

It has been suggested that an excess of excitatory amino acid (EAA) neurotransmitters such as glutamate mediates GC-induced hippocampal atrophy. GCs increase the synaptic accumulation of glutamate, possibly from an effect on its removal by glial cells. The enhanced stimulation of *N*-methyl-D-aspartate receptors will increase intracellular cytosolic calcium ions (Ca^{2+}) in postsynaptic neurons, which activates several processes, leading to increased susceptibility to injury (cell endangerment) and cell death [18,25,26]. In addition, GCs may have effects on brain-derived neurotrophin mediators such as neurotrophin, which plays a role in dendritic arborization [23]. A reduced glucose metabolism is observed on fluorine-18 fluoro-2-deoxyglucose (^{18}F-FDG) positron emission tomography (PET) scan of patients who had brain tumors taking oral dexamethasone [31]. This may be secondary to the inhibitory action of GCs on glucose transporter synthesis and translocation in neurons and glial cells [32,33]. As described previously, dexamethasone, though being anti-inflammatory, inhibits blood–brain barrier permeability and decreases cerebral edema. Thus, the cerebral morphologic changes in CS also could be secondary in part because of a loss in water content of brain tissue leading to tissue compression and ventricular enlargement [23,34,35].

Further studies are needed to better understand the mechanisms involved in human loss of brain volume. The partial reversibility of cerebral morphologic changes after correction of hypercortisolism observed by two different groups [6,7] in patients who had CS, however, seems to indicate that brain volume loss is unlikely to be only secondary to neuronal cell death.

Psychiatric disorders associated with Cushing's syndrome

Psychiatric disturbances have been associated with the exogenous administration of large amounts of steroid hormones. A substantial body of evidence suggests that depression is a major and life-threatening complication of CS [36]. In a summary of 12 studies involving 330 patients up to 1980 [37], it was observed that 45% of CS patients were depressed or suicidal. Subsequent studies used a standardized assessment of depression by specific diagnostic criteria. In his study, Haskett [38] obtained a lifetime history of psychiatric symptoms and signs from 30 patients who had proven CS. He found that most patients (83%) reported psychiatric disturbances that closely resembled typical syndromes for an episode of major affective disorder (endogenous depression, mania, or hypomania). Patients frequently attempted to minimize or conceal serious psychiatric disturbances, including suicide attempts. Schizophrenic symptoms were not evident. Indeed, major psychiatric disturbances or other mood disorders are infrequent in CS, and if psychotic symptoms occur, they are likely to be complication of mania or severe depression [39]. According to the *Diagnostic and Statistical Manual of Mental Disorders, Third Edition* (DSM-III), Hudson et al [40] also reported a high lifetime diagnosis of mood disorder in patients who had CS (81%), compared with control subjects who had rheumatoid arthritis, of whom 14% were diagnosed with major affective disorder. The rate of familial mood disorder among patients who had major depression not associated with endocrine disease was significantly higher, however, than among patients who had CS. At variance with these findings, Loosen et al [41] evaluated 20 adult patients who had CS and 20 adult patients who had major depressive disorder using the "Structured Clinical Interview" for the *Diagnostic and Statistical Manual of Mental Disorders, Revised Third Edition* (DSM-III-R). They found a major depressive disorder to be present in 68% of patients, and they obtained similar rates of depression in family members who had CS and nonendocrine major depression. In addition, this disorder frequently was associated with an anxiety disorder (generalized anxiety disorder or panic disorder), suggesting a syndrome of anxious depression in patients who had active CS. In contrast, in animal models, mutant mice for the GC receptor in the nervous system show an impaired behavioral response to stress and display reduced anxiety [42].

Sonino et al [43] reported major depressive disorders in 62% of patients who had CS. There were no significant differences between pituitary-dependent and pituitary-independent forms in the occurrence of major depression. These findings later were confirmed by an independent investigation [44]. Dorn et al [45] studied 17 patients (51.5%) who had active endogenous CS and found significant psychopathology expressed primarily by melancholic or atypical depression. In a large cohort of patients who had CS ($n = 209$), psychiatric pathologies, usually depressive illness, were present in 57% of the patients [44]. More recently, in a study focusing on demographic and clinical correlates of major depression in 162 patients who had CD, Sonino et al [46] found that the occurrence of major depression according to the *Diagnostic and Statistical Manual of Mental Disorders, Fourth Edition* (DMS-IV) criteria was present in 54% of the patients. It was associated significantly with older age, female sex, higher pretreatment urinary cortisol levels, relatively more severe clinical condition, and absence of radiologically detectable pituitary adenoma. In this study, patients who had CD and major depression appeared to suffer from a more severe form of illness, both in terms of GC production and clinical presentation, compared with those who were not depressed during the course of their disease. Interestingly, Dorn et al [47] found that atypical depressive disorders gradually improved with time after correction of hypercortisolism simultaneously with the recovery of the hypothalamic–pituitary–adrenal axis. The marked depressive symptoms, which frequently are reported by many patients who have CS, are as distressing to the patient and family as the visible cortisol-induced stigmata.

Cognitive functions in Cushing's syndrome

Although several investigations conducted in recent years have stressed the numerous effects of GCs on cognition, studies specifically studying CS and its effects on the cognitive processes are few. As mentioned earlier, Starkman et al [4] found a significant correlation between the severity of the hypercortisolism and the extent of hippocampal formation atrophy, and a correlation with the severity of the accompanying verbal learning and memory deficits in patients who have CS (this work used the logical memory test from the Wechsler Memory Scale [WMS]). There was an association between reduced hippocampal formation, verbal memory dysfunction, and elevated cortisol in patients who have CS [48]. It should be mentioned, however, that this study specifically did not document a memory deficit among patients; indeed, the performances of the CS subjects were around the average of the tests employed. This partially was confirmed by the results of Mauri et al [49], who also point to a mnesic impairment of moderate degree in CS patients relative to matched normal controls. The low performance obtained by their subjects at digit symbol tests (from the Wechsler Adult Intelligence Scales [WAIS]) may indicate an impairment of attentive and visuomotor functions. Miller et al [50] also report that CS patients scored significantly lower than normal subjects on attention (measured by tests of control and digit span from the WMS) and initial learning of verbal (measured by test of logical memory from the WMS) and visual test (measured by test of visual reproduction from the WMS) stimuli.

The memory is the function most studied in CS because of the emphasis on the hippocampus. The wide distribution of GC receptors in the cerebral cortex suggests that extrahippocampal sites also can be the target of adrenal hormones. Indeed, it is likely that multiple regions of the brain are affected to some degree by hypercortisolism. In parallel, several cognitive functions other than the commonly reported effects on memory and learning can be affected by the dysregulation of adrenal steroidogenesis. For example, Whelan et al [51] previously suggested that the pattern of neuropsychologic deficits in 35 unselected CS patients, using exhaustive Michigan Neuropsychologic Test Battery, were comparable to those seen in patients who have other types of diffuse bilateral neuropathologic processes. Impairment was more frequent and more severe in nonverbal visual–ideational and visual memory functions. It is important to mention that this pattern of more marked deficits of nonverbal functions is predominant in bilateral diffuse brain diseases such as anorexia, toxicity, aging, and some infectious diseases [52]. Starkman et al [53] also reported generalized impairment in cognitive functions (decreased concentration and memory, perceptual distortions). In a recent study [54], the authors found that untreated CS patients scored significantly lower than controls on general intellectual performance (IQ scores) and in tests of treatment of visual and spatial information, attention, reasoning, and verbal fluency. These results suggest that chronic exposure to elevated levels of cortisol is associated with deficits in several areas of cognition. The authors' results are concordant with those of Starkman et al [55], who found that in chronic hypercortisolemia caused CS, several domains of cognitive function are affected, including verbal, visuospatial, learning, and memory. The results suggest that elevated levels of GC affect the neocortex and the hippocampus.

Few studies have examined the reversibility of cognitive disorders after successful treatment objectively. Mauri et al [49] showed a significant amelioration in verbal memory performance and attentive and visuomotor functions in eight patients 6 months after the surgical cure. No changes in other cognitive functions could be detected. Martignoni et al [56] reported that 7 of 24 patients who had CS for less than 1 year had improved verbal memory after surgical treatment. Improvement was noted on only 2 of the 11 cognitive tests. On the other hand, two studies have shown no improvement in cognitive functioning in patients who have CS. Dorn and Cerrone [57] have compared the cognitive status of CS patients at the time of diagnosis and 12 months after treatment of hypercortisolism with the cognitive status of a healthy group also retested after 12 months. Overall, no statistically significant improvement occurred in cognitive functioning, as indexed by the WAIS–Revised (WAIS-R), in patients who had CS and were followed to 12 months postcure [57]. More recently, the authors evaluated 13 subjects who presented with CS with a battery of tests including of attention, visuospatial processing, memory, reasoning, and verbal fluency [58]. Except for one task of visual organization, the results showed little change in performance, suggesting that prolonged exposure to high levels of cortisol can cause long-lasting deleterious effects on cognitive function. The data suggest that correction of hypercortisolism is not necessarily correlated with short-term improvement in cognitive function. Finally, using a more qualitative approach, Gotch [59] showed that 66% of treated patients who have CS reported that the disease still had a negative influence on several dimensions of their lives such as physical, cognitive, and affective capacities.

In spite of a lack of consensus among researchers on the scope of the impaired cognitive functions in patients who have CS, they all underline the disorders of attention and memory. Following treatment of CS, the indices of improvement of cognitive processes are more parsimonious and will require longer follow-up studies.

In conclusion, loss of brain volume is observed frequently in patients who have CS and is not only limited to the hippocampus. Moreover, the loss of brain volume is at least partially reversible after the correction of hypercortisolism as in the choline metabolite. Psychiatric diseases and cognitive impairment have been documented in CS and should be taken into account when managing affected patients. Understanding neuropsychologic and cognitive disorders in CS adds to the comprehension of the effects of the GCs on the CNS and may provide clues on excessive exposure to elevated GCs levels, in particular in depression, aging, or in a prolonged stress, on various aspects of animal and human cognition.

Acknowledgments

The authors wish to express their gratitude to Mrs. Josée Baker for her secretarial assistance in preparing the manuscript.

References

[1] Momose KJ, Kjellberg RN, Kliman B. High incidence of cortical atrophy of the cerebral and cerebellar hemispheres in Cushing's disease. Radiology 1971;99:341.
[2] Trethowan WH, Cobb S. Neuropsychiatric aspects of Cushing's syndrome. AMA Arch Neurol Psychiatry 1952;67:283.
[3] Cope O, Raker JW. Cushing's disease: the surgical experience in the care of 46 cases. N Engl J Med 1955;253:119.
[4] Starkman MN, Gebarski SS, Berent S, et al. Hippocampal formation volume, memory dysfunction, and cortisol levels in patients with Cushing's syndrome. Biol Psychiatry 1992; 32:756.
[5] Simmons NE, Do HM, Lipper MH, et al. Cerebral atrophy in Cushing's disease. Surg Neurol 2000;53:72.
[6] Bourdeau I, Bard C, Noel B, et al. Loss of brain volume in endogenous Cushing's syndrome and its reversibility after correction of hypercortisolism. J Clin Endocrinol Metab 2002;87: 1949.
[7] Starkman MN, Giordani B, Gebarski SS, et al. Decrease in cortisol reverses human hippocampal atrophy following treatment of Cushing's disease. Biol Psychiatry 1999;46: 1595.
[8] Bentson J, Reza M, Winter J, et al. Steroids and apparent cerebral atrophy on computed tomography scans. J Comput Assist Tomogr 1978;2:16.
[9] Zanardi VA, Magna LA, Costallat LT. Cerebral atrophy related to corticotherapy in systemic lupus erythematosus (SLE). Clin Rheumatol 2001;20:245.
[10] Marchesi C, De Risio C, Campanini G, et al. Cerebral atrophy and plasma cortisol levels in alcoholics after short or a long period of abstinence. Prog Neuropsychopharmacol Biol Psychiatry 1994;18:519.
[11] Rothschild AJ, Benes F, Hebben N, et al. Relationships between brain CT scan findings and cortisol in psychotic and nonpsychotic depressed patients. Biol Psychiatry 1989;26:565.
[12] Sheline YI, Wang PW, Gado MH, et al. Hippocampal atrophy in recurrent major depression. Proc Natl Acad Sci U S A 1996;93:3908.
[13] Bremner JD, Narayan M, Anderson ER, et al. Hippocampal volume reduction in major depression. Am J Psychiatry 2000;157:115.
[14] Bremner JD, Randall P, Scott TM, et al. MRI-based measurement of hippocampal volume in patients with combat-related posttraumatic stress disorder. Am J Psychiatry 1995;152: 973.
[15] Khiat A, Bard C, Lacroix A, et al. Brain metabolic alterations in Cushing's syndrome as monitored by proton magnetic resonance spectroscopy. NMR Biomed 1999;12:357.
[16] Khiat A, Bard C, Lacroix A, et al. Recovery of the brain choline level in treated Cushing's patients as monitored by proton magnetic resonance spectroscopy. Brain Res 2000;862:301.

[17] Khiat A, Yared Z, Bard C, et al. Long-term brain metabolic alterations in exogenous Cushing's syndrome as monitored by proton magnetic resonance spectroscopy. Brain Res 2001;911:134.
[18] De Kloet ER, Vreugdenhil E, Oitzl MS, et al. Brain corticosteroid receptor balance in health and disease. Endocr Rev 1998;19:269.
[19] Holmes MC, Yau JL, Kotelevtsev Y, et al. 11 Beta-hydroxysteroid dehydrogenases in the brain: two enzymes two roles. Ann N Y Acad Sci 2003;1007:357.
[20] Rajan V, Edwards CR, Seckl JR. 11 Beta-hydroxysteroid dehydrogenase in cultured hippocampal cells reactivates inert 11-dehydrocorticosterone, potentiating neurotoxicity. J Neurosci 1996;16:65.
[21] Woolley CS, Gould E, McEwen BS. Exposure to excess glucocorticoids alters dendritic morphology of adult hippocampal pyramidal neurons. Brain Res 1990;531:225.
[22] Sapolsky R, Brooke S, Stein-Behrens B. Methodologic issues in studying glucocorticoid-induced damage to neurons. J Neurosci Methods 1995;58:1.
[23] Sapolsky RM. Glucocorticoids and hippocampal atrophy in neuropsychiatric disorders. Arch Gen Psychiatry 2000;57:925.
[24] Watanabe Y, Gould E, McEwen BS. Stress induces atrophy of apical dendrites of hippocampal CA3 pyramidal neurons. Brain Res 1992;588:341.
[25] McEwen BS, Sapolsky RM. Stress and cognitive function. Curr Opin Neurobiol 1995;5:205.
[26] Sapolsky RM. The physiological relevance of glucocorticoid endangerment of the hippocampus. Ann N Y Acad Sci 1994;746:294.
[27] Sloviter RS, Valiquette G, Abrams GM, et al. Selective loss of hippocampal granule cells in the mature rat brain after adrenalectomy. Science 1989;243:535.
[28] Sloviter RS, Sollas AL, Dean E, et al. Adrenalectomy-induced granule cell degeneration in the rat hippocampal dentate gyrus: characterization of an in vivo model of controlled neuronal death. J Comp Neurol 1993;330:324.
[29] Yu IT, Lee SH, Lee YS, et al. Differential effects of corticosterone and dexamethasone on hippocampal neurogenesis in vitro. Biochem Biophys Res Commun 2004;317:484.
[30] Cameron HA, McKay RD. Restoring production of hippocampal neurons in old age. Nat Neurosci 1999;2:894.
[31] Fulham MJ, Brunetti A, Aloj L, et al. Decreased cerebral glucose metabolism in patients with brain tumors: an effect of corticosteroids. J Neurosurg 1995;83:657.
[32] Masters JN, Finch CE, Sapolsky RM. Glucocorticoid endangerment of hippocampal neurons does not involve deoxyribonucleic acid cleavage. Endocrinology 1989;124:3083.
[33] Horner HC, Packan DR, Sapolsky RM. Glucocorticoids inhibit glucose transport in cultured hippocampal neurons and glia. Neuroendocrinology 1990;52:57.
[34] James HE. Effects of steroids on behavior, electrophysiology, water content and intracranial pressure in cerebral cytotoxic edema. Pharmacol Biochem Behav 1978;9:653.
[35] Andersen C, Haselgrove JC, Doenstrup S, et al. Resorption of peritumoural oedema in cerebral gliomas during dexamethasone treatment evaluated by NMR relaxation time imaging. Acta Neurochir (Wien) 1993;122:218.
[36] Sonino N, Fava GA. Psychiatric disorders associated with Cushing's syndrome. Epidemiology, pathophysiology and treatment. CNS Drugs 2001;15:361.
[37] Whitlock FA. Symptomatic affective disorders: a study of depression and mania associated with physical disease and medication. Sydney (Australia): Academic Press; 1982.
[38] Haskett RF. Diagnostic categorization of psychiatric disturbance in Cushing's syndrome. Am J Psychiatry 1985;142:911.
[39] Fava GA, Fabbri S, Sonino N. Residual symptoms in depression: an emerging therapeutic target. Prog Neuropsychopharmacol Biol Psychiatry 2002;26:1019.
[40] Hudson JI, Hudson MS, Griffing GT, et al. Phenomenology and family history of affective disorder in Cushing's disease. Am J Psychiatry 1987;144:951.
[41] Loosen PT, Chambliss B, DeBold CR, et al. Psychiatric phenomenology in Cushing's disease. Pharmacopsychiatry 1992;25:192.

[42] Tronche F, Kellendonk C, Kretz O, et al. Disruption of the glucocorticoid receptor gene in the nervous system results in reduced anxiety. Nat Genet 1999;23:99.
[43] Sonino N, Fava GA, Belluardo P, et al. Course of depression in Cushing's syndrome: response to treatment and comparison with Graves' disease. Horm Res 1993;39:202.
[44] Kelly WF. Psychiatric aspects of Cushing's syndrome. QJM 1996;89:543.
[45] Dorn LD, Burgess ES, Dubbert B, et al. Psychopathology in patients with endogenous Cushing's syndrome: atypical or melancholic features. Clin Endocrinol (Oxf) 1995;43:433.
[46] Sonino N, Fava GA, Raffi AR, et al. Clinical correlates of major depression in Cushing's disease. Psychopathology 1998;31:302.
[47] Dorn LD, Burgess ES, Friedman TC, et al. The longitudinal course of psychopathology in Cushing's syndrome after correction of hypercortisolism. J Clin Endocrinol Metab 1997;82:912.
[48] Starkman MN, Giordani B, Gebarski SS, et al. Improvement in learning associated with increase in hippocampal formation volume. Biol Psychiatry 2003;53:233.
[49] Mauri M, Sinforiani E, Bono G, et al. Memory impairment in Cushing's disease. Acta Neurol Scand 1993;87:52.
[50] Miller AC, Giordani B, Berent S, et al. Learning and memory in Cushing's disease. J Int Neuropsychol Soc 1996;2:66.
[51] Whelan TB, Schteingart DE, Starkman MN, et al. Neuropsychological deficits in Cushing's syndrome. J Nerv Ment Dis 1980;168:753.
[52] Lezak MD. Neuropathology for neuropsychologists. In: Neuropsychological assessment. 3rd edition. New York: Oxford University Press; 1995. p. 170.
[53] Starkman MN, Schteingart DE, Schork MA. Depressed mood and other psychiatric manifestations of Cushing's syndrome: relationship to hormone levels. Psychosom Med 1981;43:3.
[54] Forget H, Lacroix A, Somma M, et al. Cognitive decline in patients with Cushing's syndrome. J Int Neuropsychol Soc 2000;6:20.
[55] Starkman MN, Giordani B, Berent S, et al. Elevated cortisol levels in Cushing's disease are associated with cognitive decrements. Psychosom Med 2001;63:985.
[56] Martignoni E, Costa A, Sinforiani E, et al. The brain as a target for adrenocortical steroids: cognitive implications. Psychoneuroendocrinology 1992;17:343.
[57] Dorn LD, Cerrone P. Cognitive function in patients with Cushing's syndrome: a longitudinal perspective. Clin Nurs Res 2000;9:420.
[58] Forget H, Lacroix A, Cohen H. Persistent cognitive impairment following surgical treatment of Cushing's syndrome. Psychoneuroendocrinology 2002;27:367.
[59] Gotch PM. Cushing's syndrome from the patient's perspective. Endocrinol Metab Clin North Am 1994;23:607.

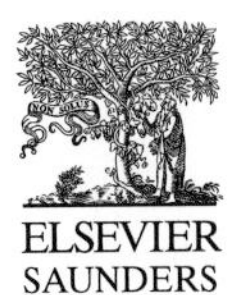
ELSEVIER
SAUNDERS

Endocrinol Metab Clin N Am
34 (2005) 371–384

ENDOCRINOLOGY
AND METABOLISM
CLINICS
OF NORTH AMERICA

Exogenous Cushing's Syndrome and Glucocorticoid Withdrawal

Rachel L. Hopkins, MD, Matthew C. Leinung, MD*

Division of Endocrinology and Metabolism, Albany Medical College, 43 New Scotland Avenue, Albany, NY 12008, USA

The first therapeutic use of glucocorticoids in 1948 resulted in dramatic clinical improvement in a patient's severe rheumatoid arthritis. Almost immediately, however, the potential adverse effects of exogenous steroid administration became evident [1]. Cushing's syndrome resulting from exogenous glucocorticoids now is well-recognized and documented. It also has been clear for some time that the discontinuation of chronic steroid use is fraught with difficulties.

Clinical presentation and diagnosis

For the most part, exogenous Cushing's syndrome presents with the same signs and symptoms as spontaneous Cushing's syndrome. There are nevertheless a few important differences in presentation [2]. Many patients who develop iatrogenic Cushing's syndrome do so after receiving high doses of steroid over long periods of time. Therefore, the clinical manifestations can be more striking than those of spontaneous Cushing's syndrome, which tend to occur more gradually. The traditional stigmata include weight gain, usually presenting as central obesity with redistribution of body fat to truncal areas and the appearance of dorsocervical and supraclavicular fat pads and the classic moon face. Plethora, easy bruising, thin skin, striae, myopathy, and muscle weakness (particularly proximal muscles) can be seen. Patients are susceptible to poor wound healing and increased incidence of infection [3] and atherosclerotic disease. The psychologic adverse effects of steroid treatment can be quite severe and include depression and psychosis.

* Corresponding author.
E-mail address: leinungm@mail.amc.edu (M.C. Leinung).

doi:10.1016/j.ecl.2005.01.013 ***endo.theclinics.com***

Although the incidence of hypertension in chronic steroid treatment is increased, these patients may have relatively less hypertension and hypokalemia compared with patients who have spontaneous Cushing's syndrome depending on the mineralocorticoid activity of the steroid they are taking. Along the same lines, patients who have iatrogenic Cushing's syndrome are unlikely to have significant increases in androgens, and therefore they have less hirsutism and other virilizing features than those who have spontaneous disease. Patients who have iatrogenic Cushing's syndrome may have an increased incidence of glaucoma and other ocular disease such as posterior subcapsular cataracts [4]. In addition, avascular necrosis is more common in iatrogenic than in spontaneous Cushing's syndrome [5]. Although rare, spinal epidural lipomatosis occurs primarily in the setting of exogenous glucocorticoid use [6].

Osteoporosis is a common and severe adverse effect of glucocorticoid excess and one of the major limitations to long-term glucocorticoid therapy. A significant number of patients on long-term steroid therapy will have at least some loss of bone density [7,8], and oral and inhaled corticosteroid use are associated with increased bone fractures [9,10]. The bone loss caused by glucocorticoids tends to be in trabecular bone as opposed to cortical bone. Therefore, most loss is in the vertebrae and ribs of the axial skeleton.

In many cases, the diagnosis of exogenous Cushing's should be fairly obvious in the setting of treatment with high-dose glucocorticoids. The diagnosis requires, first and foremost, clinical suspicion. This can be more difficult in cases caused by local delivery of steroid (eg, intra-articular and inhaled therapy) when clinicians might be less aware of Cushing's syndrome as a possible adverse result of treatment. Once the possibility of exogenous Cushing's syndrome is recognized, biochemical confirmation of the diagnosis is usually straightforward. The most striking biochemical finding is a suppressed endogenous cortisol level. Administration of hydrocortisone (cortisol) interferes with measurement of endogenous cortisol; in fact many synthetic glucocorticoids, with dexamethasone being a rare exception, can cross-react to some extent with standard cortisol assays [11]. In the authors' clinical experience, this has been especially problematic with prednisone. Nonetheless, in most cases of exogenous Cushing's syndrome, the morning serum cortisol is found to be remarkably low, especially given the setting of Cushingoid symptoms. Corticotropin (ACTH) levels also should be relatively low, as pituitary production will be suppressed by exogenous steroids. The suppression of ACTH leads to atrophy of the adrenal cortex, and thus stimulation with cosyntropin should result in a decreased or absent plasma cortisol response. In some cases, diagnosis of exogenous Cushing's syndrome has been aided or confirmed by measurement of the glucocorticoid in question, although this may require specialized laboratory analysis [12,13].

Most cases of exogenous Cushing's syndrome are iatrogenic. Glucocorticoids are used in many different forms for several neoplastic, inflammatory, and autoimmune disorders. Many of these conditions lead to high-dose or chronic steroid use that can result in Cushingoid effects. Not all cases of exogenous Cushing's syndrome come from prescribed or therapeutic use of glucocorticoids, however. It is important to be aware that numerous cases of factitious Cushing's syndrome resulting from surreptitious use of steroids have been reported. Villaneuva et al described four cases of Cushing's syndrome seen within a 2-year period in their practice caused by surreptitious glucocorticoid use [12]. As with many such patients, only one of those confronted was willing to admit to his or her surreptitious glucocorticoid use. Another situation, which might be termed occult Cushing's syndrome, is that in which a patient unknowingly receives glucocorticoid therapy. This can occur in the form of alternative remedies which, upon inspection, contain glucocorticoids. A case of Cushing's syndrome caused by an herbal remedy containing betamethasone was described recently [13]. In some communities, over-the-counter and traditional curatives contain significant amounts of potent glucocorticoids, or glucocorticoids may be prescribed by practitioners for questionable diagnoses. In a recently described case, a 32-year-old Vietnamese woman presented with an unexpected opportunistic infection [14]. Only after extensive investigation did the patient remember that she had received twice-daily subcutaneous injections of an unknown substance over 8 weeks during a visit to Vietnam. In another case, a neonate became Cushingoid after continuation for 2 months of betamethasone drops that were prescribed for an upper respiratory infection [15].

Megestrol acetate, a progestational agent used in the management of AIDS cachexia and in the treatment of breast, uterine, and prostate cancers, has been identified as having glucocorticoid activity. Megestrol acetate has been implicated in causing several cases of Cushing's syndrome, adrenal insufficiency, and hyperglycemia [16,17]. Because it is not commonly considered to have glucocorticoid activity, physicians prescribing this agent may not be aware of the associated risks. To the authors' knowledge, megestrol acetate and a related agent, medroxyprogesterone, are the only two medications not intended for therapeutic use as glucocorticoids that have glucocorticoid activity significant enough to cause Cushing's syndrome.

Factors in the development of Cushing's syndrome

Steroids with glucocorticoid activity are available in many different preparations with different modes of delivery. Glucocorticoids generally are absorbed well from various sites of application. Although the use of topical, intra-articular, or aerosol therapy has the advantage of allowing more targeted therapy and therefore theoretically fewer systemic adverse effects, every mode of exogenous glucocorticoid delivery has been implicated in the development of Cushing's syndrome.

All available forms of steroids with glucocorticoid activity are capable of producing Cushing's syndrome. Attempts at separating anti-inflammatory from metabolic effects with synthetic steroids have not been successful. The naturally occurring glucocorticoids cortisone and cortisol, and synthetic derivatives, including prednisone, prednisolone, methylprednisolone, dexamethasone, betamethasone, triamcinolone, and others are used clinically and have the potential for adverse effects. It is difficult to say which of these agents is most likely to cause Cushing's syndrome, because so many factors are involved in the generation of this disorder. Relevant properties of the steroids themselves include the formulation used, pharmacokinetics, affinity for the glucocorticoid receptor, biologic potency, and duration of action [18]. Pharmacokinetic factors include binding affinities to cortisol-binding globulin (CBG) and other plasma proteins, metabolic inactivation, and plasma half-life. Most synthetic glucocorticoids do not have significant binding to CBG and bind instead to albumin or circulate as free steroid. In contrast, synthetic glucocorticoids have a much higher affinity for the glucocorticoid receptor than cortisol itself. Potency and duration of action also are affected by rates of absorption and metabolism. Traditional assessments of potency generally have not accounted for these factors, and so published estimates of glucocorticoid activity can be taken as estimates only [18].

Whatever specific agent is involved, the development of Cushingoid signs and symptoms generally is related to dose and duration of treatment, so that even lower-potency agents with short half-lives (hydrocortisone and cortisone) can cause Cushingoid effects if given in adequate amounts with frequent delivery. Predicting doses and time courses at which Cushing's syndrome will develop is complicated by some of the issues just discussed (including the different potencies of the various glucocorticoids available), the different formulations and modes of delivery, and the fact that individual patients have different levels of sensitivity to glucocorticoids.

Some manifestations of glucocorticoid excess occur relatively quickly. Psychiatric effects, insomnia, and increased appetite can occur within hours. Generally, a Cushingoid appearance takes weeks or even months to develop, as does development of osteoporosis. With regard to dose, again there is tremendous variability between individuals. Although supraphysiologic doses usually are required before patients manifest significant Cushingoid effects, the authors' clinical experience reveals that some patients, in particular those on glucocorticoids following renal transplant, can develop Cushingoid appearance with chronic administration of as little as 5 mg/d of prednisone.

Specific modes of delivery

Oral corticosteroid therapy remains a mainstay of treatment of many inflammatory and autoimmune disorders. In the United States, prednisone is probably the most commonly used oral corticosteroid, at least for long-term use. The potential for development of Cushing's from oral steroid treatment is so well documented that most physicians are aware of the dangers. Nonetheless, there are many instances of patients who have developed unfortunate sequelae from prolonged use, most commonly in the setting of chronic disorders. In this setting, a balance must be struck between treatment of the underlying disorder and avoidance of adverse effects. In the authors' experience, many patients who present with iatrogenic Cushing's syndrome either have been lost to follow-up or treated with steroids for unclear diagnoses in the first place. Therefore, ongoing monitoring of patients and careful attention to the actual therapeutic efficacy of the steroid treatment is essential.

Although low doses of over-the-counter topical glucocorticoids are used commonly and safely, it is known that systemic absorption of steroids from topical preparations does occur and that at higher doses or with more potent preparations both adrenal axis suppression and Cushing's syndrome can occur. Breakdown of skin integrity may be an important factor. A recent report in the dermatologic literature described the case of an 11-year-old boy who has psoriasis and presented with stigmata of Cushing's syndrome after 6 months of treatment with topical halobetasol propionate and betamethasone dipropionate [19]. Signs and symptoms resolved after cessation of steroid treatment. In another case, a 72-year-old woman developed manifestations of Cushing's syndrome after long-term topical therapy with clobetasol propionate ointment. She also suffered signs of adrenal insufficiency after tapering the steroid dose and developing a urinary tract infection [20]. A 4-month-old baby developed Cushing's syndrome after his mother supplemented prescribed hydrocortisone cream with clobetasol cream [21]. Important factors in this case included use of a high-potency steroid in ointment form (as opposed to cream or lotion) and use of occlusive dressings, both of which increase the potency of topical steroids. Another case of Cushing's syndrome caused by topical steroid application was exacerbated by additional injection of periocular corticosteroids [22]. There also has been concern that over-the-counter combination preparations of steroids and antifungals may lead to unsupervised and inappropriate use of topical steroids [23]. A severe case of Cushing's syndrome was attributable to a 4-year period of Lotrisone (betamethasone dipropionate and clotrimazole) use for self-diagnosed vaginal candidiasis [24].

It once was thought that treatment with inhaled glucocorticoid therapy was relatively risk-free, because it was believed that little, if any, of the medication was absorbed systemically. It is now clear that significant systemic effects of inhaled corticosteroids can be seen, although fewer than with equivalent oral doses. These effects are dose-related and come in the form of adrenal suppression and Cushingoid stigmata, particularly bone, ocular, and skin manifestations [25]. Recent literature provides specific examples of asthmatic patients who developed both Cushing's syndrome and adrenal suppression [26,27]. In both of these cases, patients had been treated with fluticasone propionate, the most potent of the inhaled steroids currently available. This same agent has been implicated in causing adrenal insufficiency in several children treated for asthma [28,29].

Many reported cases of Cushing's syndrome resulting from inhaled glucocorticoids involved interactions with other medications. Several cases have been reported involving patients who had been on inhaled budesonide and developed Cushing's syndrome after the addition of itraconazole [30]. This has been a problem for young patients who have cystic fibrosis, for whom both inhaled corticosteroids and itraconazole have become a mainstay of therapy for management of allergic bronchopulmonary aspergillosis. At least two cases of such patients developing Cushing's syndrome have been described [31,32]. Itraconazole is a strong inhibitor of hepatic CYP3A, the same cytochrome P450 enzyme system involved in metabolism of most (and perhaps all) steroids. Therefore, it is believed that interference with P450 metabolism prolonged the systemic half-life of the glucocorticoid in these patients. The same mechanism is implicated in recently reported cases of patients who have HIV found to develop Cushing's syndrome while taking fluticasone propionate and ritonavir, another potent P450 inhibitor. One of the patients initially was diagnosed with HIV lipodystrophy [33,34]. Thus far, itraconazole and ritonavir have been the only P450 inhibiting agents implicated in Cushing's syndrome in the literature. It is plausible, however, that any agent that interferes with the cytochrome P450 system would have the potential to interfere with glucocorticoid metabolism and lead to the development of Cushing's syndrome.

Another therapeutic issue that has arisen most commonly in children is development of Cushing's syndrome and adrenal insufficiency related to the use of nasal steroid preparations. Typically, intranasal betamethasone has been the medication involved, but at least one case has been described involving dexamethasone [35,36]. Cases of Cushing's syndrome and adrenal suppression involving children have been used as warnings of the importance of carefully tailoring doses to children. Nasally induced Cushing's syndrome has been seen in adults also, with a recent case of a 28-year-old woman who developed Cushing's syndrome while using betamethasone nasal drops over a 2-year period. It was found that the patient had been taking doses far beyond those prescribed by her physician [37].

Several forms of injectable steroid therapy have been associated with signs and symptoms of Cushing's syndrome. Intravenous therapy is used almost exclusively for short-term treatment in emergency room or hospital settings. Therefore, this form of therapy is unlikely to result in Cushing's syndrome, although some patients do experience temporary adverse psychiatric effects, and certainly diabetic patients can experience blood glucose derangements even from very short courses of high-dose intravenous steroids.

Cushing's syndrome has been reported in patients taking relatively high doses of intra-articular glucocorticoids or with accidental overdose of these injections [38,39]. Pediatric cases of intra-articular and intradermal steroid injections causing Cushing's syndrome have been reported [40]. In addition, several cases of children who had received intralesional injections into keloid scars or other wounds (such as burns) have been described in the literature [41]. One of the remarkable features of these cases is the duration of Cushingoid symptoms (up to 9 months). It is proposed that the relatively avascular nature of keloids and other scars can lead to very slow absorption and thus prolonged systemic effects of steroids injected into these sites. Absorption of steroids injected into intra-articular sites can be delayed. In one case, extreme overdose likely made absorption the rate-limiting step in systemic drug disposition.

Cases of Cushing's syndrome from paraspinal depot injections also have been reported [42], and in two cases, local epidural steroid injection has lead to development of spinal epidural lipomatosis [43].

Additional unusual cases that have been reported in the literature include Cushing's syndrome induced by serial occipital nerve blocks containing triamcinolone [44] and acute adrenal crisis in a patient after withdrawal of rectal steroids [45].

Issues affecting withdrawal from steroid therapy

The discontinuation of steroid therapy can present a significant clinical challenge. Three issues exist with regard to withdrawal from steroid therapy: (1) the possibility of suppression of the hypothalamic–pituitary–adrenal (HPA) axis and resulting secondary adrenal insufficiency, (2) the possibility of worsening of the underlying disease for which steroid therapy was initiated, and (3) a phenomenon, sometimes called the steroid withdrawal syndrome, in which some patients encounter difficulty, and even significant symptoms, discontinuing or decreasing steroid doses despite having demonstrably normal HPA axes.

Treatment with supraphysiologic doses of corticosteroids at levels commonly used for treatment of inflammatory and autoimmune disorders will suppress the HPA axis. In fact, some level of suppression occurs even at physiologic doses, as ACTH secretion is decreased by the addition of exogenous steroids. At this level, however, the suppression does not appear to be clinically significant. As with exogenous Cushing's syndrome, the exact doses and duration of treatment required for significant HPA axis suppression vary between individuals. After studying the effects of various doses and different durations of treatment in glucocorticoid-treated patients, Schlaghecke et al concluded that neither dose, duration, nor basal plasma cortisol concentrations could be used reliably to predict pituitary-adrenal function in these patients [46]. Some patients who had been taking less than the equivalent of 5 mg/d of prednisone were found to have a suppressed or absent response to corticotropin-releasing hormone (CRH) stimulation. Conversely, some patients who had been on very high doses, equivalent to more than 25 mg/d of prednisone, had a normal response to CRH testing. It was not clear what the time course of treatment was that corresponded with these doses. In another study, patients who had been treated with the equivalent of 25 mg/d of prednisone for 5 to 30 days were given a low-dose (1 μg) corticotropin stimulation test [47]. Forty-five percent of the subjects were found to have a suppressed adrenal response immediately after discontinuation of steroids. All but two of these patients had recovered a normal response within 14 days. The remaining two patients continued to have a suppressed response even after 6 months. Overall, this study found no correlation between HPA axis suppression and the duration or dose of glucocorticoid treatment.

Some authors feel that glucocorticoid courses of less than 3 weeks duration will not lead to HPA axis suppression, no matter what the steroid dose, and therefore patients can be discontinued from steroid therapy immediately and safely up to that point [18]. Others believe that at relatively high doses, significant HPA suppression can occur after as little as 5 days, but that at physiologic doses, suppression is unlikely to occur in less than 1 month [48].

Despite efforts to understand the effects of long-term and high-dose steroid treatment on the HPA axis, clinicians remain unable to predict exactly which patients will have HPA suppression [49]. The actual risk of clinically significant adrenal insufficiency in patients who have been on long-term glucocorticoid therapy, however, may be somewhat overstated. A double-blind study of patients on long-term supraphysiologic glucocorticoid therapy with secondary adrenal suppression who underwent moderate to major surgical procedures found that those patients who underwent surgery on their usual dose of corticosteroids had no more complications than those given the traditional stress-dose steroids during the perioperative period [50]. Conversely, there certainly have been patients whose inability to mount an appropriate stress response after long-term glucocorticoid therapy had tragic results. Therefore caution on the side of short-term stress-dose therapy still seems prudent.

In past studies, tremendous individual variation has been found in rates of recovery from HPA axis suppression. Livanou et al [51] found that doses greater than 7.5 mg/d of prednisone (or equivalent) were more likely to result in prolonged suppression than were lower doses. There seemed to be no correlation between duration of therapy and time to recovery of the HPA axis. This study looked only at periods greater than and less than 18 months, however, and therefore, it might have missed some crucial threshold duration [51].

Controversy continues over which of the available tests of HPA function best correlates with a patient's actual ability to handle physiologic stress and which should be used in clinical practice. The gold standard is the insulin tolerance test. This is a cumbersome and somewhat risky test that needs to be performed in a monitored setting and is rarely done. The ACTH or cosyntropin stimulation test using either 1 μg [52] or 250 μg doses is a simple test that can be done easily in the office setting. There is doubt, however, that either of these is sensitive or specific enough to screen for secondary adrenal insufficiency [53]. The CRH-stimulation test is advocated by many as a relatively simple, safe test that can be performed in the office setting, although it is very expensive. The overnight metyrapone test is a test of the entire HPA axis, and although less simple than the cosyntropin test, it usually can be done with the patient at home.

Patients who have underlying inflammatory or autoimmune disorders sometimes can experience worsening of their condition as the steroid dose is decreased. This should be dealt with by increasing the glucocorticoid dose back up to a level that allows control of the underlying disease, unless increase in the glucocorticoid dose is contraindicated for some other reason (such as severe Cushingoid symptoms or osteoporosis with fractures). Only when the underlying disease is quiescent should another attempt be made to begin withdrawing the glucocorticoid. Seeking auxiliary forms of treatment for the underlying disease can aid in the ability to begin withdrawing steroid therapy.

The previously mentioned steroid withdrawal syndrome is understood poorly. It is characterized by lethargy, malaise, anorexia, myalgias, headache, fever, and can even be accompanied by desquamation of the skin. Upon testing, patients who have this syndrome can be shown to have a normal HPA axis and therefore are not suffering from adrenal insufficiency [18]. This syndrome is rare, and the exact etiology is unknown. It is important to recognize that many of these patients have become psychologically dependent upon their steroids. Whatever the cause of their symptoms, these patients do not appear to be at risk for collapse of the cardiovascular system or other extreme effects of adrenal insufficiency. Therefore, the choice of whether to continue replacement doses of steroids must be decided between the physician and the patient.

Withdrawal schemes

Given how common the use of steroid therapy is, it is surprising that there are no controlled clinical trials of methods for withdrawal from glucocorticoids. A recent systematic review examined withdrawal of therapy in patients who have chronic medical disorders but found insufficient evidence to recommend any particular withdrawal regimens [54].

Withdrawal plans therefore are based on the dual goals of treating patients who have the lowest possible steroid dose (or complete discontinuation of therapy) in order to avoid adverse effects of prolonged steroid therapy while at the same time avoiding the potential consequences of adrenal insufficiency.

Traditionally, withdrawal schemes (Fig. 1) begin by reducing the glucocorticoid incrementally from supraphysiologic to physiologic doses.

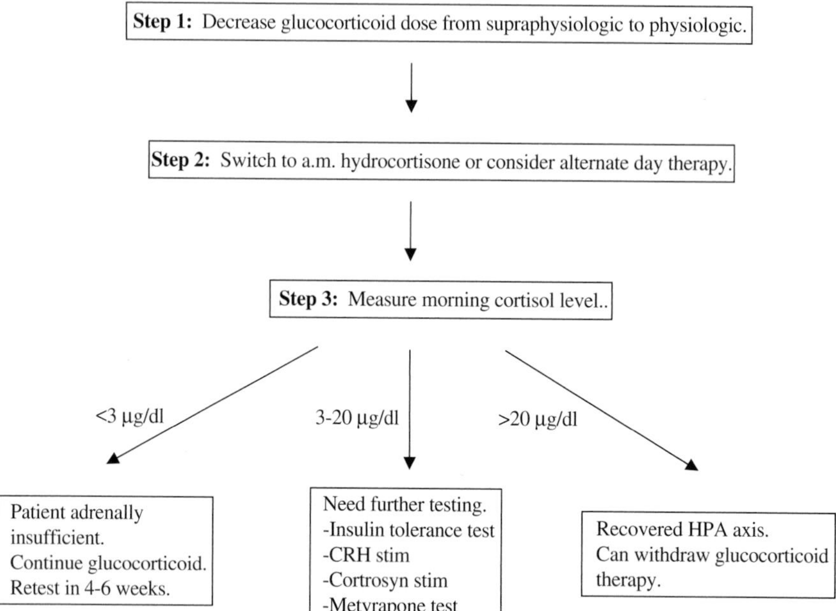

Fig. 1. A suggested algorithm for withdrawal from chronic steroid therapy. Physiologic doses of glucocorticoid are equivalent to prednisone 5 to 7.5 mg/d or hydrocortisone 15 to 20 mg/d.

The physiologic dose is approximately 5 to 7.5 mg a day of prednisone, 15 to 20 mg a day of hydrocortisone, or the equivalent. During this phase of withdrawal patients are not at risk for adrenal insufficiency, nor do most experience symptoms of withdrawal syndrome. Therefore, the greatest concern at this time will be exacerbation of underlying disease.

Once a patient is on a replacement dose of glucocorticoid, several approaches can be taken. Many practitioners like to switch to hydrocortisone if possible in order to take advantage of the short half-life of this medication. This switch may allow the HPA axis more opportunity to recover. For the same reason, some recommend switching to alternate-day therapy with an intermediate acting glucocorticoid such as prednisone being given as a single morning dose every 48 hours [48]. Although this type of regimen has been shown to work well as therapy for several diseases, it may not work as well for all patients being withdrawn from steroid therapy who have adrenal insufficiency. These patients may experience a lack of well-being during the off day of therapy.

During this stage of withdrawal it is appropriate to begin checking morning cortisol levels, which can be useful as a screening test for basal adrenal sufficiency. A cortisol level drawn at approximately 8 a.m. that measures less than 3 μg/dL indicates deficient basal cortisol secretion and the need for continued replacement therapy. If the morning cortisol is greater than 20 μg/dL, the patient can be assumed to have a recovered HPA axis and can be withdrawn entirely from glucocorticoid therapy [11].

Patients who have cortisol levels that fall between 3 and 20 μg/dL may have sufficient basal cortisol production but still be lacking in sufficient capacity to respond to significant physiologic stress. In this case an insulin tolerance test, CRH stimulation, or an overnight metyrapone test would be reasonable for assessment of the HPA axis. The authors most commonly use the overnight metyrapone test, because it is reasonably safe, convenient, and provides a reasonable assessment of the entire HPA axis.

In lieu of further testing, an alternative approach would be to continue a very gradual taper from the level of physiologic replacement [11]. If this course is chosen, the patient must be warned that supplemental glucocorticoid therapy might be needed during illness or injury for approximately 1 year after discontinuation of therapy.

For patients who have been on long-term glucocorticoid therapy, the risk for adrenal insufficiency can continue for months. Suppression can be seen for up to 9 months or even a year. Therefore, the patient and physician must discuss the potentially prolonged nature of steroid therapy withdrawal and approach the problem with patience and, sometimes, determination.

Summary

Glucocorticoid therapy in various forms is extremely common for several inflammatory, autoimmune, and neoplastic disorders. It is therefore important for the physician to be aware of the possibility of iatrogenic and factitious Cushing's syndrome. Although most common with oral therapy, it is also important to be alert to the fact that all forms of glucocorticoid delivery have the potential to cause Cushing's syndrome. Withdrawal from chronic glucocorticoid therapy presents significant challenges. These include the possibility of adrenal insufficiency after discontinuation of steroid therapy, recurrence of underlying disease as the glucocorticoid is being withdrawn, and the possibility of steroid withdrawal symptoms. Nonetheless, with patience and persistence, a reasonable approach to withdrawal of glucocorticoid therapy can be achieved.

References

[1] Kehrl JH, Fauci AS. The clinical use of glucocorticoids. Ann Allergy 1983;50(1):2–8.

[2] Chrousos GP. Glucocorticoid therapy. In: Felig P, Frohman L, editors. Endocrinology and metabolism. 4th edition. New York: McGraw-Hill, Incorporated; 2001. p. 609–32.

[3] Lionakis MS, Kontoyiannis DP. Glucocorticoids and invasive fungal infections. Lancet 2003;362(9398):1828–38.

[4] Jobling AI, Augusteyn RC. What causes steroid cataracts? A review of steroid-induced posterior subcapsular cataracts. Clin Exp Optom 2002;85(2):61–75.

[5] Mankin HJ. Nontraumatic necrosis of bone (osteonecrosis). N Engl J Med 1992;326(22): 1473–9.
[6] Kaplan JG, Barasch E, Hirschfeld A, et al. Spinal epidural lipomatosis: a serious complication of iatrogenic Cushing's syndrome. Neurology 1989;39:1031–4.
[7] Laan R, van Reil P, van de Putte L, et al. Low-dose prednisone induces rapid reversible axial bone loss in patients with rheumatoid arthritis. Ann Intern Med 1993;119(10):963–8.
[8] Israel E, Banerjee TR, Fitzmaurice GM, et al. Effects of inhaled glucocorticoids on bone density in premenopausal women. N Engl J Med 2001;345(13):941–7.
[9] Van Staa T, Leufkens H, Abenhaim L, et al. Use of oral corticosteroids and risk of fractures. J Bone Miner Res 2000;15:993–1000.
[10] Van Staa T, Leufkens H, Cooper C. Use of inhaled corticosteroids and risk of fractures. J Bone Miner Res 2001;16:581–8.
[11] Krasner AS. Glucocorticoid-induced adrenal insufficiency. JAMA 1999;282(7):671–6.
[12] Villanueva RB, Brett E, Gabrilove JL. A cluster of cases of factitious Cushing's syndrome. Endocr Pract 2000;6(2):143–7.
[13] Krapf R. Development of Cushing's syndrome after use of a herbal remedy. Lancet 2002; 360:1884.
[14] Bachmeyer C, Ciofu A, Blum L, et al. Opportunistic infections indicating factitious Cushing's syndrome: an adverse effect of cellulite treatment. Endocrinologist 2004;14(2): 54–6.
[15] Agadi S. Iatrogenic Cushing's syndrome: a different story. Lancet 2003;361(9362):1059.
[16] Mann M, Koller E, Murgo A, et al. Glucocorticoidlike activity of megestrol: a summary of food and drug administration experience and a review of the literature. Arch Intern Med 1997;157:1651–6.
[17] Leinung M, Koller EA, Fossler MJ. Corticosteroid effects of megestrol acetate. Endocrinologist 1998;8(3):153–9.
[18] Orth DN, Kovacs WJ. The adrenal cortex. In: Wilson JD, editor. Williams textbook of endocrinology. 9th edition. Philadelphia: WB Saunders Company; 1998. p. 605–10.
[19] Joe EK. Cushing's syndrome secondary to topical glucocorticoids. Dermatol Online J 2003; 9(4):16.
[20] Abma EM, Blanken R, De Heide LJ. Cushing's syndrome caused by topical steroid therapy for psoriasis. Neth J Med 2002;60(3):148–50.
[21] Ermis B, Ors R, Tastekin A, et al. Cushing's syndrome secondary to topical corticosteroids abuse. Clin Endocrinol (Oxf) 2003;58:795–7.
[22] Ozerdem U, Levi L, Cheng L, et al. Systemic toxicity of topical and periocular corticosteroid therapy in an 11-year-old male with posterior uveitis. Am J Ophthalmol 2000;130(2):240–1.
[23] Castanedo-Cazares JP, Lopez-Lucio RH, Moncada B. Cushing's syndrome following the prescription of antifungal, antibiotic, corticosteroid cream. Int J Dermatol 2003;42:318.
[24] Weber SL. Cushing's syndrome attributable to topical use of Lotrisone. Endocr Pract 1997; 3(3):140–4.
[25] Lipworth BJ. Systemic adverse effects of inhaled corticosteroid therapy: a systematic review and meta-analysis. Arch Intern Med 1999;159(9):941–55.
[26] White A, Woodmansee DP. Adrenal insufficiency from inhaled corticosteroids. Ann Intern Med 2004;140(6):W27.
[27] Wilson AM, Blumsohn A, Jung RT, et al. Asthma and Cushing's syndrome. Chest 2000; 117(2):593–4.
[28] Kennedy MJ, Carpenter JM, Lozano RA, et al. Impaired recovery of hypothalamic-pituitary-adrenal axis function and hypoglycemic seizures after high-dose inhaled corticosteroid therapy in a toddler. Ann Allergy Asthma Immunol 2002;88(5):523–6.
[29] Drake AJ, Howells RJ, Shield JP, et al. Symptomatic adrenal insufficiency presenting with hypoglycaemia in children with asthma receiving high dose inhaled fluticasone propionate. BMJ 2002;324(7345):1081–2.

[30] Bolland MJ, Bagg W, Thomas MG, et al. Cushing's syndrome due to interaction between inhaled corticosteroids and itraconazole. Ann Pharmacother 2004;38(1):46–9.

[31] De Wachter E, Vanbesien J, De Schutter I, et al. Rapidly developing Cushing's syndrome in a 4-year-old patient during combined treatment with itraconazole and inhaled budesonide. Eur J Pediatr 2003;162(7–8):488–9.

[32] Main KM, Skov M, Sillesen IB, et al. Cushing's syndrome due to pharmacological interaction in a cystic fibrosis patient. Acta Paediatr 2002;91(9):1008–11.

[33] Clevenbergh P, Corcostegui M, Gerard D, et al. Iatrogenic Cushing's syndrome in an HIV-infected patient treated with inhaled corticosteroids (fluticasone propionate) and low-dose ritonavir enhanced PI containing regimen. J Infect 2002;44(3):194–5.

[34] Gupta SK, Dube MP. Exogenous Cushing's syndrome mimicking human immunodeficiency virus lipodystrophy. Clin Infect Dis 2002;35(6):E69–71.

[35] Findlay CA, Macdonald JF, Wallace AM, et al. Childhood Cushing's syndrome induced by betamethasone nose drops and repeat prescriptions. BMJ 1998;317(7160):739–40.

[36] Perry RJ, Findlay CA, Donaldson MD. Cushing's syndrome, growth impairment, and occult adrenal suppression associated with intranasal steroids. Arch Dis Child 2002;87(1):45–8.

[37] Nutting CM, Page SR. Iatrogenic Cushing's syndrome due to nasal betamethasone: a problem not to be sniffed at! Postgrad Med J 1995;71(834):231–2.

[38] Jansen TL, Van Roon EN. Four cases of a secondary Cushingoid state following local triamcinolone acetonide (Kenacort) injection. Neth J Med 2002;60(3):151–3.

[39] Schweitzer DH, Le-Brun PP, Krishnaswami S, et al. Clinical and pharmacological aspects of accidental triamcinolone acetonide overdosage: a case study. Neth J Med 2000;56(1):12–6.

[40] Kumar S, Singh RJ, Reed AM, et al. Cushing's syndrome after intra-articular and intradermal administration of triamcinolone acetonide in three pediatric patients. Pediatrics 2004;113(6):1820–4.

[41] Teelucksingh S, Balkaran B, Ganeshmoorthi A, et al. Prolonged childhood Cushing's syndrome secondary to intralesional triamcinolone acetonide. Ann Trop Paediatr 2002;22(1):89–91.

[42] Edmonds LC, Vance ML, Hughes JM. Morbidity from paraspinal depo corticosteroid injections for analgesia: Cushing's syndrome and adrenal suppression. Anesth Analg 1991;72:820–2.

[43] Sandberg DI, Lavyne MH. Symptomatic spinal epidural lipomatosis after local epidural corticosteroid injections: case report. Neurosurgery 1999;45(1):162–5.

[44] Lavin PJ, Workman R. Cushing's syndrome induced by serial occipital nerve blocks containing corticosteroids. Headache 2001;41(9):902–4.

[45] Barlow AD, Clarke GA, Kelly MJ. Acute adrenal crisis in a patient treated with rectal steroids. Colorectal Dis 2004;6(1):62–4.

[46] Schlaghecke R, Kornely E, Santen RT, et al. The effect of long-term glucocorticoid therapy on pituitary-adrenal responses to exogenous corticotropin-releasing hormone. N Engl J Med 1992;326(4):226–30.

[47] Henzen C, Suter A, Lerch E, et al. Suppression and recovery of adrenal response after short-term, high-dose glucocorticoid treatment. Lancet 2000;355(9203):542–5.

[48] Axelrod L. Corticosteroid therapy. In: Becker KL, editor. Principles and practice of endocrinology and metabolism. 3rd edition. Philadelphia: Lippincott Williams and Wilkins; 2001. p. 751–64.

[49] Christy NP. Pituitary-adrenal function during corticosteroid therapy. Learning to live with uncertainty. N Engl J Med 1992;326(4):266–7.

[50] Glowniak JV, Loriaux DL. A double-blind study of perioperative steroid requirements in secondary adrenal insufficiency. Surgery Feb 1997;121(2):123–9.

[51] Livanou T, Ferriman D, James VH. Recovery of hypothalamo-pituitary-adrenal function after corticosteroid therapy. Lancet 1967;2(7521):856–9.

[52] Thaler LM, Blevins LS Jr. The low-dose (1 μg) adrenocorticotropin stimulation test in the evaluation of patients with suspected central adrenal insufficiency. J Clin Endocrinol Metab 1998;83(8):2726–9.

[53] Suliman AM, Smith TP, Labib M, et al. The low-dose ACTH test does not provide a useful assessment of the hypothalamic-pituitary-adrenal axis in secondary adrenal insufficiency. Clin Endocrinol (Oxf) 2002;56(4):533–9.

[54] Richter B, Neises G, Clar C. Glucocorticoid withdrawal schemes in chronic medical disorders. A systematic review. Endocrinol Metab Clin North Am 2002;31(3):751–78.

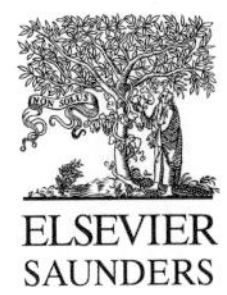

ELSEVIER
SAUNDERS

Endocrinol Metab Clin N Am
34 (2005) 385–402

ENDOCRINOLOGY
AND METABOLISM
CLINICS
OF NORTH AMERICA

Screening and Diagnosis of Cushing's Syndrome

James W. Findling, MD[a,b], Hershel Raff, PhD[b,c,*]

[a]*Endocrine–Diabetes Center, St. Luke's Medical Center, 2801 West KK River Parkway, Suite 245, Milwaukee, WI 53215, USA*
[b]*Medical College of Wisconsin, Milwaukee, WI 53226, USA*
[c]*Endocrine Research Laboratory, St. Luke's Medical Center, 2801 West KK River Parkway, Suite 245, Milwaukee, WI 53215, USA*

The diagnosis of Cushing's syndrome is the most challenging problem in clinical endocrinology. Clinical manifestations of excessive glucocorticoid exposure (either endogenous or exogenous) are protean and may be quite subtle. The observation that patients who have incidentally discovered adrenocortical adenomas and subclinical hypercortisolism frequently have improvement in their diabetes, hypertension, and obesity after adrenalectomy, increases the importance of establishing the diagnosis of even mild Cushing's syndrome [1,2]. Because the clinical syndrome is not always obvious, a low index of suspicion is needed for screening and certainly mandated in high-risk patient populations.

Epidemiology

Most epidemiologic studies have suggested that spontaneous Cushing's syndrome is an unusual disorder. A population-based study in Denmark found that the diagnosis of endogenous hypercortisolism had been established in 166 patients in an 11-year period [3]. Ninety-nine patients had Cushing's disease; 48 had adrenal-dependent Cushing's disease; 16 had ectopic corticotropin (ACTH), and three patients were unclassified. This represented an incidence of 2 cases per 1 million inhabitants per year. The patients in this study who were not cured by surgical intervention or who had malignant disease had a poor prognosis with a standard mortality ratio

* Corresponding author. Endocrine–Diabetes Center, St. Luke's Physicians Office Building, 2801 KK River Parkway, Suite 245, Milwaukee, WI 53215.
E-mail address: hraff@mcw.edu (H. Raff).

0889-8529/05/$ - see front matter
doi:10.1016/j.ecl.2005.02.001 ***endo.theclinics.com***

of 3.8 to 5.0 compared with normal controls. This study was in agreement with a similar study conducted in Vizcya, Spain, in 1994 [4]. In a Spanish population of 1.15 million, 49 patients were diagnosed with Cushing's disease in an 18-year period, yielding an incidence of 2.5 cases per 1 million inhabitants per year. The prevalence in this study population was documented at 39 cases per 1 million inhabitants at the time the study was conducted. This report also emphasized the poor prognosis in these patients, with a standard mortality ratio of 3.8. Although these data would suggest that spontaneous Cushing's syndrome is rare, other observational data and screening in high-risk populations suggest that the diagnosis frequently is overlooked. For example, the authors have evaluated 85 patients from the Milwaukee metropolitan area (population 1.5 million) over an 11-year period. Even if this represented all the patients in the area with Cushing's syndrome over that period of time (and the authors estimate that it probably represents 30% to 50%), this would represent an incidence of approximately 5 patients per million inhabitants per year.

Screening studies performed in high-risk populations recently have suggested an unexpectedly high incidence of occult Cushing's syndrome. In 1996, Leibowitz et al performed screening studies in 90 obese subjects who had poorly controlled diabetes mellitus (hemoglobin A1C > 9%) and found three patients (3.3%) who had surgically confirmed Cushing's syndrome [5]. More recently, Catargi et al [6] carefully studied 200 obese patients who had type 2 diabetes mellitus and hemoglobin A1C values greater than 8%. Four patients (2%) had definite Cushing's syndrome and seven had subclinical hypercortisolism with unilateral adrenal adenomas demonstrating uptake on iodocholesterol scintigraphy and elevated late-night cortisol levels. Another study performed in Turkey screened 100 consecutive obese subjects (body mass index > 25 kg/m^2) and found 9 subjects who had surgically proven Cushing's syndrome (5 pituitary and 4 adrenal) [7]. Moreover, subclinical hypercortisolism has been shown in at least 10% of patients who have adrenal incidentalomas [8], a finding that is seen in approximately 2% of the adult population. These studies suggest that spontaneous Cushing's syndrome is more common than previously appreciated.

Who should be screened?

Endogenous hypercortisolism may occur at any age and usually has an insidious onset, with a usual duration of illness before clinical diagnosis of 3 to 5 years. The disorder appears to be more common in women, particularly in patients who have pituitary- and adrenal-dependent Cushing's syndrome; however, the ratio may be fairly equal in patients who have ectopic ACTH-dependent Cushing's syndrome [8]. The authors believe that screening tests should be performed in subjects who have relatively specific signs and symptoms of hypercortisolism or in patients who have clinical diagnoses that may be caused by endogenous cortisol excess.

Specific signs and symptoms

Signs and symptoms that should provoke a biochemical evaluation for possible Cushing's syndrome are shown in Box 1. Weight gain with redistribution of fat centrally affecting the face, neck, trunk, and abdomen is one of the most common clinical findings. Unfortunately, this type of weight gain is very common and may be indistinguishable from those patients who have the metabolic syndrome. The weight gain is often insidious, and frequent review of old photographs may help the clinician better appreciate the physical changes that may have occurred in patients who have weight gain. The physical changes that may occur in a patient over a period of 12 years are illustrated in Fig. 1. Although patients who have Cushing's syndrome may have the classic moon facies, the facial rounding can be quite subtle. The patient in Fig. 1 was examined by many clinicians (including several endocrinologists) before the diagnosis of spontaneous Cushing's syndrome was considered. The presence of significant supraclavicular

Box 1. Who should be screened for Cushing's syndrome?

Signs and symptoms
Central obesity with:
- Facial rounding with plethora
- Increased supraclavicular and dorsocervical fat
- Cutaneous wasting with ecchymoses
- Wide violaceous striae (greater than 1 cm)
- Proximal myopathy
- Increased lanugo hair
- Superficial fungal infections
- Growth retardation (in children)

Clinical diagnosis
Metabolic syndrome X
- Diabetes mellitus (Hgb A1C > 8%)
- Hypertension
- Hyperlipidemia
- Polycystic ovary syndrome (PCOS)

Hypogonadotropic hypogonadism
- Oligomenorrhea/amenorrhea/infertility
- Decreased libido and impotence

Osteoporosis (especially rib fracture)
- Patients aged < 65 y

Incidental adrenal mass

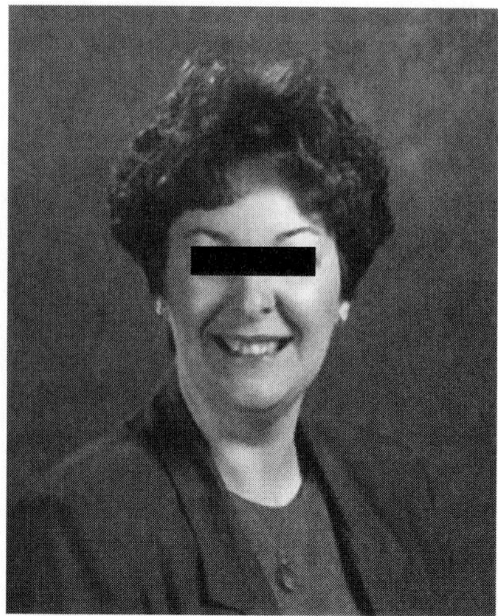
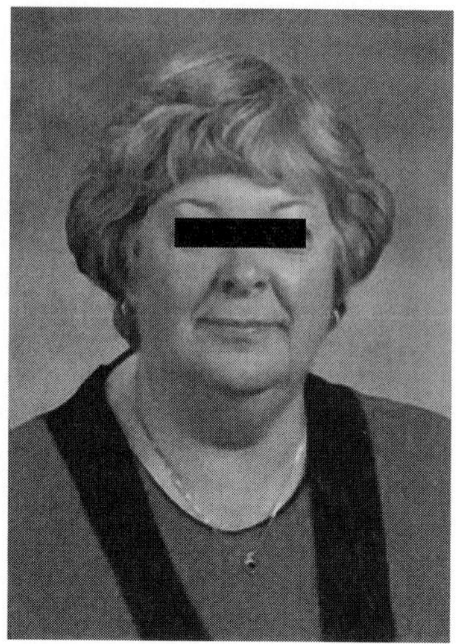

Fig. 1. Progression of facial features before (*left*) and after a period of 12 years (*right*) of Cushing's disease.

fullness and dorsocervical fat accumulation should generate a screening test for hypercortisolism.

The catabolic effects of glucocorticoid excess frequently lead to cutaneous wasting from atrophy of the epidermis and underlying connective tissue. These changes result in the thin appearance of the skin with the typical plethoric facial appearance and easy bruisability. The skin is fragile and, when removing adhesive tape, may peel off like damp tissue paper. Most women who have Cushing's syndrome have skin fold thickness less than 2 mm in the dorsum of the hand, compared with greater than 2 mm with PCOS [9]. The significant weight gain and the skin changes often result in violaceous depressed and wide striae (usually > 1 cm in diameter). These striae usually occur on the abdomen but also may occur over the breasts, hips, buttocks, thighs, and axilla. Striae usually are observed in patients who have significant hypercortisolism, and rarely in patients over the age of 40 [10]. Minor wounds or abrasions may heal poorly. In addition, because of the immunosuppressive effects of hypercortisolism, superficial mucocutaneous fungal infections such as tinea versicolor also may be seen [11]. Although androgen excess may be present and result in facial hirsutism, vellus hypertrichosis (lanugo hair) that is glucocorticoid-dependent is probably more common in women who have Cushing's syndrome. In addition, papular acne may occur in younger patients who have Cushing's syndrome.

The catabolic effects of hypercortisolism also may result in type II muscle fiber atrophy with significant weakness in the proximal musculature [12]. Patients frequently complain of difficulty climbing stairs or rising from a chair. The myopathy may be particularly problematic in older adults and may be misdiagnosed as amyotrophic lateral sclerosis or multiple sclerosis. Body composition studies have demonstrated reduced body cell mass, indicating a true protein loss in these patients [13].

Glucocorticoid excess also is known to blunt somatic growth. The impairment of somatic growth is mostly caused by direct action of glucocorticoids in the growing long bones in children, arresting the development of epiphysial cartilage [14,15]. Hypercortisolism also blunts growth hormone secretion, but insulin-like growth factor-1 levels are usually normal [15]. Growth retardation associated with progressive, and frequently generalized, obesity is the hallmark of Cushing's syndrome in children. After correction of hypercortisolism, children who have retarded linear growth rate should be treated with growth hormone, because there is a limited window of opportunity to promote an increase in growth to obtain normal adult height [16]. Impaired growth hormone responses to provocative stimuli also are observed in adult patients who have Cushing's syndrome and may persist for up to 2 years after treatment [17]. The authors are unaware of studies evaluating the efficacy of growth hormone replacement therapy in these patients.

Nonspecific signs and symptoms

Cushing's syndrome is associated with a range of psychologic and cognitive problems (see article by Bourdeau et al elsewhere in this issue). Most patients who have Cushing's syndrome meet criteria for depression, and a few patients have other neuropsychiatric problems including mania, anxiety, and cognitive dysfunction [18]. Psychosis may even occur, and suicidal tendency often has been reported in patients who have endogenous hypercortisolism. Children who have Cushing's syndrome often exhibit obsessive–compulsive behavior and do extremely well in their schoolwork [19]. Cognitive dysfunction with reversible loss of brain volume also has been reported [20].

Less common and unappreciated clinical features of Cushing's syndrome may involve the eyes. In Cushing's original report, 4 of 12 patients were described with exophthalmos [21]. A recent study demonstrated that 45% of patients who have active Cushing's syndrome had exophthalmos (> 16 mm) compared with 20% of treated Cushing's syndrome patients and 2% of normal controls [22]. The proptosis in patients who have Cushing's syndrome is asymptomatic and presumably caused by retro-orbital fat accumulation. Two other unique eye findings have been reported in patients who have Cushing's syndrome. Lisch nodules, thought to be specific for neurofibromatosis, but rare in the general population, are melanocytic hamartomas of the iris. These yellow or brown, dome-shaped elevations projecting from the surface of the iris recently were observed in 2 of 14 consecutive patients evaluated for endogenous hypercortisolism [23]. It was speculated that the underlying mechanism leading to the overgrowth of the melanocytes in the iris may be similar to the corticotroph adenomatous change in the pituitary. The same group also reported the presence of central serous chorioretinopathy in 3 of 60 consecutive patients who have Cushing's syndrome [24]. This unusual condition represents the accumulation of subretinal fluid at the posterior pole of the fundus, causing an area of retinal detachment and some decrease in visual acuity. These findings also have been reported in patients receiving high-dose glucocorticoid therapy.

Clinical diagnoses associated with hypercortisolism

There are a few clinical disorders that alone should stimulate a consideration for the presence of Cushing's syndrome (see Box 1). Cushing's syndrome results in the entire clinical spectrum of the metabolic syndrome including obesity, diabetes, hypertension, and gonadal dysfunction. This phenotype has a high prevalence, and, with the increasing recognition of mild or subclinical hypercortisolism, it is clear that these two syndromes are clinically indistinguishable. The higher mortality rate observed in patients who have Cushing's syndrome seems to be related to the cardiovascular complications associated with the metabolic syndrome [4] as discussed in the article by Pivonello et al elsewhere in this issue.

The insulin resistance that accompanies hypercortisolism results in a decrease in glucose use by peripheral tissues; impaired glucose tolerance may occur in 30% to 60% of patients, and frank diabetes may occur in 25% to 50% of patients [25]. As previously mentioned, 2% to 3% of patients who have poorly controlled type 2 diabetes may have unrecognized Cushing's syndrome [5,6]. Glucocorticoid excess also plays an essential role in the accumulation of abdominal body fat. Thus, obesity is an independent risk factor for reduced life expectancy and correlates well with all of the metabolic sequelae and atherosclerosis associated with the metabolic syndrome. The importance of cortisol in the generation of abdominal obesity recently has been highlighted by targeted overexpression of 11β-hydroxysteroid dehydrogenase type 1 in transgenic mice [26]. This resulted in increased visceral fat, presumably because of local production of active glucocorticoid within the adipocyte.

Arterial hypertension occurs in at least 80% of patients who have Cushing's syndrome and is a major contributing factor to cardiovascular morbidity. Although the hypertension may be mild, organ damage such as cardiac hypertrophy with left ventricular concentric remodeling may occur as a result [27]. The mechanism for the hypertension presumably is related to the mineralocorticoid activity of cortisol. In the presence of severe hypercortisolism, there is a failure to completely metabolize cortisol to the inactive cortisone by the renal enzyme 11β-hydroxysteroid dehydrogenase type 2. This allows cortisol binding to the mineralocorticoid receptor in the distal nephron, resulting in hypertension and hypokalemia. Other possible mechanisms of hypertension in patients who have Cushing's syndrome include enhancement of the inotropic pressor effects of vasoactive substances including catecholamines, vasopressin, and angiotensin II, and possible suppression of vasodilatory mechanisms including nitric oxide and prostacyclin production [28].

The hyperlipidemia seen in patients who have Cushing's syndrome appears to be similar to the dyslipidemia associated with the metabolic syndrome. There is an increase in very low density lipoprotein (LDL) and LDL with a decrease in high density lipoprotein (HDL) levels. This results in elevation of total triglyceride and cholesterol levels [29,30].

Less appreciated is the hypercoagulability in patients who have Cushing's syndrome leading to an increased risk for thromboembolic events mostly after surgery or during inferior petrosal sinus sampling [31]. Hypercortisolism stimulates the synthesis of several clotting factors such as fibrinogen by the liver and von Willebrand factor by endothelial cells. In addition, glucocorticoids also increase the synthesis of plasminogen activator inhibitor type 1, the main inhibitor of the fibrinolytic system [32]. The general consensus is that patients who have Cushing's syndrome should be given heparin during inferior petrosal sinus sampling and that anticoagulation should be considered in the postoperative period in many patients.

Because women who have Cushing's syndrome may present with menstrual irregularities or signs and symptoms of androgen excess, the diagnosis of PCOS often is considered. Kaltsas et al recently showed that most women who have Cushing's syndrome also have PCOS and suggested that women who have PCOS should undergo screening studies for hypercortisolism [33]. Interestingly, the menstrual irregularity in these women appears to be more closely related to the degree of cortisol excess than the actual circulating androgen concentrations [34]. Male patients frequently present with diminished libido or impotence associated with subnormal testosterone concentration. Hypogonadotropic hypogonadism is not an uncommon finding in men who have hypercortisolism and is underappreciated. Therefore, Cushing's syndrome should be considered in men who have hypogonadotropic hypogonadism, particularly if they have other phenotypic characteristics of hypercortisolism.

The diagnosis of Cushing's syndrome should be considered in patients who have unexplained osteoporosis, particularly in those younger than 65 years. Glucocorticoids influence bone and calcium homeostasis at many levels (see article by Shaker and Lukert elsewhere in this issue). Pathologic fractures may be the presenting feature of Cushing's syndrome, and rib fractures seem to be especially common. There is also an increased risk of nephrolithiasis in patients who have Cushing's syndrome. A recent study found kidney stones in 50% of patients who have active Cushing's syndrome, 27% of patients in remission, and 6.5% of controls [35]. Patients who have active Cushing's syndrome and nephrolithiasis had a significantly increased prevalence of arterial hypertension, hypercalciuria, hypocitraturia, and hyperuricosuria.

In light of the evidence that 6% to 10% of patients who have incidentally discovered adrenal masses (of at least 2 cm) have subclinical hypercortisolism, it seems obvious that screening studies for Cushing's syndrome are needed in this fairly common group of patients [36]. Information concerning evaluation and treatment of these patients is found in the article by Terzolo et al elsewhere in this issue.

Nonspecific routine laboratory abnormalities

There are no routine laboratory abnormalities that are specific for Cushing's syndrome. Thyrotropin (TSH) levels are lower in patients who have Cushing's syndrome and increase after remission [37]. Rarely, patients who have Cushing's syndrome will be referred to an endocrinologist because of a subnormal TSH (usually between 0.1 and 0.4). It is also well appreciated that successful cure of Cushing's syndrome may unmask a preexisting autoimmune thyroid disorder with the appearance of hypothyroidism or hyperthyroidism [38]. Other more routine laboratory studies are rarely helpful. High normal values of hemoglobin, hematocrit, and red blood cell count may be seen because of androgen excess, but elevations into the polycythemic range are very rare. Leukocytosis, usually with depressed percentages of lymphocyte and eosinophils, may be seen occasionally. Electrolyte disturbances are quite uncommon with the exception of hypokalemia in patients who have prodigious hypercortisolism. Routine radiographs may be helpful in showing low bone density in the axial skeleton. Rarely, chest roentgenograms may show widening of the mediastinum because of mediastinal lipomatosis.

Screening tests

The choice of tests in the initial evaluation of a patient suspected of endogenous hypercortisolism can be difficult. Even more problematic is the interpretation of the results of these tests, particularly if they are not in agreement with each other. This is particularly so in mild Cushing's syndrome; if the symptoms are subtle, the biochemical abnormalities are likely to be subtle as well. The authors recently published several extensive reviews of biochemical tests useful in the diagnosis of Cushing's syndrome [8,39–42]. Therefore, this section will focus on newer studies and conclude with an exposition on studies recently published that compare tests by modern statistical analyses.

Urine free cortisol

The measurement of free cortisol in a 24-hour urine collection has been the mainstay of the diagnosis of endogenous hypercortisolism [43]. The concept is that if the daily production of cortisol is increased, the free cortisol filtered and not reabsorbed or metabolized in the kidney will be increased measurably. Mild Cushing's syndrome often results from small, but significant increases in nighttime cortisol secretion (Fig. 2). Because most of the cortisol secreted during any 24-hour period is usually between 4 AM and 4 PM, subtle increases in nighttime cortisol secretion may not be detected in standard 24-hour urine free cortisol measurements. It also requires an adequate urine collection that must be verified with a measurement of urinary creatinine.

The other problem with this test in the past was the different methods used to measure cortisol in urine. There are still laboratories that use direct immunoassay of cortisol without chromatographic separation. Although this assay lacks specificity, it may be useful if the patient is excreting an unusual pattern of cortisol metabolites that cross-react with the cortisol antibody. Most, however, consider the gold standard for urine free cortisol to involve some type of chromatographic separation, usually high-performance liquid chromatography (HPLC) [44–47]. Assuming the chromatography is done properly, the next issue is the method of detection. Immunoassay can be done after HPLC, although tandem mass spectrometry provides more specific results [45]. There are substances that will interfere with some of these chromatographic methods including carbamazepine [46] and fenofibrate [47].

Several recent studies found the sensitivity of urine-free cortisol (UFC) to range from 45% to 71% at 100% specificity [48–52]. That is, it is not uncommon for patients who have mild Cushing's syndrome to have at least one or more normal urine free cortisol measurements. Moreover, UFC may be increased in patients who have so-called "pseudo-Cushing's syndrome,"

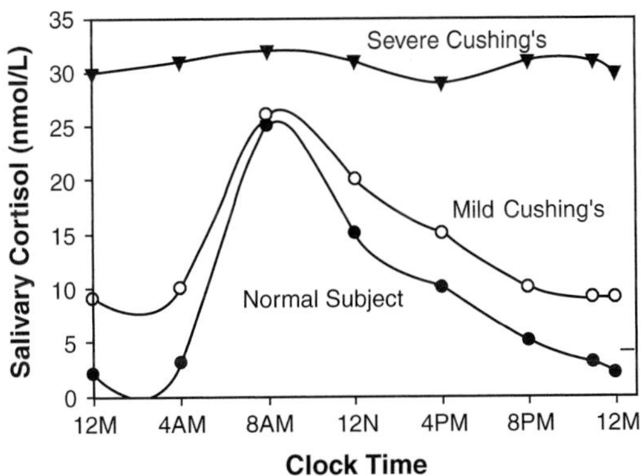

Fig. 2. Theoretical salivary cortisol levels during a typical day in a normal subject, a patient who has mild Cushing's disease, and a patient who has severe Cushing's syndrome. Note that the 11 PM–3 AM time period is the best to discriminate between mild Cushing's disease and normal subjects. For diagnostic purposes, salivary cortisol is usually sampled at 11 PM. (*Reprinted from* Raff H. Role of salivary cortisol determinations in the diagnosis of Cushing's syndrome. Curr Opin Endocrinol Diabetes 2004;11:271–5; with permission.)

which includes alcoholism, endogenous depression, and eating disorders [51,52]. When UFC is compared with other available screening tests using objective statistical analyses, its sensitivity and specificity are less than ideal (Table 1).

Circadian rhythm studies

One of the first biochemical disturbances that patients develop with mild Cushing's syndrome is a failure to decrease cortisol secretion to its normal nadir at night (see Fig. 2). This phenomenon has been exploited in the diagnosis of Cushing's syndrome with several different approaches.

Measurement of an elevated serum cortisol at midnight has a very high sensitivity and specificity for Cushing's syndrome of any etiology [51,53]. The main problem with this approach is the logistical problem of obtaining an unstressed blood sample in a routine clinical setting at midnight. This has made the widespread application of this test impractical.

A solution to this sampling problem is the measurement of salivary cortisol at bedtime as a surrogate for serum cortisol [40,41,50,52,54–57]. The authors' initial study with this test demonstrated a sensitivity and specificity of approximately 95% [54]. There now have been many major studies validating this approach to screen for Cushing's syndrome [49,50,52,54–57], and this method will continue to increase in popularity as salivary cortisol assays become readily available [58,59]. A potential drawback of this test, however, is its specificity. There are many factors that can elevate cortisol secretion falsely at bedtime including proximal stress, sleep disturbances, psychoneuroendocrine factors, and contamination of the saliva sample [40]. Therefore, whereas 24-hour UFC lacks reliable sensitivity, salivary cortisol under certain circumstances may be too sensitive.

Another approach has been to perform urine collections for the measurement of free cortisol just from the overnight period [60]. The concept is that if one collects urine during and just after the circadian nadir, the sensitivity of the test might be improved. It also would require only one or two urine collections. This approach requires a very accurate

Table 1
Diagnostic characteristics of different biochemical tests at 100% sensitivity or 100% specificity

Diagnostic characteristic	LDDST: cortisol			Nighttime: cortisol	
	Serum [48]	Salivary [49]	24-h UFC [48]	Serum [48,51]	Salivary [50]
Sensitivity at 100% specificity	54%	NC	71%	75%, 96%	93%
Specificity at 100% sensitivity	41%	93%	73%	77%	96%

Abbreviation: NC, not calculated (sensitivity was 100% at 93% specificity).
Data from Refs. [48–51].

measurement of urinary creatinine to which the free cortisol measurement is normalized.

Suppression tests

The authors have reviewed the physiologic basis of using the sensitivity to glucocorticoid negative feedback to diagnose endogenous hypercortisolism [39]. Briefly, the theory is that a small enough dose of dexamethasone will not inhibit ACTH release from corticotroph adenomas or occult ectopic ACTH-secreting tumors, while suppressing ACTH from normal pituitary tissue. (Obviously, ACTH-independent [adrenal] Cushing's syndrome should be unaffected by dexamethasone administration). It is now clear that neither the overnight nor the 2-day, low-dose dexamethasone suppression tests (LDDST) are of sufficient reliability to be used to rule out Cushing's syndrome [61–63]. The authors recently demonstrated that 18% of patients who have proven Cushing's disease suppressed serum cortisol to the standard cut-off of 5 μg/dL (135 nmol/L), while 8% showed suppression to less than 2 μg/dL (< 54 nmol/L) [62]. The performance of the 2-day LDDST was even worse. Therefore, there was no cut-off that identified all patients who have Cushing's syndrome.

Most reference laboratories with high volumes use direct serum cortisol assays using platforms that employ chemiluminescent or electrochemiluminescent immunoassays. It recently has been shown that the performance of different assays introduces significant intermethod variability when performing the LDDST to detect patients who have mild or preclinical Cushing's syndrome [64]. Because a reliable LDDST requires accuracy at low serum cortisol concentrations, variability between reference laboratories is likely to introduce even more uncertainty in the usefulness of this test. This variability would not be included in the lack of sensitivity and specificity identified in a well-controlled study in which the same assay methodology is used.

Despite these limitations, the overnight LDDST remains widely employed. A recent consensus statement recommended that patients who have plasma cortisol greater than 1.8 μg/dL (50 nmol/L) after overnight 1 mg dexamethasone administration merit further evaluation [65]. It is predicted that this more stringent criterion will yield a diagnostic sensitivity of 95% to 98% [62], but that specificity (ie, false-positives) will suffer as a result.

Stimulation tests

The secretion of ACTH from the pituitary, in addition to being under negative glucocorticoid feedback control, is stimulated primarily by hypothalamic corticotropin-releasing hormone (CRH) and, to a lesser extent, arginine vasopressin (AVP). The CRH test has been used to attempt to identify patients who have mild ACTH-dependent Cushing's syndrome

[66]. The theory is that corticotroph adenomas will display exaggerated ACTH responses compared with normal subjects as long as they continue to express receptors for CRH. Furthermore, a V2 analog of vasopressin, DDAVP (desmopressin), also has been used to attempt to identify patients who have mild Cushing's disease [58,59]. The theory is that corticotroph adenomas will have an exaggerated response to vasopressin compared with normal subjects. Neither test appears to possess the adequate sensitivity or specificity to merit their expense [66–68].

Combined testing

Different diagnostic tests can be performed on separate occasions to attempt to improve the overall reliability compared with each test alone [39]. Because each of the standard tests for the diagnosis of Cushing's syndrome has merit but also some weaknesses, another approach to improve overall performance could be to perform two tests simultaneously in each patient. Recent examples of this are the combination LDDST–CRH test and the combination of late-night salivary cortisol and LDDST.

Low-dose dexamethasone suppression–corticotropin-releasing hormone test

The logic of the LDDST–CRH is that one can improve the discriminatory potential of each test for mild Cushing's disease by performing them simultaneously. The theory is that only abnormal corticotrophs will respond to CRH while suppressed with dexamethasone [69,70]. In this test, starting at noon, dexamethasone (0.5 mg) is administered every 6 hours for a total of eight doses, with the last given at 6 AM before dynamic studies. CRH (1 μg/kg) is then given intravenously at 8 AM with measurement of cortisol and ACTH every 15 minutes for 1 hour. A serum cortisol greater than 1.4 μg/dL (> 38.6 nmol/L) is considered abnormal. There are no currently accepted criteria for an abnormal plasma ACTH response to LDDST–CRH.

The initial studies with the LDDST–CRH test were promising but required great attention to detail and compliance with the rather sophisticated protocol. Its main strength was its ability to distinguish mild Cushing's syndrome from the so-called pseudo-Cushing's syndrome. The criteria for pseudo-Cushing's syndrome included a failure for symptoms to progress for 17 months. It would be interesting to see if any of those patients from 1993 [69] subsequently have been discovered to have Cushing's disease. A recent study in patients who have anorexia nervosa found about half with abnormal LDDST–CRH tests, raising a concern that it does not reliably discriminate Cushing's syndrome from every form of endogenous pathophysiologic activation of the hypothalamic-pituitary-adrenal axis [71].

The LDDST–CRH test requires measurement of serum cortisol, thereby using endogenous adrenocortical amplification of an ACTH signal for success [69–71]. To accomplish this, the test requires a very sensitive serum cortisol measurement that is not the standard reference laboratory assay. It also, again, raises the possibility of variable reliability between reference laboratories [64]. The LDDST–CRH test is very expensive in terms of material and labor, and it usually is reserved only for patients who have mild Cushing's syndrome or to confirm the diagnosis when other screening tests are equivocal [39].

Late-night salivary cortisol–low-dose dexamethasone suppression

When the authors first published results with late-night salivary cortisol to screen for Cushing's, they hypothesized that the high sensitivity of the test combined with better specificity of the LDDST might be exploited by a combined test [54]. The theory is that almost all patients who have Cushing's syndrome have elevated late-night salivary (or serum) cortisol, but a fair number of patients who have pseudo-Cushing's syndrome do also (ie, low specificity). The LDDST, however, while having low sensitivity, may have a better specificity. Castro et al recently evaluated this concept by showing an increase in specificity from 88% with late-night salivary cortisol alone to 100% using the combined test but only when using nonobese subjects as the control group [49]. The problem was that the specificity for Cushing's syndrome compared with obese patients who presumably did not have it was not increased by the combined test. In a follow-up study, it was suggested that perhaps a higher dose of dexamethasone might improve the specificity of the test [72]. Most importantly, they clearly showed that measurement of salivary cortisol after an overnight LDDST was significantly better than measuring serum cortisol, presumably because salivary cortisol is a much better estimate of free, biologically active cortisol [40].

Comparison of diagnostic characteristics

Because each diagnostic test for Cushing's syndrome has liabilities, it is helpful to perform an objective comparison using well-defined diagnostic criteria. Table 1 focuses on several recent studies that meet the evidence-based criteria of comparing several tests within one group of patients, and performing careful step-wise analysis of sensitivity versus specificity. This table shows the sensitivity at a cut-off that provides 100% specificity, and the specificity at a cut-off that provides 100% sensitivity. Obviously, there is always a tradeoff between the two. Generally, high sensitivity is preferred for screening tests, but combinations of tests may improve both criteria.

The first characteristic that is clear from this table is that the LDDST using the measurement of serum cortisol had the poorest performance of all of the tests [48]. Again, either sensitivity or specificity can be improved at the expense of the other by adjusting cut-off levels. Of all the tests, nighttime salivary cortisol has the highest sensitivity and specificity [50,55]. It is important to point out that the authors purposefully did not use their own data in this analysis; these were independent evaluations of these tests with no apparent bias. It is also important to note that UFC performed better than the LDDST but still not as well as night-time salivary cortisol.

Probably the most important information for clinical endocrinologists is the practical nature of measuring salivary cortisol at 11 PM. There are now several assay methods available and reference laboratories that routinely perform this analysis [58,59]. The patient obtains the saliva at home thereby minimizing extraneous stress. The approach does not require the cumbersome collection of complete 24-hour urine samples, nor does it require taking (and absorbing) dexamethasone at the correct time. Salivary cortisol can be assessed in small children and the elderly without difficulty [40]. The authors have found this approach to be extremely useful and expect that its use will become accepted widely with the increased need for inexpensive, convenient, and reliable ways to screen the increasingly obese population for Cushing's syndrome.

Diagnostic strategy

Fig. 3 shows a strategy for screening patients for Cushing's syndrome. Salivary cortisol is obtained at 11 PM, usually on at least two separate nights. If both results are below the reference range (less than 4.3 nmol/L), Cushing's syndrome is unlikely. If both results are above twice the reference range cut-off (8.6 nmol/L), Cushing's syndrome is likely, particularly if the sampling times are verified, and other confounding factors (like contami-

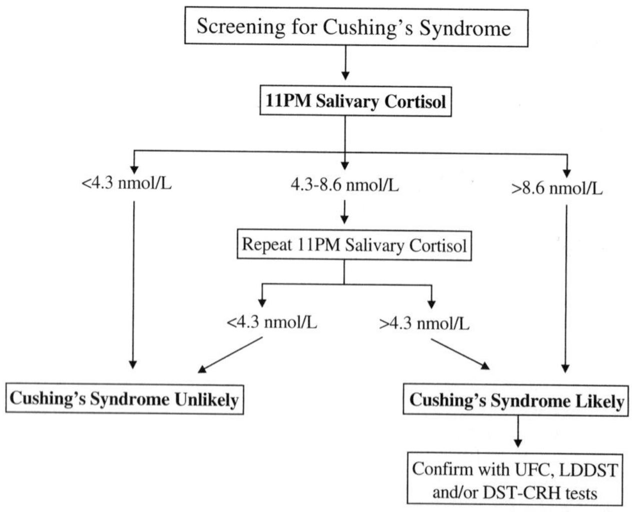

Fig. 3. A simple paradigm for screening patients for Cushing's syndrome using late-night salivary cortisol (cutoff values from Ref. [39]). This approach takes advantage of the excellent sensitivity of this test.

nation with steroid hand creams) are excluded. If the results are equivocal or not consistent between the two samples, two additional salivary cortisol samples should be obtained. It is also important to verify consistently abnormal salivary cortisol levels with other tests as indicated to confirm the diagnosis before entering the differential diagnostic strategy (described by Lindsay and Nieman elsewhere in this issue).

Summary

The recognition of mild or subclinical Cushing's syndrome and the protean nature of its clinical presentation are changing the diagnostic approach. Recent screening studies in high-risk populations have suggested that spontaneous Cushing's syndrome is more common than appreciated, and its incidence/prevalence has been underestimated. The authors believe that patients who have specific signs and symptoms or clinical diagnoses should be considered for screening (see Box 1). Currently, late-night salivary cortisol measurements provide the best sensitivity with reasonable specificity to recommend it as the initial screening test. In fact, trying to diagnose mild Cushing's syndrome without measuring late-night salivary cortisol may be like trying to diagnose mild primary hypothyroidism without obtaining a TSH. Despite their limitations, urine free cortisol and LDDST will continue to be used to confirm the presence and magnitude of endogenous hypercortisolism.

References

[1] Terzolo M, Pia A, Ali A, et al. Adrenal incidentaloma: a new cause of the metabolic syndrome? J Clin Endocrinol Metab 2002;87(3):998–1003.

[2] Reincke M, Nieke J, Krestin GP, et al. Preclinical Cushing's syndrome in adrenal incidentalomas: comparison with adrenal Cushing's syndrome. J Clin Endocrinol Metab 1992;75(3):826–32.

[3] Lindholm J, Juul S, Jorgensen JO, et al. Incidence and late prognosis of Cushing's syndrome: a population-based study. J Clin Endocrinol Metab 2001;86(1):117–23.

[4] Etxabe J, Vazquez JA. Morbidity and mortality in Cushing's disease: an epidemiological approach. Clin Endocrinol 1994;40(4):479–84.

[5] Leibowitz G, Tsur A, Chayen SD, et al. Preclinical Cushing's syndrome: an unexpected frequent cause of poor glycaemic control in obese diabetic patients. Clin Endocrinol 1996; 44(6):717–22.

[6] Catargi B, Rigalleau V, Poussin A, et al. Occult Cushing's syndrome in type-2 diabetes. J Clin Endocrinol Metab 2003;88(12):5808–13.

[7] Kadioglu P, Tiryakioglu O, Yirmibescik S, et al. Screening for Cushing's syndrome in obese patients: is it really necessary? Presented at the Endocrine Society Meeting. New Orleans, Louisiana, June 16–19, 2004.

[8] Findling JW, Raff H. Diagnosis and differential diagnosis of Cushing's syndrome. Endocrinol Metab Clin North Am 2001;30(3):729–47.

[9] Corenblum B, Kwan T, Gee S, et al. Bedside assessment of skin-fold thickness. A useful measurement for distinguishing Cushing's disease from other causes of hirsutism and oligomenorrhea. Arch Intern Med 1994;154(7):777–81.

[10] Urbanic RC, George JM. Cushing's disease—18 years' experience. Medicine 1981;60(1): 14–24.
[11] Findling JW, Tyrrell JB, Aron DC, et al. Fungal infections in Cushing's syndrome. Ann Intern Med 1981;95(3):392.
[12] Rebuffe-Scrive M, Krotkiewski M, Elfverson J, et al. Muscle and adipose tissue morphology and metabolism in Cushing's syndrome. J Clin Endocrinol Metab 1988;l67(6):1122–8.
[13] Pirlich M, Biering H, Gerl H, et al. Loss of body cell mass in Cushing's syndrome: effect of treatment. J Clin Endocrinol Metab 2002;87(3):1078–84.
[14] Giustina A, Wehrenberg WB. The role of glucocorticoids in the regulation of growth hormone secretion. Trends Endocrinol Metab 1992;3:306–11.
[15] Lebrethon MC, Grossman AB, Afshar F, et al. Linear growth and final height after treatment for Cushing's disease in childhood. J Clin Endocrinol Metab 2000;85(9):3262–5.
[16] Magiakou MA, Mastorakos G, Chrousos GP. Final stature in patients with endogenous Cushing's syndrome. J Clin Endocrinol Metab 1994;79(4):1082–5.
[17] Feldt-Rasmussen U, Abs R, Bengtsson BA, et al. KIMS International Study Board on behalf of KIMS Study Group. Growth hormone deficiency and replacement in hypopituitary patients previously treated for acromegaly or Cushing's disease. Eur J Endocrinol 2002;146(1):67–74.
[18] Dorn LD, Burgess ES, Dubbert B, et al. Psychopathology in patients with endogenous Cushing's syndrome: atypical or melancholic features. Clin Endocrinol 1995;43(4):433–42.
[19] Magiakou MA, Mastorakos G, Oldfield EH, et al. Cushing's syndrome in children and adolescents. Presentation, diagnosis, and therapy. N Engl J Med 1994;331(10):629–36.
[20] Bourdeau I, Bard C, Noel B, et al. Loss of brain volume in endogenous Cushing's syndrome and its reversibility after correction of hypercortisolism. J Clin Endocrinol Metab 2002; 87(5):1949–54.
[21] Cushing H. The basophil adenomas of the pituitary body and their clinical manifestations (pituitary basophilism). Bull Johns Hopkins Hosp 1932;50:137–95.
[22] Kelly W. Exophthalmos in Cushing's syndrome. Clin Endocrinol 1996;45(2):167–70.
[23] Bouzas EA, Mastorakos G, Chrousos GP, et al. Lisch nodules in Cushing's disease. Arch Ophthalmol 1993;111(4):439–40.
[24] Bouzas EA, Scott MH, Mastorakos G, et al. Central serous chorioretinopathy in endogenous hypercortisolism. Arch Ophthalmol 1993;111(9):1229–33.
[25] Biering H, Knappe G, Gerl H, et al. Prevalence of diabetes in acromegaly and Cushing's syndrome. Acta Med Austriaca 2000;27(1):27–31.
[26] Masuzaki H, Paterson J, Shinyama H, et al. A transgenic model of visceral obesity and the metabolic syndrome. Science 2001;294(5549):2166–70.
[27] Fallo F, Budano S, Sonino N, et al. Left ventricular structural characteristics in Cushing's syndrome. J Hum Hypertens 1994;8(7):509–13.
[28] Danese RD, Aron DC. Cushing's syndrome and hypertension. Endocrinol Metab Clin North Am 1994;23(2):299–324.
[29] Taskinen MR, Nikkila EA, Pelkonen R, et al. Plasma lipoproteins, lipolytic enzymes, and very low density lipoprotein triglyceride turnover in Cushing's syndrome. J Clin Endocrinol Metab 1983;57(3):619–26.
[30] Friedman TC, Mastorakos G, Newman TD, et al. Carbohydrate and lipid metabolism in endogenous hypercortisolism: shared features with metabolic syndrome X and NIDDM. Endocr J 1996;43(6):645–55.
[31] Boscaro M, Sonino N, Scarda A, et al. Anticoagulant prophylaxis markedly reduces thromboembolic complications in Cushing's syndrome. J Clin Endocrinol Metab 2002; 87(8):3662–6.
[32] Casonato A, Pontara E, Boscaro M, et al. Abnormalities of von Willebrand factor are also part of the prothrombotic state of Cushing's syndrome. Blood Coagul Fibrinolysis 1999; 10(3):145–51.

[33] Kaltsas GA, Korbonits M, Isidori AM, et al. How common are polycystic ovaries and the polycystic ovarian syndrome in women with Cushing's syndrome? Clin Endocrinol 2000; 53(4):493–500.
[34] Lado-Abeal J, Rodriguez-Arnao J, Newell-Price JD, et al. Menstrual abnormalities in women with Cushing's disease are correlated with hypercortisolemia rather than raised circulating androgen levels. J Clin Endocrinol Metab 1998;83(9):3083–8.
[35] Faggiano A, Pivonello R, Melis D, et al. Nephrolithiasis in Cushing's disease: prevalence, etiopathogenesis, and modification after disease cure. J Clin Endocrinol Metab 2003;88(5): 2076–80.
[36] Invitti C, Giraldi FP, de Martin M, et al. Diagnosis and management of Cushing's syndrome: results of an Italian multi-centre study. Study Group of the Italian Society of Endocrinology on the Pathophysiology of the Hypothalamic-Pituitary-Adrenal Axis. J Clin Endocrinol Metab 1999;84(2):440–8.
[37] Invitti C, Manfrini R, Romanini BM, et al. High prevalence of nodular thyroid disease in patients with Cushing's disease. Clin Endocrinol 1995;43(3):359–63.
[38] Colao A, Pivonello R, Faggiano A, et al. Increased prevalence of thyroid autoimmunity in patients successfully treated for Cushing's disease. Clin Endocrinol 2000;53(1):13–9.
[39] Raff H, Finding JW. A physiological approach to diagnosis of Cushing's syndrome. Ann Intern Med 2003;138:980–91.
[40] Raff H. Salivary cortisol: a useful measurement in the diagnosis of Cushing's syndrome and the evaluation of the hypothalamic-pituitary-adrenal axis. Endocrinologist 2000;10:9–17.
[41] Raff H. Role of salivary cortisol determinations in the diagnosis of Cushing's syndrome. Current Opinion in Endocrinology and Diabetes 2004;11:271–5.
[42] Findling JW, Raff H. Newer diagnostic techniques and problems in Cushing's disease. Endocrinol Metab Clin North Am 1999;28:191–210.
[43] Murphy BEP. Urinary free cortisol determinations: what they measure. Endocrinologist 2002;12:143–50.
[44] Lin CL, Wu TJ, Machacek DA, et al. Urinary free cortisol and cortisone determined by high performance liquid chromatography in the diagnosis of Cushing's syndrome. J Clin Endocrinol Metab 1997;82:151–5.
[45] Taylor RL, Machacek D, Singh RJ. Validation of a high-throughput liquid chromatography-tandem mass spectrometry method for urinary cortisol and cortisone. Clin Chem 2002;48: 1511–9.
[46] Findling JW, Pinkstaff SM, Shaker JL, et al. Pseudohypercortisoluria: spurious elevation of urinary cortisol due to carbamazepine. Endocrinologist 1998;8:51–4.
[47] Meikle AW, Findling J, Kushnir MM, et al. Pseudo-Cushing's syndrome caused by fenofibrate interference with urinary cortisol assayed by high-performance liquid chromatography. J Clin Endocrinol Metab 2003;88:3521–4.
[48] Gorges R, Knappe G, Gerl H, et al. Diagnosis of Cushing's syndrome: re-evaluation of midnight plasma cortisol vs urinary free cortisol and low-dose dexamethasone suppression test in a large patient group. J Endocrinol Invest 1999;22:241–9.
[49] Castro M, Elias PCL, Quidute ARP, et al. Outpatient screening for Cushing's syndrome: the sensitivity of the combination of circadian rhythm and overnight dexamethasone suppression salivary cortisol tests. J Clin Endocrinol Metab 1999;84:878–82.
[50] Yaneva M, Mosnier-Pudar H, Dugue MA, et al. Midnight salivary cortisol for the initial diagnosis of Cushing's syndrome of various causes. J Clin Endocrinol Metab 2004;89: 3345–51.
[51] Papanicolaou DA, Yanovski JA, Cutler GB, et al. A single midnight cortisol measurement distinguishes Cushing's syndrome from pseudo-Cushing's states. J Clin Endocrinol Metab 1998;83:1163–7.
[52] Papanicolaou DA, Mullen N, Kyrou I, et al. Nighttime salivary cortisol: a useful test for the diagnosis of Cushing's syndrome. J Clin Endocrinol Metab 2002;87:4515–21.

[53] Newell-Price J, Trainer P, Perry L, et al. A single sleeping midnight cortisol has 100% sensitivity for the diagnosis of Cushing's syndrome. Clin Endocrinol 1995;43:545–50.
[54] Raff H, Raff JL, Findling JW. Late-night salivary cortisol as a screening test for Cushing's syndrome. J Clin Endocrinol Metab 1998;83:2681–6.
[55] Putignano P, Toja P, Dubini A, et al. Midnight salivary cortisol versus urinary free and midnight serum cortisol as screening tests for Cushing's syndrome. J Clin Endocrinol Metab 2003;88:4153–7.
[56] Gafni RI, Papanicolaou DA, Nieman LK. Nighttime salivary cortisol measurement as a simple, noninvasive, outpatient screening test for Cushing's syndrome in children and adolescents. J Pediatr 2000;137:30–5.
[57] Martinelli CE, Sader SL, Oliveira EB, et al. Salivary cortisol for screening of Cushing's syndrome in children. Clin Endocrinol 1999;51:67–71.
[58] Raff H, Homar PJ, Burns EA. Comparison of two methods for measuring salivary cortisol. Clin Chem 2002;48:207–8.
[59] Raff H, Homar PJ, Skoner DP. A new enzyme immunoassay for salivary cortisol. Clin Chem 2003;49:203–4.
[60] Corcuff JB, Tabarin A, Rashedi M, et al. Overnight urinary free cortisol determination: a screening test for the diagnosis of Cushing's syndrome. Clin Endocrinol 1998;48:503–8.
[61] Wood PJ, Barth JH, Friedman DB, et al. Evidence for the low dose dexamethasone suppression to screen for Cushing's syndrome—recommendations for a protocol for biochemistry laboratories. Ann Clin Biochem 1997;34:222–9.
[62] Findling JW, Raff H, Aron DC. The low-dose dexamethasone suppression test: a reevaluation in patients with Cushing's syndrome. J Clin Endocrinol Metab 2004;89:1222–6.
[63] Isidori AM, Kaltsas GA, Mohammed S, et al. Discriminatory value of the low-dose dexamethasone suppression test in establishing the diagnosis and differential diagnosis of Cushing's syndrome. J Clin Endocrinol Metab 2003;88:5299–306.
[64] Odagiri E, Naruse M, Terasaki K, et al. The diagnostic standard of preclinical Cushing's syndrome: evaluation of the dexamethasone suppression test using various cortisol kits. Endocr J 2004;51:295–302.
[65] Arnaldi G, Angeli A, Atkinson AB, et al. Diagnosis and complications of Cushing's syndrome: a consensus statement. J Clin Endocrinol Metab 2003;88:5593–602.
[66] Giraldi FP, Invitti C, Cavagnini F. The corticotropin-release hormone test in the diagnosis of ACTH-dependent Cushing's syndrome: a reappraisal. Clin Endocrinol 2001;54:601–7.
[67] Tsagarakis S, Vasiliou V, Kokkoris P, et al. Assessment of cortisol and ACTH responses to the desmopressin test in patients with Cushing's syndrome and simple obesity. Clin Endocrinol 1999;51:473–7.
[68] Scott LV, Medbak S, Dinan TG. ACTH and cortisol release following intravenous desmopressin: a dose–response study. Clin Endocrinol 1999;51:653–8.
[69] Yanovski JA, Cutler GB Jr, Chrousos GP, et al. Corticotropin-releasing hormone stimulation following low-dose dexamethasone administration. JAMA 1993;269:2232–8.
[70] Yanovski JA, Cutler GB Jr, Chrousos GP, et al. The dexamethasone-suppressed corticotropin-releasing hormone stimulation test differentiates mild Cushing's disease from normal physiology. J Clin Endocrinol Metab 1998;83:348–52.
[71] Duclos M, Corcuff JB, Rober P, et al. The dexamethasone-suppressed corticotrophin-releasing hormone stimulation test in anorexia nervosa. Clin Endocrinol 1999;51:725–31.
[72] Castro M, Elias LLK, Elias PCL, et al. A dose–response study of salivary cortisol after dexamethasone suppression test in Cushing's disease and its potential use in the differential diagnosis of Cushing's syndrome. Clin Endocrinol 2003;59:800–5.

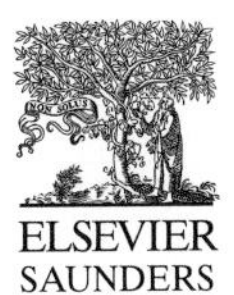

ELSEVIER
SAUNDERS

Endocrinol Metab Clin N Am
34 (2005) 403–421

ENDOCRINOLOGY
AND METABOLISM
CLINICS
OF NORTH AMERICA

Differential Diagnosis and Imaging in Cushing's Syndrome

John R. Lindsay, MD, Lynnette K. Nieman, MD*

Reproductive Biology and Medicine Branch,
National Institute for Child Health and Human Development, National Institutes of Health,
10 Center Drive, Building 10, CRC 1-3140, Bethesda, MD 20892-1109, USA

Establishing the cause of Cushing's syndrome (CS) should be undertaken only after the clinical and biochemical diagnosis has been confirmed. This process of differential diagnosis relies on a combination of dynamic endocrine testing and directed radiologic imaging. The causes of CS can be divided broadly into adrenocorticotropin (ACTH)–dependent or –independent forms (Box 1). Sustained exposure to excess cortisol suppresses the normal production of corticotropin-releasing hormone (CRH) and ACTH. As a result, circulating plasma ACTH concentrations are low in primary adrenal disorders, and normal or increased in patients with excess ACTH secretion from a pituitary tumor (Cushing's disease [CD]) or an ectopic source. These physiologic differences lead to measurement of plasma ACTH as the initial focus of differential diagnosis.

Noninvasive biochemical testing

Basal plasma adrenocorticotropin

Plasma ACTH should be measured by sensitive assay to differentiate ACTH-dependent from ACTH-independent hypercortisolism [1]. A two-site immunometric assay (IRMA) is the method of choice because it more reliably discriminates low or suppressed ACTH levels (< 10 pg/mL; 2.2 pmol/L) compared with radioimmunoassay (RIA) [1,2]. Specimens may be collected at any time because the normal evening nadir of ACTH and cortisol are lost in CS [3]. It is prudent to measure ACTH on multiple occasions to ensure diagnostic accuracy. To avoid falsely low results, collect

* Corresponding author.
E-mail address: niemanl@mail.nih.gov (L.K. Nieman).

0889-8529/05/$ - see front matter. Published by Elsevier Inc.
doi:10.1016/j.ecl.2005.01.009

Box 1. Frequency of the causes of Cushing's syndrome

ACTH-dependent CS
Pituitary-dependent CS: 68%
Ectopic ACTH syndrome: 12%
Ectopic CRH syndrome: rare (< 1%)

ACTH-independent CS
Adrenal adenoma: 10%
Adrenal carcinoma: 8%
Macronodular adrenal hyperplasia: rare (1%)
Micronodular adrenal hyperplasia: rare (< 1%)

the sample in prechilled EDTA tubes, with transport in an ice bath and prompt refrigerated centrifugation and plasma separation.

Plasma ACTH suppression (< 5 pg/mL; 1.1 pmol/L) identifies ACTH-independent primary adrenal causes of CS. No further biochemical testing is needed and imaging of the adrenal glands then will localize the abnormality to a unilateral adrenal adenoma or carcinoma or bilateral adrenal disorders (see later discussion of imaging) [1]. A normal or elevated ACTH (> 15 pg/mL; 3.3 pmol/L) level is consistent with an ACTH-producing tumor [2]. Intermediate ACTH concentrations between 5 and 15 pg/mL (1.1–3.3 pmol/L) are generally consistent with ACTH-dependent CS. In these patients, suboptimal cortisol responses to CRH stimulation may identify the few cases of ACTH-independent CS with borderline basal ACTH values [4]. Additionally, a suppressed plasma dehydroepiandrosterone sulfate level supports the diagnosis of an ACTH-independent disorder [5].

ACTH levels identify patients with ACTH-dependent disorders, but cannot distinguish reliably between CD and ectopic ACTH secretion (EAS) [6,7]. ACTH precursors resulting from incomplete cleavage of the peptide are demonstrated in EAS by small-cell carcinoma and carcinoid tumors [8,9]. Further comparison with CD patients is needed to determine if this measurement can discriminate the two groups.

Tests used to discriminate between adrenocorticotropin-dependent causes

Hypokalemia

The presence of hypokalemia suggests the possibility of EAS [10,11]. The severity of hypercortisolism in these cases likely leads to saturation of 11β-hydroxysteroid-dehydrogenase (11β-HSD2), which inactivates cortisol in the renal tubule, allowing cortisol to act as a mineralocorticoid. The degree of hypercortisolism, as measured by urinary free cortisol (UFC), correlates closely with the degree of hypokalemia. Thus hypokalemia reflects the extent and not the cause of hypercortisolism, so that as with ACTH levels, it does not discriminate reliably between CD and EAS [10].

High-dose dexamethasone suppression test

High-dose dexamethasone suppression testing (HDDST) relies on the concept that pituitary corticotroph tumor cells retain sensitivity to negative feedback effects of glucocorticoids, but not in EAS. The reported sensitivity of the two-day 8-mg HDDST for detection of CD varies from 65% to 100% with specificity for EAS or adrenal disorders ranging from 67% to 100% [12–16]. Liddle [14] described the original 6-day test, and set a criterion of 50% suppression of urinary 17-hydroxysteroid on day 2 (following dexamethasone 2 mg/6 h ×48 h), consistent with CD.

Several investigators since have attempted to improve the diagnostic efficacy of the test using UFC or more conservative criteria for interpretation. Flack [17] demonstrated that the accuracy of UFC as an endpoint in HDDST was equivalent to that of 17-hydroxysteroid excretion. Using combined criteria of greater than 90% suppression of UFC and greater than 64% suppression of 17-hydroxysteroid excretion, the test achieved 100% specificity and 83% sensitivity for the diagnosis of CD [17]. In a follow-up study, a more stringent criterion for suppression of 17 hydroxysteroids (69%) was required to maintain specificity of 100%, with a reduction in sensitivity to 79% [18].

The 8-mg overnight dexamethasone suppression test was developed to be more cost-effective than the original 6-day test described by Liddle [14,19]. Tyrrell [19] demonstrated that the overnight test had high diagnostic accuracy using criteria of 50% suppression of serum cortisol. The diagnostic accuracy of the test can be improved further using criterion for suppression of serum cortisol of more than 68% [18]. By this criterion the sensitivity and specificity of the test were 71% and 100%, respectively, in a study of 34 patients who had CD and seven who had EAS [18]. The 8-mg overnight test had equivalent sensitivity compared with the 6-day test and improved diagnostic accuracy was achieved using combined criteria from the 8-mg overnight and 6-day tests [18].

Aron and colleagues [12] recently questioned the incremental benefit of the HDDST added to other biochemical tests for prediction of EAS. Based on Liddle's criterion, the sensitivity and specificity of the HDDST for the diagnosis of CD were 81% and 67%, respectively. Although the mean percent suppression was significantly greater for patients who had CD than for those who had EAS (72% versus 41%, respectively), the range of suppression was 0% to 99% for each diagnosis [12]. Although the HDDST can detect patients who have CD with relatively high sensitivity, it does not exclude accurately those who have EAS. Factors that influence the poor diagnostic accuracy of the test include reliance on urinary measures with possible incomplete urine collections, interfering substances, episodic cortisol secretion leading to apparent suppression and effects of drugs, and interindividual variability in clearance, which alters dexamethasone bioavailability. As a result, the HDDST should not be used as the sole test for the differential diagnosis of ACTH-dependent CS.

Metyrapone and desmopressin stimulation tests

Metyrapone and desmopressin are potentially useful for the differential diagnosis because of the enhancement of ACTH and cortisol release in CD compared with EAS. Metyrapone acts by blocking *CYP11B1* (11β-hydroxylase) and preventing conversion of 11-deoxycortisol to cortisol. In CD the subsequent decrease in cortisol feedback leads to a temporary rise in ACTH and cortisol precursors because these tumors, and not those of EAS, respond to negative feedback. The metyrapone test has limited efficacy when used alone, but the diagnostic accuracy of the test can be improved when combined with the HDDST [20].

Desmopressin stimulates ACTH and cortisol release in CD by selective stimulation of the V2- and V3-vasopressin receptors. Desmopressin used alone also has limited usefulness for discriminating CD from EAS because of an overlap in cortisol and ACTH responses [21]. Combined with CRH, desmopressin may have improved diagnostic accuracy for the differential diagnosis, but this remains controversial [21]. Desmopressin testing remains an experimental agent in the evaluation of CS. Neither metyrapone nor desmopressin are recommended for diagnostic use [2].

Corticotropin-releasing hormone stimulation test

In CD, the pituitary tumor corticotrophs remain responsive to CRH stimulation, whereas adrenal tumors and most ectopic ACTH-producing tumors do not respond [22–24]. The CRH stimulation test involves basal sampling for cortisol and ACTH followed by administration of 1 μg/kg or 100 μg of CRH. Early studies gave ovine CRH (oCRH) between 1900 and 2100 hours, with sampling for ACTH and cortisol over 75 minutes [22]. Since then the test has been validated with human CRH (hCRH) as a morning test with a shorter sampling period of 65 minutes that can be undertaken at any time of day in patients with persistent hypercortisolism [25]. The test usually is well tolerated, except for flushing in approximately 20% of patients and occasional metallic taste [25].

Table 1 summarizes the diagnostic criteria and accuracy for the test from five international centers with extensive experience [23,25–28] that used a range of protocols. Sensitivities ranged from 70% to 93% and 50% to 91% for ACTH and cortisol criteria, respectively, for a range of specificity of 88% to 100%. Apart from inherent differences in the patient populations, the timing of the samples and type of CRH may influence these different results. The National Institutes of Health series, the largest individual series

Table 1
Summary of corticotropin-releasing hormone stimulation test results for differential diagnosis of Cushing's syndrome in international series

	Studies				
Diagnostic utility	Kaye and Crapo, 1990 [23]	Nieman, 1993 [25]	Invitti, 1999 [28]	Giraldi, 2001 [26]	Newell-Price, 2002 [27]
No. of patients and diagnosis	142 CD 21 EAS 19 AA	99 CD 17 EAS —	158 CD 13 EAS 41 ACTH-independent	148 CD 14 EAS —	101 CD 14 EAS —
CRH dose and species (%)	1 μg/kg BW *or* 100 μg oCRH	1 μg/kg BW oCRH	100 μg hCRH *or* oCRH	100 μg hCRH (36) oCRH (64)	100 μg oCRH
ACTH criteria % (rise above basal)	**50**	**35**	**50**	**50**	**105**
Sensitivity %	86	93	85	87 [hCRH] 85 [oCRH]	70
Specificity	95	100	100	100	100
Cortisol criteria % (rise above basal)	**20**	**20**	**50**	**50**	**14**
Sensitivity %	91	91	59	50 [hCRH] 67 [oCRH]	85
Specificity %	95	88	92	100	100

Abbreviations: AA, adrenal adenoma; BW, body weight.

to date, set criteria for CD of 35% increase in ACTH and 20% increase in cortisol following 1 μg/kg of oCRH, measuring both hormones at −5 and 0 minutes before CRH, ACTH at 15 and 30 minutes, and cortisol at 30 and 45 minutes afterwards in 101 patients who had CD and 17 patients who had EAS [25]. In that study the test had a sensitivity and specificity of 91% and 88%, respectively, using cortisol criteria [25]. Using ACTH criteria, the sensitivity and specificity of the test for detection of CD improved to 93% and 100%, respectively. The present sensitivity and specificity for the test using ACTH criteria are approximately 90%, derived from unpublished data in addition to the authors' original observations (see Table 1).

The original ACTH criterion for the CRH test was based on RIA methodology, which has been replaced largely by a more sensitive and reproducible IRMA [1]. A recent multicenter Italian study demonstrated similar diagnostic accuracy for each assay technique, but this issue remains to be validated in additional large series [26]. Furthermore, the diagnostic approach between Europe and the United States varies regarding use of hCRH and dosing with weight-based or 100-μg fixed-dose CRH regimens

[26]. It is difficult to evaluate directly these potential variables because there have been no direct trials of fixed versus weight-adjusted dosing and limited direct comparisons of hCRH versus oCRH [26,27,29,30]. The available data suggest reduced hCRH versus oCRH responses, which is not surprising given the pharmacokinetics of hCRH. As a result the criteria for identification of CD are lower for the human analog.

In summary, the CRH stimulation test is a useful noninvasive test for the differential diagnosis of ACTH-dependent CS, but has limited usefulness when used alone. The main controversies regard variability in testing schedules and a wide range of diagnostic cut-off point criteria. The overall positive and negative predictive values (PPV and NPV) of the test range between 98% and 100% and 33% and 57%, respectively, using ACTH criteria. Using cortisol criteria, the PPV is similar and NPV ranges from 20% to 50% [23,25–27]. Combining the results of positive CRH and dexamethasone testing improves the diagnostic performance of either test alone because up to 98% of cases of CD may be identified using this approach [31]. In four series, however, 18% to 65% of patients who have CD lacked a response to one or both tests [4,22,32–34]. Significantly, because of the presence of limited apparently CRH-responsive ectopic ACTH tumors, 100% specificity may not be achievable even if using increased cut-off levels for responses [2]. Additional modalities for the differential diagnosis usually are required, including IPSS and imaging techniques (see later discussion).

Invasive testing for the differential diagnosis of adrenocorticotropin-dependent Cushing's syndrome

Inferior petrosal sinus sampling

IPSS is the single best diagnostic test for differentiation of ACTH-dependent CS [35,36]. IPSS offers diagnostic sensitivity, specificity, and accuracy that is substantially greater than the pretest probability of 85% to 90% for CD [7,35,36]. This invasive technique involves catheterization of both petrosal sinuses and measurement of ACTH in blood obtained from each sinus and a peripheral vein (Fig. 1). Serial samples for central and peripheral plasma ACTH concentrations then are drawn at −1 and 0 minutes before and at 3, 5, and 10 minutes after CRH administration (1 μg/kg body weight or 100 μg given intravenously). In CD, a central-to-peripheral ACTH gradient results from high ACTH levels in venous drainage from the pituitary, and contrasts with the absence of a gradient in EAS. IPSS should be considered only for patients who have confirmed consistent hypercortisolism because the test cannot discriminate between normal subjects and patients who have CD. Overall, IPSS is technically successful in 85% to 99% of procedures [36]. When performed by a radiologist experienced in the technique, serious complications such as venous thrombosis, pulmonary embolism, cranial nerve palsy, and brain stem vascular damage may be minimized [37–41].

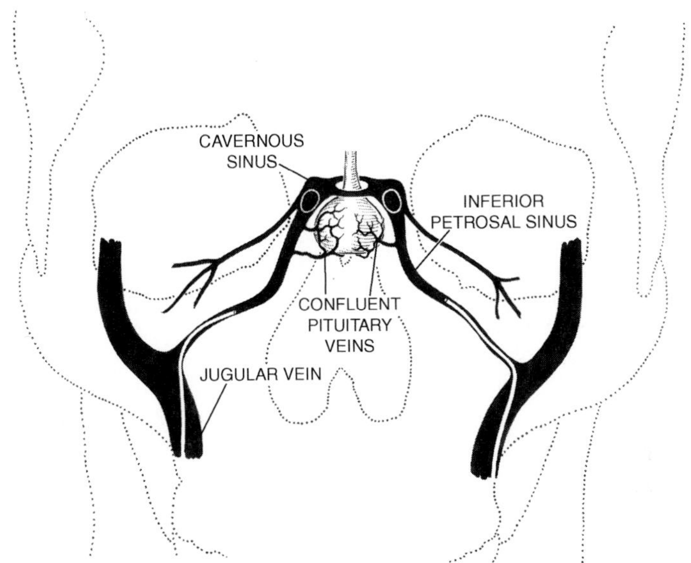

Fig. 1. Inferior petrosal sinus sampling. Line drawing representing the anatomy of the petrosal sinuses. (*Reproduced from* Oldfield EH, Chrousos GP, Schultze HM, et al. N Eng J Med 1985;312:100. Copyright 1985, Massachusetts Medical Society; with permission.)

A central-to-peripheral ACTH ratio greater than 3.0 following the administration of oCRH is consistent with CD (Fig. 2) [36,42]. Most patients who have EAS have a central-peripheral ratio of less than 2.0 before and after CRH administration [36]. With increasing use of IPSS worldwide, reports of false negative and false positive results have reduced the originally reported diagnostic accuracy of 100% [35,36]. By combining various reports of 726 patients who had CD and 112 who had EAS, there were 41 false negatives and seven false positives, providing a diagnostic sensitivity and specificity for IPSS of 94% (Table 2) [10,32,35–37,42–50].

The validity of the test relies on successful cannulation of the petrosal sinuses. Digital subtraction angiography should be performed to ensure correct catheter placement and to evaluate venous anatomy. A hypoplastic or anomalous inferior petrosal sinus in 0.8% of a large series of 501 patients was believed to underlie false-negative results in patients subsequently found to have surgically proven CD [43]. Other causes of false results include IPSS undertaken during a normocortisolemic period in patients with intermittent ectopic ACTH-secretion and false positives caused by CRH-secreting tumors [50,51]. Efforts to improve the diagnostic accuracy include additional sampling during IPSS for other anterior pituitary hormones, including prolactin for normalization of ACTH ratios [52].

In the authors' view, patients with a definite pituitary tumor on imaging (see later discussion) and CRH results consistent with CD, or who have

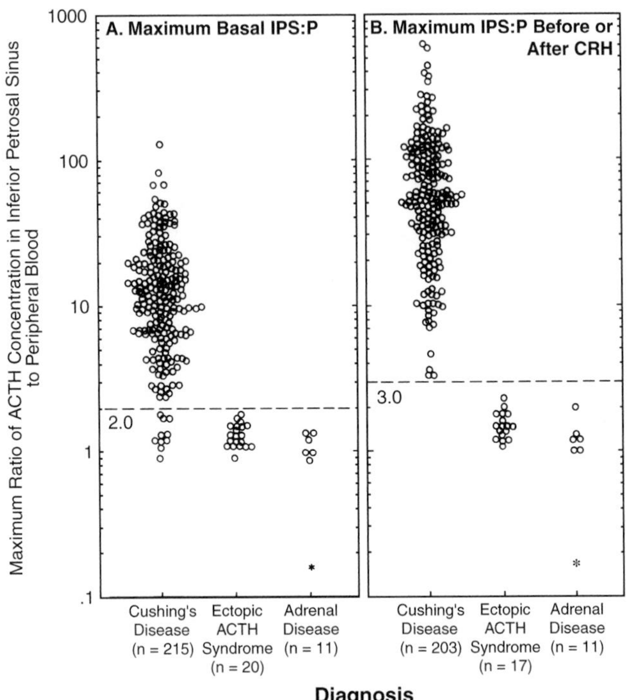

Fig. 2. Maximal central-peripheral ratio of plasma ACTH in patients who have CS. (*A*) The maximal ratio was > 2.0 in 205 of 215 patients who had confirmed CD but < 2.0 in patients who had EAS or primary adrenal disease. (*B*) Patients who had CD who received CRH had maximal ratios of > 3.0, whereas patients who had EAS had ratios < 3.0. (*Reproduced from* Oldfield EH, Doppman JL, Nieman LK, et al. N Engl J Med 1991;325(13):897–905. Copyright 1991, Massachusetts Medical Society; with permission.)

HDDST and CRH results consistent with CD, have a near 100% probability of having CD and do not need IPSS for diagnosis (Fig. 3). All other patients who have ACTH-dependent CS benefit from IPSS [2]. IPSS can be particularly helpful in determining the relevance of a small pituitary adenoma in a patient with biochemical tests that do not favor CD, given a prevalence of pituitary incidentaloma in up to 10% of the normal population. In summary, although IPSS remains the best single test for the differential diagnosis of ACTH-dependent CS, factors such as local radiologic expertise, CRH availability, and cost may influence its use in clinical practice.

IPSS has limited usefulness for localizing an ACTH-secreting pituitary adenoma within the gland, which has been a matter of controversy [53]. A combined literature review of 313 cases with lateralization studies using pituitary surgery as the criterion standard until 1998 revealed a range of diagnostic accuracy of IPSS for localization between 50% and 100% [54].

Table 2
Summary of international series of inferior Petrosal Sinus Sampling

	No. of				%		
First author, year [Ref. no.]	CD	EAS	False neg	False pos	Sens	Spec	Tech OK
Findling, 1991 [35]	20	9	0	0	100	100	93
Oldfield, 1991 [36][a]	(215)	(20)	0	0	100	100	99
Yamamoto, 1995 [50]	—	2	—	2	—	—	—
Lopez, 1996 [49]	32	0	1	—	95	—	—
Booth, 1998 [48][b]	37	0	7	—	81	—	86
Kaltsas, 1999 [42][b]	107	6	2	0	97	100	65→88
Invitti, 1999 [28]	85	10	11	0	85	100	—
Doppman, 1999 [43]	510	—	4	—	99	—	—
Bonelli, 2000 [37]	82	10	6	1	92	90	93
Tsagarakis, 2000 [46][b]	30	4	0	0	87; 100[b]	100	85
Wiggam, 2000 [32][c]	44	1	8	—	82	—	84
Findling, 2001 [7]	—	2	—	2	—	—	—
Colao, 2001 [45]	74	10	2	1	90	100	—
Ilias, 2002 [89]	—	60	—	1	—	98	—
Total	**726**	**112**	**41**	**7**	**94**	**94**	—

Abbreviations: Tech OK, technically successful; False neg, false negative; False pos, false positive.

IPSS is the only diagnostic test for CD with a sensitivity > 85%–90% pretest probability of the condition. Importantly, the test also has very high specificity for EAS. The excellent diagnostic accuracy of IPSS, however, is achieved only at centers with experienced interventional radiologists and even then it is technically successful only 85%–99% of the time. With widespread worldwide use of IPSS, reports of false-negative and -positive results have decreased the initially reported diagnostic accuracy of 100% to a sensitivity and specificity of about 94%, as shown in this Table.

[a] This series is counted in Ref. [43], thus these numbers are not included in the total number of patients who have CD or EAS (see parenthetical data above).

[b] CRH ± desmopressin.

[c] No CRH.

A gradient of 1.4 or greater across both sides of the pituitary correctly predicted tumor location in 78% [54]. This should be compared with a pretest probability for localization of 33% to 50% based on whether a tumor is situated right, left, or midline. Booth and colleagues [48] compared the efficacy of IPSS and imaging for prediction of localization of the pituitary tumor. They demonstrated successful localization in 70% using IPPS compared with 49% using imaging. In contrast, in an Italian multicenter study, IPSS was less reliable than MRI and CT (65% versus 75% and 79%, respectively) [45].

Jugular venous sampling

Jugular venous sampling (JVS) was developed as a simpler and possibly safer alternative for localizing ACTH-secreting tumors, given the technical demands of IPSS [55]. A comparison of JVS was undertaken recently to

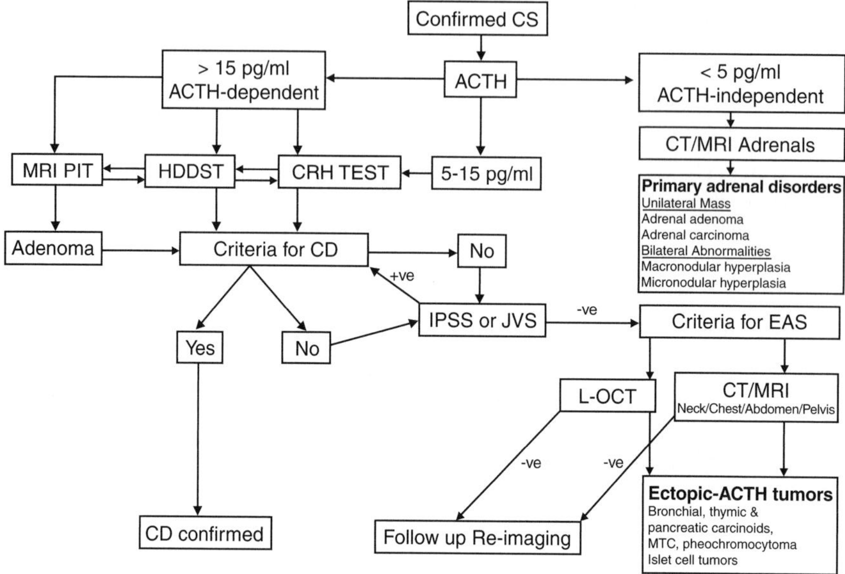

Fig. 3. Algorithm for the differential diagnosis of CS. L-OCT, 6-mCi octreotide imaging; MTC, medullary thyroid carcinoma; PIT, pituitary.

determine its diagnostic efficacy compared with the criterion standard [31]. Seventy-four patients who had surgically confirmed CD and 11 patients who had EAS were studied. At 100% specificity IPSS had 94% sensitivity compared with JVS, which had a sensitivity of 83%. JVS was conducted without serious adverse sequelae, although one subject developed transient arm numbness as a result of anesthetic infiltration in the neck.

A previous study of JVS using a central-peripheral ACTH ratio criteria of greater than 2.0 at baseline and greater than 3.0 after CRH demonstrated sensitivity of 81% compared with 93% using IPSS [56]. Diagnostic cut-off point criteria using JVS will need further validation in larger series in individual centers. Importantly, ACTH values and central-peripheral ratios from jugular samples are generally lower than IPSS ratios as a result of dilution within the jugular vein [31]. CRH administration is required to improve diagnostic performance and separation between the patient groups [31]. Although IPSS had better diagnostic accuracy, JVS may be considered in centers with limited IPSS experience. In the event of a negative JVS study the authors would recommend subsequent referral for IPSS at an experienced center [31].

Cavernous sinus sampling

Teramoto and colleagues [57] originally examined the role of cavernous sinus sampling (CVS) as an alternative to IPSS for the differential diagnosis of ACTH-dependent CS. Because the cavernous sinuses are closer to the pituitary gland than the petrosal sinus, it is possible that CVS would provide greater central-to-peripheral ACTH gradients so that CRH administration would not be needed for accurate diagnosis. Several groups, however, including the authors', have concluded that CVS offers no additional advantage over IPSS. Doppman and colleagues [58] demonstrated a 20% false negative rate in the absence of CRH stimulation.

Given the potential risk for further complications from entering the cavernous sinus and the extra cost, the authors consider the technique inferior to IPSS. One of the purported advantages of CVS is a success regarding tumor localization [59–61]. This issue remains controversial in light of previous and recent reports demonstrating a lack of usefulness of the technique for localization compared with IPSS [58,62,63]. In the most recent study, IPSS demonstrated 86% accuracy for lateralization in patients with both catheters in the inferior petrosal sinuses compared with 50% in patients with both catheters in the cavernous sinuses [63]. CVS did not improve the results and was associated with neurologic complications on two occasions, resulting in transient sixth cranial nerve palsies [63]. The authors do not recommend the use of CVS on the basis of diagnostic usefulness, cost, or safety compared with IPSS alone.

Imaging modalities

Pituitary

Pituitary MRI should be obtained in all patients who have ACTH-dependent CS [2]. The technique replaced CT as the first-line imaging modality because it has improved sensitivity for detection of microadenomas [23]. It is essential to obtain a pituitary (not brain) study, which uses a smaller field of view, and to acquire the images using a 1.5-T magnet to improve resolution. Corticotroph adenomas are characteristically hypodense on MRI and fail to enhance following administration of gadopentetate dimeglumine (Gd-DPTA) contrast. A small proportion of pituitary microadenomas (5%) will absorb Gd-DTPA, becoming isointense with the enhancing pituitary gland on the immediate postgadolinium scan [7]. Therefore, precontrast scans and contrast-enhanced studies always should be performed to improve diagnostic accuracy.

Although T1-weighted spin echo (SE) pituitary MRI is superior to CT, the technique has limited sensitivity, between 50% and 60% [64–66]. A false negative study may result from small tumor size or signal characteristics of the ACTH-secreting tissue that are similar to normal pituitary tissue [44,65,67–70]. Added to the limitations of sensitivity, the specificity of SE MRI is limited by the presence of incidental pituitary lesions in up to 10% of the normal population, many of which range in size up to 6 mm [71–73]. Consequently, many institutions, including the authors', previously opted to rely on IPSS for differentiating pituitary from ectopic sources of ACTH. A recent consensus statement, which reflects the authors' current practice, concluded that pituitary MRI may provide a definitive diagnosis without the need for further invasive testing in the setting of a greater than 6-mm pituitary adenoma with classic clinical and dynamic biochemical results (ie, responses to CRH and dexamethasone consistent with CD) [2].

A recent series evaluated the possibility for improved tumor detection using MRI with 1-mm spoiled gradient recalled acquisition in the steady state (SPGR) sequences compared with SE [68]. This technique has potential benefits, such as faster acquisition, provision of thinner slices, and better soft tissue enhancement [68,74]. Compared with SE for detection of tumor, SPGR had superior sensitivity (80% versus 49%) but a higher false positive rate (2% versus 4%). The authors recommend the addition of coronal postcontrast SPGR to conventional SE pituitary imaging protocols to improve MRI detection of ACTH-secreting pituitary tumors. This technique should be used in combination, not alone, however, to minimize false positives [68].

Adrenal imaging

Thin-section CT or MRI of the adrenal glands is often the final diagnostic test in patients who have ACTH-independent causes of CS [75,76]. Both modalities help identify adrenal carcinoma [77]. The differential diagnosis and imaging features of adrenal tumors have been reviewed previously [76,78]. Features suggestive of a benign adenoma include tumor size less than 4 cm, attenuation values of < 10 Hounsfield units on unenhanced CT, homogeneity, and regular tumor margins [77]. Features compatible with an autonomously functioning adrenal adenoma include atrophy of the contralateral gland. In the absence of atrophy of the contralateral gland or the remaining involved gland, the biochemical diagnosis should be reconsidered. If the diagnosis is affirmed, ACTH-dependent micronodular or macronodular adrenal hyperplasia should be considered [54]. Bilateral micronodular disease, with or without Carney's complex, is suggested by classic clinical features or paradoxical responsiveness to dexamethasone [79]. In these patients, imaging of the adrenal glands may reveal slightly enlarged glands with or without discernable nodules, but a proportion will have normal adrenal glands.

Ectopic adrenocorticotropin syndrome

Localization of ectopic ACTH-secreting tumors is challenging and primarily relies on CT, MRI, and nuclear medicine imaging. The most common tumors causing EAS are lung, bronchial, pancreatic, and thymic carcinoid tumors. Medullary thyroid carcinoma, pheochromocytoma, gastrinoma, and small-cell lung carcinoma also should be sought, however

Table 3
Biochemical markers for ectopic sources of Cushing's syndrome

Causes of EAS	Markers
Medullary thyroid carcinoma	Calcitonin
Pheochromocytoma	Plasma-free metanephrines and 24-h urine cathecholamines/metanephrines
Gastrinoma	Gastrin
Neuroendocrine/carcinoid tumors	Urine 5-HIAA, chromogranin A, and serotonin

(Table 3). Many of these tumors express somatostatin receptors on their cell surface, thereby facilitating localization using nuclear imaging modalities such as somatostatin receptor scintigraphy (SRS) [80]. The usefulness of SRS in EAS compared with conventional CT or MRI has been debated.

Somatostatin receptor scintigraphy

SRS was developed to facilitate localization of ectopic ACTH-secreting tumors, which often can remain occult because of their small size during follow-up. The preferred clinical endpoint is accurate tumor localization and definitive surgical therapy. In persistent occult EAS, however, medical therapy or bilateral adrenalectomy may be required in a significant portion of cases. SRS offers the potential for more accurate tumor localization and identification of functional neuroendocrine tissue [81].

An analysis of seven recent studies examining the usefulness of SRS in EAS demonstrated diagnostic sensitivity ranging from 33% to 80% for tumor localization [11,82–88]. Comparison of these series is not straightforward given variable study design and whether outcomes were based on single or multiple imaging procedures or even on final histologic diagnosis [11,82–88]. Early studies of SRS in EAS were disappointing in view of similar sensitivity for tumor detection compared with conventional imaging [82,85].

SRS always should be correlated with conventional imaging because of false positive results observed with follicular thyroid adenoma, inflammation, radiation fibrosis, and accessory spleen [82,85]. Although more recent series demonstrate higher sensitivity for tumor localization, some observed differences likely are accounted for partially by differences in study design and referral practices [84]. There have been a few reports of negative SRS becoming positive, and repeat SRS should be considered during long-term follow-up in persistent occult disease [84]. SRS has limited sensitivity for identifying tumors less than 1 cm, perhaps reflecting the concentration or type of somatostatin receptor expression [82]. Using a range of dosing regimens (6–18 mCi), the smallest tumor size detected using SRS was 0.6 cm [83,88]. A recent prospective blinded study was undertaken to evaluate whether the diagnostic yield for SRS could be improved by using a higher dose of octreotide to account for differences in tumor size, receptor expression, or radioactivity [83]. High-dose octreotide imaging (18 mCi) identified a tumor in one patient with otherwise negative imaging, leading the authors to conclude that high-dose octreotide imaging be considered only when other imaging modalities fail to localize the ectopic ACTH tumor in patients who have EAS [83]. This approach must be considered investigational, however.

In summary, the combination of SRS and conventional CT/MRI probably facilitates the best overall localization in these difficult cases [83]. The authors advocate the use of all three modalities in combination to improve sensitivity for detection of occult lesions, given limitations of individual modalities used alone [82,83]. If a tumor is not found, repeat imaging should be performed every 6 to 12 months.

Florine-18–fluorodeoxyglucose PET

Functional imaging using SRS has provided mixed results for localization of EAS tumors. To improve on the sensitivity of nuclear imaging modalities the authors recently examined the potential of florine-18–fluorodeoxyglucose PET ([^{18}F]-FDG–PET) for tumor localization in 17 patients [83]. ACTH-secreting tumors were localized in 13 patients and were occult in four. [^{18}F]-FDG–PET detected 6 of 17 cases but failed to identify tumors that were occult on CT/MRI. The sensitivity of CT and combined 6- or 18-mCi SRS was higher than that of MRI or [^{18}F]-FDG–PET. This small series suggests that [^{18}F]-FDG–PET confers no additional benefit for detection of ectopic ACTH-secreting tumors beyond existing modalities [83].

Summary

The evaluation of a patient who has confirmed CS is a challenging process that requires a combined biochemical and imaging strategy for effective tumor localization. The first step in the diagnostic algorithm (see Fig. 3) is to determine whether the patient has ACTH-dependent or independent hypercortisolism, using a two-site IRMA ACTH assay. In ACTH-independent CS, imaging of the adrenal glands is usually sufficient to localize the adrenal pathology and provide a diagnosis. In ACTH-dependent CS, however, no noninvasive biochemical strategy offers sufficient sensitivity or sensitivity for diagnosis when used alone. Most patients require a combination of pituitary MRI with dexamethasone suppression and CRH stimulation or petrosal sinus sampling for diagnosis. Focused imaging using MRI, CT, or nuclear imaging can facilitate tumor localization in patients who have EAS.

References

[1] Raff H, Findling JW. A new immunoradiometric assay for corticotropin evaluated in normal subjects and patients with Cushing's syndrome. Clin Chem 1989;35(4):596–600.

[2] Arnaldi G, Angeli A, Atkinson AB, et al. Diagnosis and complications of Cushing's syndrome: a consensus statement. J Clin Endocrinol Metab 2003;88(12):5593–602.
[3] Weitzman ED, Fukushima D, Nogeire C, et al. Twenty-four hour pattern of the episodic secretion of cortisol in normal subjects. J Clin Endocrinol Metab 1971;33(1):14–22.
[4] Hermus AR, Pieters GF, Pesman GJ, et al. The corticotropin-releasing-hormone test versus the high-dose dexamethasone test in the differential diagnosis of Cushing's syndrome. Lancet 1986;2(8506):540–4.
[5] Flecchia D, Mazza E, Carlini M, et al. Reduced serum levels of dehydroepiandrosterone sulphate in adrenal incidentalomas: a marker of adrenocortical tumour. Clin Endocrinol (Oxf) 1995;42(2):129–34.
[6] Howlett TA, Drury PL, Perry L, et al. Diagnosis and management of ACTH-dependent Cushing's syndrome: comparison of the features in ectopic and pituitary ACTH production. Clin Endocrinol (Oxf) 1986;24(6):699–713.
[7] Findling JW, Raff H. Diagnosis and differential diagnosis of Cushing's syndrome. Endocrinol Metab Clin North Am 2001;30(3):729–47.
[8] Himsworth RL, Bloomfield GA, Coombes RC, et al. 'Big ACTH' and calcitonin in an ectopic hormone secreting tumour of the liver. Clin Endocrinol (Oxf) 1977;7(1):45–62.
[9] Stewart PM, Gibson S, Crosby SR, et al. ACTH precursors characterize the ectopic ACTH syndrome. Clin Endocrinol (Oxf) 1994;40(2):199–204.
[10] Torpy DJ, Mullen N, Ilias I, et al. Association of hypertension and hypokalemia with Cushing's syndrome caused by ectopic ACTH secretion: a series of 58 cases. Ann N Y Acad Sci 2002;970:134–44.
[11] Loli P, Vignati F, Grossrubatscher E, et al. Management of occult adrenocorticotropin-secreting bronchial carcinoids: limits of endocrine testing and imaging techniques. J Clin Endocrinol Metab 2003;88(3):1029–35.
[12] Aron DC, Raff H, Findling JW. Effectiveness versus efficacy: the limited value in clinical practice of high dose dexamethasone suppression testing in the differential diagnosis of adrenocorticotropin-dependent Cushing's syndrome. J Clin Endocrinol Metab 1997;82(6): 1780–5.
[13] Orth DN. Cushing's syndrome. N Engl J Med 1995;332(12):791–803.
[14] Liddle GW. Tests of pituitary-adrenal suppressibility in the diagnosis of Cushing's syndrome. J Clin Endocrinol Metab 1960;20:1539–60.
[15] Crapo L. Cushing's syndrome: a review of diagnostic tests. Metabolism 1979;28(9):955–77.
[16] Grossman AB, Howlett TA, Perry L, et al. CRF in the differential diagnosis of Cushing's syndrome: a comparison with the dexamethasone suppression test. Clin Endocrinol (Oxf) 1988;29(2):167–78.
[17] Flack MR, Oldfield EH, Cutler GB Jr, et al. Urine free cortisol in the high-dose dexamethasone suppression test for the differential diagnosis of the Cushing syndrome. Ann Intern Med 1992;116(3):211–7.
[18] Dichek HL, Nieman LK, Oldfield EH, et al. A comparison of the standard high dose dexamethasone suppression test and the overnight 8-mg dexamethasone suppression test for the differential diagnosis of adrenocorticotropin-dependent Cushing's syndrome. J Clin Endocrinol Metab 1994;78(2):418–22.
[19] Tyrrell JB, Findling JW, Aron DC, et al. An overnight high-dose dexamethasone suppression test for rapid differential diagnosis of Cushing's syndrome. Ann Intern Med 1986;104(2):180–6.
[20] Avgerinos PC, Yanovski JA, Oldfield EH, et al. The metyrapone and dexamethasone suppression tests for the differential diagnosis of the adrenocorticotropin-dependent Cushing syndrome: a comparison. Ann Intern Med 1994;121(5):318–27.
[21] Tsagarakis S, Tsigos C, Vasiliou V, et al. The desmopressin and combined CRH-desmopressin tests in the differential diagnosis of ACTH-dependent Cushing's syndrome: constraints imposed by the expression of V2 vasopressin receptors in tumors with ectopic ACTH secretion. J Clin Endocrinol Metab 2002;87(4):1646–53.

[22] Nieman LK, Chrousos GP, Oldfield EH, et al. The ovine corticotropin-releasing hormone stimulation test and the dexamethasone suppression test in the differential diagnosis of Cushing's syndrome. Ann Intern Med 1986;105(6):862–7.
[23] Kaye TB, Crapo L. The Cushing syndrome: an update on diagnostic tests. Ann Intern Med 1990;112(6):434–44.
[24] Dickstein G, DeBold CR, Gaitan D, et al. Plasma corticotropin and cortisol responses to ovine corticotropin-releasing hormone (CRH), arginine vasopressin (AVP), CRH plus AVP, and CRH plus metyrapone in patients with Cushing's disease. J Clin Endocrinol Metab 1996;81(8):2934–41.
[25] Nieman LK, Oldfield EH, Wesley R, et al. A simplified morning ovine corticotropin-releasing hormone stimulation test for the differential diagnosis of adrenocorticotropin-dependent Cushing's syndrome. J Clin Endocrinol Metab 1993;77(5):1308–12.
[26] Giraldi FP, Invitti C, Cavagnini F. The corticotropin-releasing hormone test in the diagnosis of ACTH-dependent Cushing's syndrome: a reappraisal. Clin Endocrinol (Oxf) 2001;54(5): 601–7.
[27] Newell-Price J, Morris DG, Drake WM, et al. Optimal response criteria for the human CRH test in the differential diagnosis of ACTH-dependent Cushing's syndrome. J Clin Endocrinol Metab 2002;87(4):1640–5.
[28] Invitti C, Giraldi FP, de Martin M, et al. Diagnosis and management of Cushing's syndrome: results of an Italian multicentre study. Study Group of the Italian Society of Endocrinology on the Pathophysiology of the Hypothalamic-Pituitary-Adrenal Axis. J Clin Endocrinol Metab 1999;84(2):440–8.
[29] Nieman LK, Cutler GB Jr, Oldfield EH, et al. The ovine corticotropin-releasing hormone (CRH) stimulation test is superior to the human CRH stimulation test for the diagnosis of Cushing's disease. J Clin Endocrinol Metab 1989;69(1):165–9.
[30] Trainer PJ, Faria M, Newell-Price J, et al. A comparison of the effects of human and ovine corticotropin-releasing hormone on the pituitary-adrenal axis. J Clin Endocrinol Metab 1995;80(2):412–7.
[31] Ilias I, Chang R, Pacak K, et al. Jugular venous sampling: an alternative to petrosal sinus sampling for the diagnostic evaluation of adrenocorticotropic hormone-dependent Cushing's syndrome. J Clin Endocrinol Metab 2004;89(8):3795–800.
[32] Wiggam MI, Heaney AP, McIlrath EM, et al. Bilateral inferior petrosal sinus sampling in the differential diagnosis of adrenocorticotropin-dependent Cushing's syndrome: a comparison with other diagnostic tests. J Clin Endocrinol Metab 2000;85(4): 1525–32.
[33] Tabarin A, San Galli F, Dezou S, et al. The corticotropin-releasing factor test in the differential diagnosis of Cushing's syndrome: a comparison with the lysine-vasopressin test. Acta Endocrinol (Copenh) 1990;123(3):331–8.
[34] Reimondo G, Paccotti P, Minetto M, et al. The corticotrophin-releasing hormone test is the most reliable noninvasive method to differentiate pituitary from ectopic ACTH secretion in Cushing's syndrome. Clin Endocrinol (Oxf) 2003;58(6):718–24.
[35] Findling JW, Kehoe ME, Shaker JL, et al. Routine inferior petrosal sinus sampling in the differential diagnosis of adrenocorticotropin (ACTH)-dependent Cushing's syndrome: early recognition of the occult ectopic ACTH syndrome. J Clin Endocrinol Metab 1991;73(2): 408–13.
[36] Oldfield EH, Doppman JL, Nieman LK, et al. Petrosal sinus sampling with and without corticotropin-releasing hormone for the differential diagnosis of Cushing's syndrome. N Engl J Med 1991;325(13):897–905.
[37] Bonelli FS, Huston J III, Carpenter PC, et al. Adrenocorticotropic hormone-dependent Cushing's syndrome: sensitivity and specificity of inferior petrosal sinus sampling. AJNR Am J Neuroradiol 2000;21(4):690–6.
[38] Obuobie K, Davies JS, Ogunko A, et al. Venous thrombo-embolism following inferior petrosal sinus sampling in Cushing's disease. J Endocrinol Invest 2000;23(8):542–4.

[39] Lefournier V, Gatta B, Martinie M, et al. One transient neurological complication (sixth nerve palsy) in 166 consecutive inferior petrosal sinus samplings for the etiological diagnosis of Cushing's syndrome. J Clin Endocrinol Metab 1999;84(9):3401–2.
[40] Sturrock ND, Jeffcoate WJ. A neurological complication of inferior petrosal sinus sampling during investigation for Cushing's disease: a case report. J Neurol Neurosurg Psychiatry 1997;62(5):527–8.
[41] Miller DL, Doppman JL, Peterman SB, et al. Neurologic complications of petrosal sinus sampling. Radiology 1992;185(1):143–7.
[42] Kaltsas GA, Giannulis MG, Newell-Price JD, et al. A critical analysis of the value of simultaneous inferior petrosal sinus sampling in Cushing's disease and the occult ectopic adrenocorticotropin syndrome. J Clin Endocrinol Metab 1999;84(2):487–92.
[43] Doppman JL, Chang R, Oldfield EH, et al. The hypoplastic inferior petrosal sinus: a potential source of false-negative results in petrosal sampling for Cushing's disease. J Clin Endocrinol Metab 1999;84(2):533–40.
[44] Lienhardt A, Grossman AB, Dacie JE, et al. Relative contributions of inferior petrosal sinus sampling and pituitary imaging in the investigation of children and adolescents with ACTH-dependent Cushing's syndrome. J Clin Endocrinol Metab 2001;86(12):5711–4.
[45] Colao A, Faggiano A, Pivonello R, et al. Inferior petrosal sinus sampling in the differential diagnosis of Cushing's syndrome: results of an Italian multicenter study. Eur J Endocrinol 2001;144(5):499–507.
[46] Tsagarakis S, Kaskarelis IS, Kokkoris P, et al. The application of a combined stimulation with CRH and desmopressin during bilateral inferior petrosal sinus sampling in patients with Cushing's syndrome. Clin Endocrinol (Oxf) 2000;52(3):355–61.
[47] Invitti C, Giraldi FP, Cavagnini F. Inferior petrosal sinus sampling in patients with Cushing's syndrome and contradictory responses to dynamic testing. Clin Endocrinol (Oxf) 1999;51(2):255–7.
[48] Booth GL, Redelmeier DA, Grosman H, et al. Improved diagnostic accuracy of inferior petrosal sinus sampling over imaging for localizing pituitary pathology in patients with Cushing's disease. J Clin Endocrinol Metab 1998;83(7):2291–5.
[49] Lopez J, Barcelo B, Lucas T, et al. Petrosal sinus sampling for diagnosis of Cushing's disease: evidence of false negative results. Clin Endocrinol (Oxf) 1996;45(2):147–56.
[50] Yamamoto Y, Davis DH, Nippoldt TB, et al. False-positive inferior petrosal sinus sampling in the diagnosis of Cushing's disease. Report of two cases. J Neurosurg 1995;83(6):1087–91.
[51] Young J, Deneux C, Grino M, et al. Pitfall of petrosal sinus sampling in a Cushing's syndrome secondary to ectopic adrenocorticotropin-corticotropin releasing hormone (ACTH-CRH) secretion. J Clin Endocrinol Metab 1998;83(2):305–8.
[52] Findling J, Kehoe ME, Raff H. Identification of patients with Cushing's disease with negative pituitary adrenocorticotropin (ACTH) gradients during inferior petrosal sinus sampling: prolactin as an index of pituitary venous effluent. J Clin Endocrinol Metab 2004; 89:6005–9.
[53] Miller DL, Doppman JL, Nieman LK, et al. Petrosal sinus sampling: discordant lateralization of ACTH-secreting pituitary microadenomas before and after stimulation with corticotropin-releasing hormone. Radiology 1990;176(2):429–31.
[54] Newell-Price J, Trainer P, Besser M, et al. The diagnosis and differential diagnosis of Cushing's syndrome and pseudo-Cushing's states. Endocr Rev 1998;19(5):647–72.
[55] Doppman JL, Oldfield EH, Nieman LK. Bilateral sampling of the internal jugular vein to distinguish between mechanisms of adrenocorticotropic hormone-dependent Cushing syndrome. Ann Intern Med 1998;128(1):33–6.
[56] Erickson D, Huston J III, Young WF Jr, et al. Internal jugular vein sampling in adrenocorticotropic hormone-dependent Cushing's syndrome: a comparison with inferior petrosal sinus sampling. Clin Endocrinol (Oxf) 2004;60(4):413–9.
[57] Teramoto A, Nemoto S, Takakura K, et al. Selective venous sampling directly from cavernous sinus in Cushing's syndrome. J Clin Endocrinol Metab 1993;76(3):637–41.

[58] Doppman JL, Nieman LK, Chang R, et al. Selective venous sampling from the cavernous sinuses is not a more reliable technique than sampling from the inferior petrosal sinuses in Cushing's syndrome. J Clin Endocrinol Metab 1995;80(8):2485–9.

[59] Graham KE, Samuels MH, Nesbit GM, et al. Cavernous sinus sampling is highly accurate in distinguishing Cushing's disease from the ectopic adrenocorticotropin syndrome and in predicting intrapituitary tumor location. J Clin Endocrinol Metab 1999;84(5):1602–10.

[60] Oliverio PJ, Monsein LH, Wand GS, et al. Bilateral simultaneous cavernous sinus sampling using corticotropin-releasing hormone in the evaluation of Cushing disease. AJNR Am J Neuroradiol 1996;17(9):1669–74.

[61] Teramoto A, Yoshida Y, Sanno N, et al. Cavernous sinus sampling in patients with adrenocorticotrophic hormone-dependent Cushing's syndrome with emphasis on inter- and intracavernous adrenocorticotrophic hormone gradients. J Neurosurg 1998;89(5):762–8.

[62] Mamelak AN, Dowd CF, Tyrrell JB, et al. Venous angiography is needed to interpret inferior petrosal sinus and cavernous sinus sampling data for lateralizing adrenocorticotropin-secreting adenomas. J Clin Endocrinol Metab 1996;81(2):475–81.

[63] Lefournier V, Martinie M, Vasdev A, et al. Accuracy of bilateral inferior petrosal or cavernous sinuses sampling in predicting the lateralization of Cushing's disease pituitary microadenoma: influence of catheter position and anatomy of venous drainage. J Clin Endocrinol Metab 2003;88(1):196–203.

[64] Boscaro M, Barzon L, Fallo F, et al. Cushing's syndrome. Lancet 2001;357(9258):783–91.

[65] Dwyer AJ, Frank JA, Doppman JL, et al. Pituitary adenomas in patients with Cushing disease: initial experience with Gd-DTPA-enhanced MR imaging. Radiology 1987;163(2): 421–6.

[66] Doppman JL, Frank JA, Dwyer AJ, et al. Gadolinium DTPA enhanced MR imaging of ACTH-secreting microadenomas of the pituitary gland. J Comput Assist Tomogr 1988; 12(5):728–35.

[67] Tabarin A, Laurent F, Catargi B, et al. Comparative evaluation of conventional and dynamic magnetic resonance imaging of the pituitary gland for the diagnosis of Cushing's disease. Clin Endocrinol (Oxf) 1998;49(3):293–300.

[68] Patronas N, Bulakbasi N, Stratakis CA, et al. Spoiled gradient recalled acquisition in the steady state technique is superior to conventional postcontrast spin echo technique for magnetic resonance imaging detection of adrenocorticotropin-secreting pituitary tumors. J Clin Endocrinol Metab 2003;88(4):1565–9.

[69] Colombo N, Loli P, Vignati F, et al. MR of corticotropin-secreting pituitary microadenomas. AJNR Am J Neuroradiol 1994;15(8):1591–5.

[70] de Herder WW, Uitterlinden P, Pieterman H, et al. Pituitary tumour localization in patients with Cushing's disease by magnetic resonance imaging. Is there a place for petrosal sinus sampling? Clin Endocrinol (Oxf) 1994;40(1):87–92.

[71] Elster AD. Sellar susceptibility artifacts: theory and implications. AJNR Am J Neuroradiol 1993;14(1):129–36.

[72] Hall WA, Luciano MG, Doppman JL, et al. Pituitary magnetic resonance imaging in normal human volunteers: occult adenomas in the general population. Ann Intern Med 1994; 120(10):817–20.

[73] Arnaldi G, Mancini T, Kola B, et al. Cyclical Cushing's syndrome in a patient with a bronchial neuroendocrine tumor (typical carcinoid) expressing ghrelin and growth hormone secretagogue receptors. J Clin Endocrinol Metab 2003;88(12):5834–40.

[74] Stadnik T, Stevenaert A, Beckers A, et al. Pituitary microadenomas: diagnosis with two-and three-dimensional MR imaging at 1.5 T before and after injection of gadolinium. Radiology 1990;176(2):419–28.

[75] Perry RR, Nieman LK, Cutler GB Jr, et al. Primary adrenal causes of Cushing's syndrome. Diagnosis and surgical management. Ann Surg 1989;210(1):59–68.

[76] NIH state-of-the-science statement on management of the clinically inapparent adrenal mass ("incidentaloma"). NIH Consens State Sci Statements 2002;19(2):1–25.

[77] Grumbach MM, Biller BM, Braunstein GD, et al. Management of the clinically inapparent adrenal mass ("incidentaloma"). Ann Intern Med 2003;138(5):424–9.
[78] Mansmann G, Lau J, Balk E, et al. The clinically inapparent adrenal mass: update in diagnosis and management. Endocr Rev 2004;25(2):309–40.
[79] Doppman JL, Travis WD, Nieman L, et al. Cushing syndrome due to primary pigmented nodular adrenocortical disease: findings at CT and MR imaging. Radiology 1989;172(2): 415–20.
[80] Doppman JL, Nieman L, Miller DL, et al. Ectopic adrenocorticotropic hormone syndrome: localization studies in 28 patients. Radiology 1989;172(1):115–24.
[81] Granberg D, Sundin A, Janson ET, et al. Octreoscan in patients with bronchial carcinoid tumours. Clin Endocrinol (Oxf) 2003;59(6):793–9.
[82] Torpy DJ, Chen CC, Mullen N, et al. Lack of utility of (111)In-pentetreotide scintigraphy in localizing ectopic ACTH producing tumors: follow-up of 18 patients. J Clin Endocrinol Metab 1999;84(4):1186–92.
[83] Pacak K, Ilias I, Chen CC, et al. The role of [(18)F]fluorodeoxyglucose positron emission tomography and [(111)In]-diethylenetriaminepentaacetate-D-Phe-pentetreotide scintigraphy in the localization of ectopic adrenocorticotropin-secreting tumors causing Cushing's syndrome. J Clin Endocrinol Metab 2004;89(5):2214–21.
[84] Tsagarakis S, Christoforaki M, Giannopoulou H, et al. A reappraisal of the utility of somatostatin receptor scintigraphy in patients with ectopic adrenocorticotropin Cushing's syndrome. J Clin Endocrinol Metab 2003;88(10):4754–8.
[85] Tabarin A, Valli N, Chanson P, et al. Usefulness of somatostatin receptor scintigraphy in patients with occult ectopic adrenocorticotropin syndrome. J Clin Endocrinol Metab 1999; 84(4):1193–202.
[86] Granberg D, Sundin A, Janson ET, et al. Octreoscan in patients with bronchial carcinoid tumours. Clin Endocrinol (Oxf) 2003;59(6):793–9.
[87] Catargi B, Rigalleau V, Poussin A, et al. Occult Cushing's syndrome in type-2 diabetes. J Clin Endocrinol Metab 2003;88(12):5808–13.
[88] Phlipponneau M, Nocaudie M, Epelbaum J, et al. Somatostatin analogs for the localization and preoperative treatment of an adrenocorticotropin-secreting bronchial carcinoid tumor. J Clin Endocrinol Metab 1994;78(1):20–4.
[89] Ilias I, Nieman LK. Cushing Syndrome due to ectopic ACTH secretion: two decades' experience at a single center. Presented at the Endocrine Society 84th Annual Meeting, San Francisco, California, June 19–22, 2002. 2002: Program and abstracts, OR 49–4, p. 131.

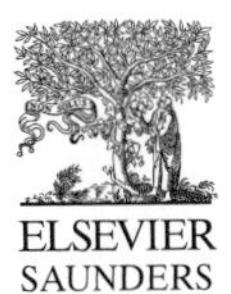

ELSEVIER
SAUNDERS

Endocrinol Metab Clin N Am
34 (2005) 423–439

ENDOCRINOLOGY
AND METABOLISM
CLINICS
OF NORTH AMERICA

Subclinical Cushing's Syndrome in Adrenal Incidentalomas

Massimo Terzolo, MD[a,*], Silvia Bovio, MD[a], Giuseppe Reimondo, MD[a], Anna Pia, MD[b], Giangiacomo Osella, MD[a], Giorgio Borretta, MD[b], Alberto Angeli, MD[a]

[a]*Division of Internal Medicine, University of Turin, Azienda Sanitaria Ospedaliera San Luigi, Regione Gonzole, 10, 10043 Orbassano, Italy*
[b]*Division of Endocrinology, Azienda Ospedaliera Santa Croce e Carle, Cuneo, Italy*

Subclinical Cushing's syndrome is a topic of recent interest and controversy, because the serendipitous discovery of an adrenal mass has become an increasingly frequent event owing to the routine use of sophisticated radiologic techniques. Clinically inapparent adrenal masses are detected inadvertently, in the course of work-up or treatment of unrelated disorders, and they commonly are referred to as adrenal incidentalomas [1–3]. The term adrenal incidentaloma is an umbrella definition encompassing a spectrum of different pathologic entities that share the same path of discovery; adrenal adenoma is the most frequent type of incidental mass [1–3].

That adrenal incidentaloma and the related condition of subclinical Cushing's syndrome are receiving broader attention is justified by the fact that adrenal adenoma is one of the most common tumors in people, and its prevalence increases with age. Therefore, appropriate management of adrenal incidentalomas will be a growing public health challenge for society as it ages, also because there is increased attention toward subclinical diseases [2,3]. Accordingly, the identification of patients who have subclinical Cushing's syndrome may provide an opportunity for early treatment of a notoriously dangerous disease, while recent refinements in the field of minimally invasive surgery have rendered adrenalectomy easier to perform. The financial aspect of

This work was partially funded by the Ministero dell'Università e della Ricerca Scientifica e Tecnologica (grant no. 2001062719_004).

* Corresponding author.
E-mail address: terzolo@usa.net (M. Terzolo).

doi:10.1016/j.ecl.2005.01.008 *endo.theclinics.com*

the problem has to be evaluated carefully, because the serendipitous detection of an adrenal mass will be growing in the future because of further advances in radiologic techniques [4,5].

Definition

Subclinical Cushing's syndrome occurs in patients who have clinically nonfunctioning adrenal adenomas when cortisol secretion becomes autonomous and dysregulated, not fully restrained by pituitary feedback. Previously, the term preclinical Cushing's syndrome often was used interchangeably with subclinical Cushing's syndrome in the literature. As proposed by Ross [6], the term subclinical Cushing's syndrome is probably more accurate, not implying any assumption on the evolution toward clinically overt hypercortisolism. It is unlikely that subclinical hypercortisolism is a preclinical state of a patent glucocorticoid excess, because the prevalence data of Cushing's syndrome caused by adrenal adenoma and silent hypercortisolism in clinically inapparent adrenal adenoma greatly differ [6].

At the recent National Institutes of Health (NIH) State-of-the-Science Conference, it was concluded that a better term for this condition might be "subclinical autonomous glucocorticoid hypersecretion" [2]. Notwithstanding semantic discussions, the definition of subclinical Cushing's syndrome is based upon fulfillment of two criteria.

First, the patient should not present a clear Cushing phenotype, even if some physical stigmata suggestive of hypercortisolism (eg, facial fullness and central obesity) can be identified with a careful second examination after detection of an adrenal mass [7]. This is a critical issue that escapes standardization but depends on individual clinical judgment and personal practice. It may be anticipated that physicians who have less expertise with Cushing's syndrome patients might overlook (mild) signs of hypercortisolism and pursue evaluation of adrenal function only following the (incidental) discovery of an adrenal mass. In the authors' experience, a few patients referred for an adrenal incidentaloma actually displayed a previously unrecognized Cushingoid habitus; in a couple of such patients, Cushing's syndrome was even corticotropin (ACTH)-dependent.

Second, the patient should harbor an adrenal mass detected serendipitously. Although argumentation concerning the clinical consequences of subclinical hypercortisolism may be pertinent also to pituitary incidentaloma [8] and over-replacement of adrenal steroid therapy [9], subclinical Cushing's syndrome commonly is associated with adrenal incidentaloma. Cortical adenoma is by far the leading cause of subtle glucocorticoid excess; however, it also may be demonstrated in some patients who have adrenocortical carcinoma [10,11] and, exceptionally, noncortical mass such as myelolipoma [12]. The study of subclinical endocrine dysfunction is usually less attractive in patients who have adrenocortical carcinoma because of the natural history of the tumor [13]. In the case of myelolipoma, pathologic examination demonstrates a mixed tumor with interspersed adrenocortical cells [12].

Diagnostic strategies

Although the pathophysiologic concept of autonomous cortisol secretion by an adrenal adenoma is straightforward, demonstration of subclinical Cushing's syndrome remains an elusive goal. The diagnostic process of subclinical cortisol excess may prove to be challenging for physicians and their patients for biologic or methodologic reasons.

First, the degree of hypercortisolism only slightly exceeds the physiologic daily production rate of cortisol and is distributed continuously among different patients, because there is a spectrum of variability from non-functioning adenoma to autonomous cortisol-producing adrenal adenoma [2,7]. As a consequence, several different alterations in the endocrine tests aimed at assessing the function of the hypothalamic–pituitary–adrenal (HPA) axis may be found in such patients [7,14–16].

Second, the study of subclinical cortisol excess is pursued by means of the standard biochemical tests used in the screening of Cushing's syndrome that are ill-suited to assessing patients who have only aspecific signs of hypercortisolism, such as hypertension, diabetes, or obesity, if any [6,17]. In the absence of reliable clinical clues, it is hard to distinguish between true-positive and false-positive test results. Moreover, the frequency of subclinical hypercortisolism among patients who have adrenal incidentaloma is roughly comparable with the false-positive rate of the tests used for screening for overt Cushing's syndrome. Therefore, confusion because of methodologic issues adds to the intrinsic biologic variability of silent cortisol excess precluding definition of a uniform entity.

In the literature, the prevalence of subclinical Cushing's syndrome ranged from 5% to 20% [2,14–16,18–22]. This discrepancy is hardly surprising, because the percentage of patients who qualify for this endocrine disorder is highly dependent on the endocrine protocols (testing methods) and criteria used to define subclinical cortisol excess (Table 1). Various endocrine algorithms with disparate assumptions can be found in different series that are also heterogeneous as to sample size and inclusion criteria [1–3,7,22]. Some conclusions, however, can be drawn from the larger series.

Loss of the physiologic circadian rhythm of cortisol, with a blunted nyctohemeral variation, was reported frequently, despite normal baseline cortisol levels [14,16,19,30]. An increase in urinary-free cortisol (UFC) excretion was found less frequently [15,16,21,26,30,33], and this confirms the view that measurement of UFC has insufficient sensitivity to detect mild hypercortisolism [51]. Cortisol excess might be minimal but sufficient to suppress ACTH secretion, as low-to-undetectable ACTH levels were reported repeatedly in clinically inapparent adrenal tumors [14–16,19–21].

Table 1
Alterations of the hypothalamic–pituitary–adrenal axis and prevalence of subclinical Cushing's syndrome in patients who have adrenal incidentaloma

		%				
First author, year [Ref. no.]	No. of patients	Increased UFC	Low ACTH	High cortisol after DST[a]	Low ACTH after CRH	SCS prevalence
Virkkala, 1989 [23]	20	NA	NA	NA	NA	25
Hensen, 1990 [24]	13	0	15	23	100	8.0
Herrera, 1991 [25]	172	NA	NA	1.1[b]	NA	1.1
Jockenhövel, 1992 [26]	18	5.5	5.5	50[b]	NR	5.5
Reincke, 1992 [14]	66	1.5	7.5	12[c]	7.5	12
Aso, 1992 [27]	210	NR	NR	NR	NR	3.3
Kobayashi, 1993 [28]	14	50[d]	NR	50[b]	NR	50
Siren, 1993 [29]	36	NA	NA	NA	NA	5.5
Caplan, 1994 [20]	26	NA	11	NA	NA	11
Osella, 1994 [30]	45	2	NA	15	22	16
Seppel, 1994 [31]	52	NA	NA	NA	NA	1.9
Flecchia, 1995 [32]	24	21	25	17	NR	29
Ambrosi, 1995 [15]	32	12	3	14	33	12
Bencsik, 1996 [33]	63	NA	NA	NA	NA	21
Bardet, 1996 [34]	35	11	21	13[b]	33	8.5
Linos, 1996 [35]	57	0	NR	13	NR	8.8
Bastounis, 1997 [36]	86	NA	NA	NA	NA	3.5
Bondanelli, 1997 [11]	38	2.6	18	10[c]	8	10
Kasperlik-Zaluska, 1997 [37]	208	5.2[d]	34	3.0[c]	17	2.9
Proye, 1998 [38]	103	NR	NR	NR	NR	0
Terzolo, 1998 [16]	53	7.5	9.4	17	NR	6.0
Murai, 1999 [39]	59	NR	NR	NR	NR	1.7
Tutuncu, 1999 [40]	33	NR	NR	NR	NR	6.1
Rossi, 2000 [41]	65	17	23	25	NR	18.4
Mantero, 2000 [42]	1004	11	15	10	17	9.2
Morioka, 2000 [43]	56	3.6[d]	7.1	11	33	12.5
Favia, 2000 [44]	158	NR	NR	5.1	NR	5.1
Tanabe, 2001 [45]	38	NR	26	47[e]	31	47
Midorikawa, 2001 [46]	20	20[d]	15	25	62	20
Grossrubatscher, 2001 [47]	53	4.0[d]	15	11	NR	5.7
Valli, 2001 [48]	31	61	26	39	NR	31.4
Barzon, 2002 [49]	284	NR	NR	NR	NR	11.3
Bulow, 2002 [50]	381	0.8	NR	1.0	NR	1.0

Abbreviations: DST, dexamethasone suppression test; NA, not available; NR, not reported; SCS, subclinical Cushing's syndrome.

[a] DST is the 1 mg overnight test with a threshold for cortisol suppression at 5.0 μg/dL unless specified otherwise.

[b] 2 mg DST.

[c] 8 mg DST.

[d] Urinary 17-hydroxycorticosteroid.

[e] Threshold for cortisol suppression at 3.0 μg/dL.

Technical problems concerning measurement of ACTH concentrations close to the detection limits of the assay should be recognized [51]. The response of ACTH and cortisol to CRH also may be blunted in these patients, but CRH challenge did not add significant information to baseline ACTH levels [14–16,30]. In the authors' experience, interpretation of CRH test is confounded by the wide scattering of ACTH and cortisol responses and by their divergent patterns in some patients [30,52]. A reduction in dehydroepiandrosterone sulfate (DHEAS) concentration, which is possibly the most frequent hormonal finding in patients who have adrenal incidentalomas [15,30,32–34,53], was thought to reflect suppression of ACTH secretion by autonomous cortisol production [32,30]. Conflicting data, however, have come from the studies that correlated DHEAS concentration with other test results [33,52,53]. At present, there is insufficient information to conclude that low DHEAS concentration is a reliable, indirect marker of autonomous cortisol secretion [30,53]. Moreover, DHEAS secretion declines with age physiologically, and this may hamper recognition of reduced DHEAS concentrations in an aged population [30].

Dexamethasone suppression tests (DSTs) were employed extensively to screen for subclinical hypercortisolism in patients who had adrenal incidentaloma. Test protocols, however, differed with regard to dexamethasone dose and threshold value for adequate cortisol suppression. The NIH state-of-the-science conference panel recommended the 1 mg DST as the standard for screening autonomous cortisol secretion [2]. Previously, most endocrinologists used either an overnight 1 mg or a standard low-dose suppression test [28,53]. The classical 2-day test may be more accurate than the overnight test [54], but it is also more difficult to perform in everyday practice. Definition of adequate cortisol suppression to dexamethasone is arguably one of the most controversial issues. The traditional threshold of 5 μg/dL (138 nmol/L) was recommended in the NIH consensus statement [2]; however, some experts proposed using lower cut points to increase the detection of subclinical hypercortisolism [55]. The rationale for this choice is that in most healthy subjects, cortisol is barely detectable following 1 mg of dexamethasone [55,56]; thus, in a recent consensus statement on the diagnosis of Cushing's syndrome, the cut-off level was reduced to below 1.8 μg/dL (50 nmol/L) [51]. Specificity, however, decreases when lower postdexamethasone cortisol values are used, which may yield more false-positive test results; thus, other authors suggested employing high-dose dexamethasone tests (3 or even 8 mg), because the diagnosis of pituitary Cushing's syndrome is not a consideration [14,17]. At present, there is insufficient evidence to solve these controversies. Using the overnight 1 mg suppression test for screening purposes seems sound, however, because this test is designed specifically for diagnosing hypercortisolism, while there is less experience in using high-dose dexamethasone tests in settings other than the differential diagnosis of Cushing's syndrome.

Functional autonomy of clinically inapparent adrenal adenomas may be depicted in vivo by iodocholesterol scintigraphy with a typical imaging pattern of unilateral tracer uptake in the adenoma and absent uptake in the contralateral adrenal gland. Several studies correlated the scintigraphic pattern of unilateral uptake with cortisol hypersecretion by the adenoma and consequent pituitary ACTH suppression [1,10,34,57]. Scintigraphic uptake represents a very precocious sign of functional autonomy, because NP-59 uptake on the side of the mass with nonvisualization of the contralateral adrenal gland (concordant uptake) may occur despite overall normal biochemical tests [16,30]. The specificity of this finding was questioned, as it was argued that increased uptake simply reflects the presence of enlarged adrenal tissue [30,58]. Adrenal scintigraphy, however, is a time-consuming and expensive technique that is not widely available; thus, its use has not gained general acceptance outside research settings.

To circumvent the problem of false positivity of biochemical testing, some experts advocated that two concomitant alterations should be demonstrated to diagnose a patient who has subclinical Cushing's syndrome [10,15,16,42]. Several possible combinations of abnormal tests may be found when the HPA axis is studied in detail [14–16,30], and it remains difficult, even with this approach, to define the entity of cortisol excess truly relevant to assume subclinical Cushing's syndrome. The current debate and confusion on what strategy is best suited to detect adrenal cortical autonomy might be concluded by finding at what point cortisol excess does lead to clinical morbidity. The response is shrouded in uncertainty, because there is only limited knowledge on the natural history of adrenal incidentalomas [17].

Long-term consequences

There is a wealth of data on the endocrine features of clinically inapparent adrenal adenomas, but there is still scant information on the detrimental effects, if any, of silent hypercortisolism [7,59–61]. Notwithstanding uncertainty regarding ascertainment of subclinical Cushing's syndrome, there is no doubt that many patients who have clinically inapparent adrenal adenoma can be exposed to a chronic, albeit slight, cortisol excess [5]. Thus, it is biologically plausible to assume that they should suffer, at least to some extent, from the classic long-term complications of full-blown Cushing's syndrome, such as arterial hypertension, obesity, or diabetes, which cluster in the metabolic syndrome [51,62].

The relationship between these diseases and unsuspected adrenal adenomas was investigated in autopsy studies that produced controversial results [1]. In a multi-institutional survey performed in Italy, which collected 1004 patients who had adrenal incidentaloma, the prevalence of arterial hypertension, diabetes, and obesity was remarkably high, with a rate of 41%, 10%, and 28%, respectively [42]. However, the interpretation of these data is partially confounded by the retrospective nature of the study, the possibility

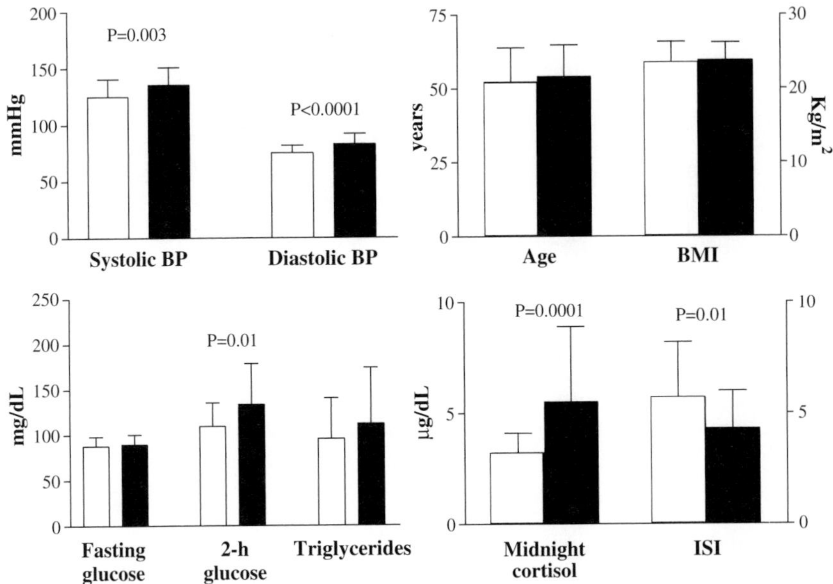

Fig. 1. Comparison of 41 patients who have clinically inapparent adrenal adenoma (*solid bar*) and 41 patients who have euthyroid multinodular goiter, who served as controls (*open bar*), in terms of clinical and biochemical variables. (*Data from* Terzolo M, Pia A, Alì A, et al. Adrenal incidentaloma: a new cause of the metabolic syndrome? Clin Endocrinol Metab 2002;87:998–1003.) BP, blood pressure.

of referral bias, and the large prevalence of these diseases in the general population. In a cross-sectional study, the authors recently demonstrated that nonobese, normoglycemic patients who had clinically inapparent adrenal adenoma had frequent occurrence of impaired glucose tolerance (IGT), elevated blood pressure, and reduced insulin sensitivity compared with matched controls (Fig. 1) [63]. Such alterations were not restricted to patients who had subclinical Cushing's syndrome; however, they were more marked in such patients than in those harboring nonfunctioning adenoma (Fig. 2). A significant inverse correlation was found between values of the OGTT-derived insulin sensitivity index and midnight serum cortisol concentrations [63].

The results of this study confirm and extend those previously obtained by Fernandez-Real et al [64] in an uncontrolled study, and by Garrapa et al [65] in a case–control study. Fernandez-Real et al [64] found a remarkably high prevalence of IGT or unknown diabetes among patients who had non-functioning adrenal tumors, whereas Garrapa et al [65] found increased visceral fat mass along with IGT and hyperinsulinemia in an analogous cohort of patients. They reported that the degree of metabolic and body fat alterations was intermediate between that of controls and patients who had overt Cushing's syndrome [65]. More recently, Tauchmanova et al [66] found

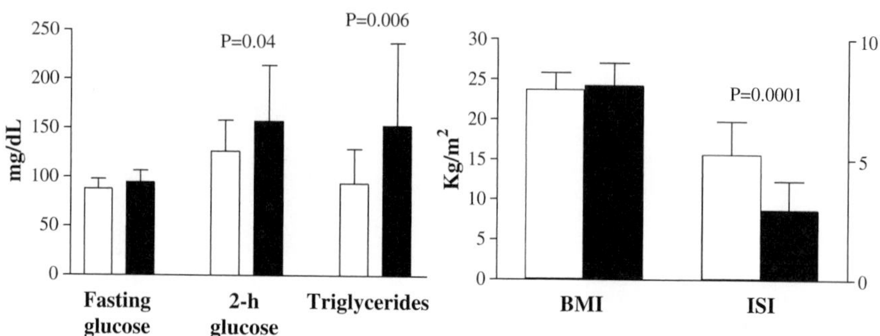

Fig. 2. Comparison of patients who have clinically inapparent adrenal adenoma by the functional status, subclinical Cushing's syndrome (n = 12, *solid bar*) and nonfunctioning adrenal adenoma (n = 29, *open bar*). (*Data from* Terzolo M, Pia A, Alì A, et al. Adrenal incidentaloma: a new cause of the metabolic syndrome? Clin Endocrinol Metab 2002;87:998–1003.)

that 28 of 126 subjects who adrenal incidentaloma and met the criteria for subclinical Cushing's syndrome, sustained an adverse cardiovascular and metabolic risk profile because of elevated blood pressure, greater waist-to-hip ratio, higher triglycerides, total and low-density lipoprotein (LDL) cholesterol and fibrinogen levels, elevation of the homeostasis model assessment (HOMA) index, and an exceedingly high prevalence of IGT or diabetes mellitus compared with matched controls. The impact of these abnormalities upon the vascular system was documented by significant changes in carotid intimal–medial thickness [66].

Overall, several lines of evidence from different studies consistently support the view that subclinical Cushing's syndrome may be associated with the clinical phenotype of the insulin resistance syndrome that fosters several unwanted metabolic and vascular manifestations [5]. There are limitations, however, in the studies that should be addressed for a meaningful appraisal of the data. First, caution should be taken in generalizing results from series gathered in academic centers. Additionally, referral bias is an obvious issue, because they are not population-based studies. Second, there is the potential of confounding because of the case–control design. The complexity of an accurate matching between patients and controls for the many factors that may affect cardiovascular risk should be disclosed. Third, in none of the studies was assessment of insulin sensitivity based on the use of the glucose clamp technique, which is considered the gold standard [67]. The surrogate markers employed, however, were validated previously for epidemiologic studies. Fourth, the published series are not large, but protocols are similar, and data are remarkably consistent across studies. An alternative hypothesis that adrenal incidentaloma itself may be an unrecognized manifestation of the metabolic syndrome cannot be ruled out [68], even if a causal link between subclinical Cushing's syndrome and insulin resistance is the most plausible explanation for the available data [5].

Demonstration of end-organ complications linked to silent hypercortisolism adds strength to the concept of subclinical Cushing's syndrome, which otherwise remains a condition whose definition is somewhat arbitrary, being established only on a biochemical basis [5]. In this line of research, the authors tried to correlate endocrine data and clinical phenotype of patients who had incidentally detected adrenal adenoma. Preliminary results suggest that some features of the metabolic syndrome cluster in the patients who have elevated midnight cortisol concentration [69]. The presence of a relationship between elevated midnight cortisol concentration and metabolic and vascular alterations does not establish causality; however, these data are in agreement with previous observations of the authors' group, suggesting that midnight serum cortisol may be viewed as a surrogate marker of insulin sensitivity in patients who have clinically inapparent adrenal adenoma [63]. Interestingly, the authors found that elevation of midnight serum cortisol was one of the most frequent alterations of the HPA axis in such patients. This is biologically plausible, because high late-night cortisol levels appear to be the earliest and most sensitive marker for Cushing's syndrome, so that it has been exploited as a diagnostic tool [51,70–72]. Moreover, silent hypercortisolism may be characterized more frequently by a qualitative rather than quantitative alteration of cortisol secretion [30].

There is evidence that the slight amount of cortisol excess caused by clinically inapparent adrenal adenomas, even if insufficient to give a full-blown Cushingoid phenotype, may promote development of insulin resistance and its attendant clinical manifestations. Subclinical hypercortisolism may prove to be harmful, particularly to individuals who express other (genetically determined or acquired) risk factors, and it may play an important role in accelerating the atherosclerosis process [5]. Even if it is held that the metabolic syndrome is associated with enhanced all-cause and cardiovascular mortality [73,74], evidence of increased morbidity and mortality in patients who have clinically inapparent adrenal adenoma and subclinical Cushing's syndrome or not, is lacking. The (scarce) available data suggest that most patients who have adrenal incidentaloma remain asymptomatic throughout life [7,75], but the existing follow-up studies have focused almost exclusively on imaging and endocrine work-up protocols. Prospective studies addressing more appropriate outcome measures, such as disease-specific or all-cause mortality, are needed. These studies may be unfeasible, however, if not by means of multi-institutional collaboration, because of the low frequency of disease-specific outcomes.

Osteoporosis is another established consequence of overt cortisol excess [51], but data on bone mineral density in patients who have clinically inapparent adrenal adenoma are controversial. A research group reported that patients who have subclinical Cushing's syndrome have reduced bone mass in eugonadal and hypogonadal subjects [76–78], while another research group published conflicting data [41,79]. Additionally, the authors did not find any difference in bone mass density between patients and controls, or between patients who had or did not have subclinical hypercortisolism [80]. Differences in the devices used to estimate bone density and in selection criteria of either patients or controls, along with the small number of subjects studied, are likely explanations for the divergent results. There is limited evidence that women who have subclinical Cushing's syndrome are exposed to a higher risk of vertebral fractures independent of their gonadal status [81]. Longitudinal studies of adequate statistical power are mandatory to estimate the risk of osteoporotic fractures that affect outcome and quality of life.

The studies that evaluated the risk of progression from subclinical to overt Cushing's syndrome are as a whole reassuring and demonstrate that the clinical evolution of silent hypercortisolism occurs rarely, if ever. Development of the overt clinical syndrome during follow-up was observed in a negligible number of cases, while appearance of silent biochemical alterations was reported in a percentage ranging from 0% to 11% across different studies [22]. Masses of 3 cm or greater are more likely to develop silent hyperfunction than smaller tumors, and the risk seems to plateau after 3 to 4 years, even if it does not subside completely [75,82]. On the other hand, the authors observed spontaneous normalization of subclinical hypercortisolism in some patients, and this finding raises the possibility that cortisol output by an adrenal adenoma may be variable over the course of time [16]. Interpretation of these follow-up studies is affected by their small sample size, variable length of follow-up, and variable follow-up strategies. The potential for ascertainment bias also should be disclosed, because many of these observations are made in small, retrospective series. The limited and incomplete evidence available precludes making any stringent recommendation for periodic hormonal testing. One current approach is an overnight 1 mg DST at yearly intervals, or earlier if clinically indicated [2]. Also the issue of progression over time of metabolic derangements that could be attributable to subclinical Cushing's syndrome remains unsolved by the available studies.

Management strategies

In the era of evidence-based medicine, the long-term complications of incidentally discovered adrenal adenomas remain virtually unknown and, consequently, the management of such tumors is largely empirical. There is little evidence of a relatively high mortality rate caused by cardiovascular disease in patients who have adrenal incidentaloma, but the studies have limited power and suffer from several methodologic limits [83,84]. Either adrenalectomy or careful observation was suggested as a treatment option in patients who have clinically inapparent adrenal adenoma. Patients who have subclinical hypercortisolism should receive perioperative glucocorticoids after removal of the functioning mass, because they are at risk for hypoadrenalism [1–3]. They should be monitored for subsequent HPA axis recovery and clinical improvement. It is difficult, however, to predict the risk of postoperative adrenal insufficiency on the basis of endocrine and scintigraphic data; thus, a short course of steroid coverage is recommended in all patients after adrenalectomy [60]. Steroids should be discontinued after demonstration of an intact HPA axis according to established work-up protocols [85]. Guidelines for follow-up of patients who do not undergo adrenalectomy have not been defined.

Although adrenalectomy has been demonstrated to correct the biochemical abnormalities, its effect on long-term outcome and quality of life is unknown [4]. Preliminary results suggest that adrenalectomy may ameliorate the cardiovascular risk profile of patients who have subclinical Cushing's syndrome, but data remain inconsistent [7,46,66]. Even if these data were confirmed in larger prospective series, it is unlikely that any patient who has subclinical Cushing's syndrome would benefit from surgery [5,60].

As previously mentioned, autonomous cortisol secretion by the tumor and its attendant detrimental effects may vary greatly across different individuals. Moreover, if the aim is to prevent metabolic and cardiovascular events, surgery should be compared in terms of risk, cost, and outcome with the other possible interventions, including life-style changes and pharmacologic intervention. An optimal preventive measure should be harmless for patients, but this is not the case with adrenalectomy, even when performed by laparoscopic technique. Indeed, in experienced hands laparoscopic adrenalectomy has relatively little morbidity and minimal (but not zero) mortality, but experience is critical, and there is a learning curve [86]. Thus, performing surgery on more people has the potential to cause considerable morbidity, even if it is a safe procedure [4]. Conversely, there is ample evidence of the benefits of drug intervention for treating several clinical manifestations of the metabolic syndrome.

Until the risks and benefits of surgical removal of silent hyperfunctioning adrenal adenomas are elucidated, clinicians should elect to surgery patients who have subclinical Cushing's syndrome who display diseases potentially attributable to cortisol excess that are of recent onset or are resistant to medical intervention. This strategy is based purely on pragmatism and not evidence. The time course of the attendant disorders may be important for the surgical choice, however, because it is held that established complications of overt Cushing's syndrome do not resolve fully after successful surgery [87]. Patients who are not candidates for surgery (possibly most patients) should be enrolled in a program of regular and careful follow-up to detect, treat, and control hypertension, diabetes, dyslipidemia, and other manifestations of the metabolic syndrome. These disorders should be treated aggressively with drugs that are of proven benefit in preventing cardiovascular events [5]. Because the metabolic syndrome is directly responsible for the cardiovascular risk of patients who have clinically inapparent adrenal adenoma, therapeutic efforts should be directed toward the real culprit.

Summary

The incidental discovery of an adrenal mass is a frequent event owing to the routine use of sophisticated radiologic techniques. The potential harm to health associated with incidentally discovered cortical adenoma, the most frequent tumor among adrenal incidentalomas, is unclear at present. As a consequence, diagnostic algorithms and management strategies vary widely across different centers. Incidentally discovered adrenal adenoma may secrete cortisol autonomously, in a way that is no longer under close control by pituitary feedback in 5% to 20% of cases. Exhaustive endocrine evaluation may provide a wide spectrum of results, because subclinical Cushing's syndrome is a heterogeneous condition.

Data are insufficient to estimate the outcome of patients who have subclinical Cushing's syndrome. Evidence, however, is gathering that subclinical Cushing's syndrome may contribute to developing the phenotype of insulin resistance, thus portending to atherosclerosis and relevant cardiovascular complications. It is tempting to speculate that subclinical Cushing's syndrome represents a very mild variant of endogenous glucocorticoid excess syndrome sharing similar target organ damages and long-term complications with the full-blown variant (Fig. 3). Even if progression to overt glucocorticoid excess is rare, subclinical Cushing's syndrome has the potential to carry an adverse prognosis. A critical issue, however, is whether precocious diagnosis and treatment are more effective in paucisymptomatic patients and whether the beneficial effects justify the costs incurred. Data are insufficient to indicate the superiority of a surgical

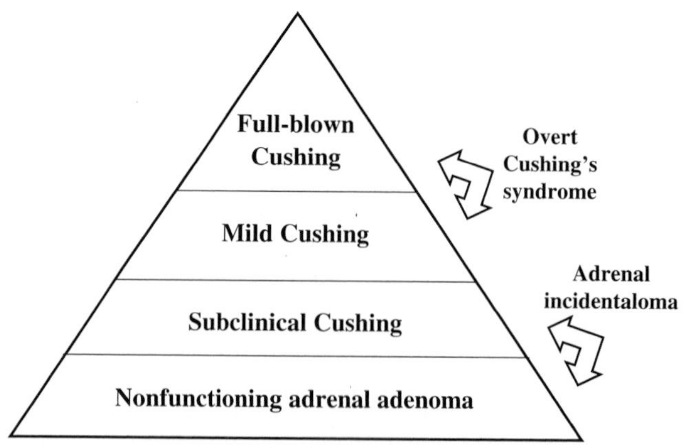

Fig. 3. The spectrum of hypercortisolism.

Box 1. Research agenda

- Identify biochemical markers of cortisol excess predictive of target-organ damage
- Identify a subset of patients at increased risk of adverse outcome
- Compare surgery versus medical treatment on predefined outcomes (cardiovascular morbidity or surrogate endpoints)
- Establish cost-effective follow-up schedules for imaging and biochemical work-up of patients managed conservatively

or nonsurgical approach to manage patients who have subclinical hyperfunctioning adrenal cortical adenoma.

As was concluded at the NIH consensus conference, additional research is needed to guide practice [2]. It is of the utmost importance to establish collaborative prospective studies with clearly defined entry criteria and standardized evaluation protocols and treatment modalities to appraise the natural history and long-term morbidity of clinically inapparent adrenal adenoma and subclinical Cushing's syndrome. A possible research agenda is drafted in (Box 1).

References

[1] Kloos RT, Gross MD, Francis IR, et al. Incidentally discovered adrenal masses. Endocr Rev 1995;16:460–84.
[2] Grumbach MM, Biller BMK, Braunstein GD, et al. Management of the clinically inapparent adrenal mass (incidentaloma). Ann Intern Med 2003;138:424–9.
[3] Mansmann G, Lau J, Balk E, et al. The clinically inapparent adrenal mass: update in diagnosis and management. Endocr Rev 2004;25(2):309–40.
[4] Aron DC. The adrenal incidentaloma: disease of modern technology and public health problem. Rev Endocr Metab Disord 2001;2:335–42.
[5] Angeli A, Terzolo M. Adrenal incidentaloma—a modern disease with old complications [editorial comment]. J Clin Endocrinol Metab 2002;87:4869–71.
[6] Ross NS. Epidemiology of Cushing's syndrome and subclinical disease. Endocrinol Metab Clin North Am 1994;23:539–46.
[7] Reincke M. Subclinical Cushing's syndrome. Endocrinol Metab Clin North Am 2000;29: 42–56.
[8] Feldkamp J, Santen R, Harms E, et al. Incidentally discovered pituitary lesions: high frequency of macro-adenomas and hormone-secreting adenomas - results of a prospective study. Clin Endocrinol (Oxf) 1999;51:109–13.
[9] Agha A, Liew A, Finucane F, et al. Conventional glucocorticoid replacement overtreats adult hypopituitary patients with partial ACTH deficiency. Clin Endocrinol (Oxf) 2004;60: 688–93.
[10] Barzon L, Scaroni C, Sonino N, al. Incidentally discovered adrenal tumors: endocrine and scintigraphic correlates. J Clin Endocrinol Metab 1988;83:55–62.
[11] Bondanelli M, Campo M, Trasforini G, et al. Evaluation of hormonal function in a series of incidentally discovered adrenal masses. Metabolism 1997;46:107–13.

[12] Boronat M, Moreno A, Ramon y Cajal S, et al. Subclinical Cushing's syndrome due to adrenal myelolipoma. Arch Pathol Lab Med 1997;121:735–7.
[13] Crucitti F, Bellantone R, Ferrante A, et al. The Italian Registry for Adrenal Cortical Carcinoma: analysis of a multi-institutional series of 129 patients. The ACC Italian Registry Study Group. Surgery 1996;119:161–70.
[14] Reincke M, Nieke J, Krestin GP, et al. Preclinical Cushing's syndrome in adrenal incidentalomas: comparison with adrenal Cushing's syndrome. J Clin Endocrinol Metab 1992;75:826–32.
[15] Ambrosi B, Peverelli S, Passini E, et al. Abnormalities of endocrine function in patients with clinically silent adrenal masses. Eur J Endocrinol 1995;132:422–8.
[16] Terzolo M, Alì A, Osella G, et al. Subclinical Cushing's syndrome in adrenal incidentaloma. Clin Endocrinol (Oxf) 1998;48:89–97.
[17] Chidiac RM, Aron DC. Incidentalomas A disease of modern technology. Endocrinol Metab Clin North Am 1997;26:233–53.
[18] Huiras CM, Pehlig GB, Caplan RH. Adrenal insufficiency after operative removal of apparently nonfunctioning adrenal adenomas. JAMA 1989;261:894–8.
[19] Mc Leod M, Thompson N, Gross M, et al. Subclinical Cushing's syndrome in patients with adrenal gland incidentalomas. Pitfalls in diagnosis and management. Am Surg 1990; 56:398–403.
[20] Caplan RH, Strutt PJ, Wickus GG. Subclinical hormone secretion by incidentally discovered adrenal masses. Arch Surg 1994;129:291–6.
[21] Fernandez-Real JM, Ricart-Engel W, Simò R. Preclinical Cushing's syndrome: report of three cases and literature review. Horm Res 1994;41:230–5.
[22] Barzon L, Sonino N, Fallo F, et al. Prevalence and natural history of adrenal incidentalomas. Eur J Endocrinol 2003;149:273–85.
[23] Virkkala A, Valimaki M, Pelkonen R, et al. Endocrine abnormalities in patients with adrenal tumours incidentally discovered on computed tomography. Acta Endocrinol 1989;121: 67–72.
[24] Hensen J, Buhl M, Bahr V, et al. Endocrine activity of the silent adrenocortical adenoma is uncovered by response to corticotropin-releasing hormone. Klin Wochenschr 1990;68: 608–14.
[25] Herrera MF, Grant CS, Van Heerden JA, et al. Incidentally discovered adrenal tumors: an institutional perspective. Surgery 1991;110:1014–21.
[26] Jockenhövel F, Kuck W, Hauffa B, et al. Conservative and surgical management of incidentally discovered adrenal tumors (incidentalomas). J Endocrinol Invest 1992;15: 331–7.
[27] Aso Y, Homma Y. A survey on incidental adrenal tumors in Japan. J Urol 1992;147:1478–81.
[28] Kobayashi S, Seki T, Nonomura K, et al. Clinical experience of incidentally discovered adrenal tumor with particular reference to cortical function. J Urol 1993;150:8–12.
[29] Siren J, Haapiainen R, Huikuri K, et al. Incidentalomas of the adrenal gland: 36 operated patients and review of literature. World J Surg 1993;17:634–9.
[30] Osella G, Terzolo M, Borretta G, et al. Endocrine evaluation of incidentally discovered adrenal masses (incidentalomas). J Clin Endocrinol Metab 1994;79:1532–9.
[31] Seppel T, Schlaghecke R. Augmented 14α-hydroxyprogesterone response to ACTH stimulation as evidence of decreased 21-hydroxylase activity in patients with incidentally discovered adrenal tumours (incidentalomas). Clin Endocrinol (Oxf) 1994;41: 445–51.
[32] Flecchia D, Mazza E, Carlini M, et al. Reduced serum levels of dehydroepiandrosterone sulphate in adrenal incidentalomas: a marker of adrenocortical tumour. Clin Endocrinol (Oxf) 1995;42:129–34.
[33] Bencsik Z, Szabolcs I, Kovacs Z, et al. Low dehydroepiandrosterone sulfate (DHEA-S) level is not a good predictor of hormonal activity in nonselected patients with incidentally detected adrenal tumors. J Clin Endocrinol Metab 1996;81:1726–9.

[34] Bardet S, Rohmer V, Murat A, et al. ^{131}I-6-β-iodomethylnorcholesterol scintigraphy: an assessment of its role in the investigation of adrenocortical incidentalomas. Clin Endocrinol (Oxf) 1996;44:587–96.
[35] Linos DA, Stylopoulos N. How accurate is computed tomography in predicting the real size of adrenal tumors? Arch Surg 1997;132:740–3.
[36] Bastounis EA, Karayiannakis AJ, Anapliotou MLG, et al. Incidentalomas of the adrenal gland: diagnostic and therapeutic implications. Am Surg 1997;63:356–60.
[37] Kasperlik-Zaluska AA, Roslonowska E, Slowinska-Srzednicka J, et al. Incidentally discovered adrenal mass (incidentaloma): investigation and management of 208 patients. Clin Endocrinol (Oxf) 1997;46:29–37.
[38] Proye C, Jafari Manjili M, Combemale F, et al. Experience gained from operation of 103 adrenal incidentalomas. Langenbeck's Arch Surg 1998;383:330–3.
[39] Murai M, Baba S, Nakashima J, et al. Management of incidentally discovered adrenal masses. World J Urol 1999;17:9–14.
[40] Tutuncu NB, Gedik O. Adrenal incidentaloma: report of 33 cases. J Surg Oncol 1999;70: 247–50.
[41] Rossi R, Tauchmanova L, Luciano A, et al. Subclinical Cushing's syndrome in patients with adrenal incidentaloma: clinical and biochemical features. J Clin Endocrinol Metab 2000;85: 1440–8.
[42] Mantero F, Terzolo M, Arnaldi G, et al. A survey on adrenal incidentaloma in Italy. J Clin Endocrinol Metab 2000;85:637–44.
[43] Morioka M, Fujii T, Matsuki T, et al. Preclinical Cushing's syndrome: report on seven cases and review of the literature. Int J Urol 2000;7:126–32.
[44] Favia G, Lumachi F, D'Amico DF. Adrenocortical carcinoma: is prognosis different in nonfunctioning tumors? Results of surgical treatment in 31 patients. World J Surg 2001;25: 735–8.
[45] Tanabe A, Naruse M, Nishikawa T, et al. Autonomy of cortisol secretion in clinically silent adrenal incidentaloma. Horm Metab Res 2001;33:444–50.
[46] Midorikawa S, Sanada H, Hashimoto S, et al. The improvement of insulin resistance in patients with adrenal incidentaloma by surgical resection. Clin Endocrinol (Oxf) 2001;49: 311–6.
[47] Grossrubatscher E, Vignati F, Possa M, et al. The natural history of incidentally discovered adrenocortical adenomas: a retrospective evaluation. J Endocrinol Invest 2001;24:846–55.
[48] Valli N, Catargi B, Ronci N, et al. Biochemical screening for subclinical cortisol-secreting adenomas amongst adrenal incidentalomas. Eur J Endocrinol 2001;144:401–8.
[49] Barzon L, Fallo F, Sonino N, et al. Development of overt Cushing's syndrome in patients with adrenal incidentalomas. Eur J Endocrinol 2002;146:61–6.
[50] Bulow B, Ahren B. Adrenal incidentaloma—experience of a standardized diagnostic programme in the Swedish prospective study. J Intern Med 2002;252:239–46.
[51] Arnaldi G, Angeli A, Atkinson AB, et al. Diagnosis and complications of Cushing's syndrome: a consensus statement. J Clin Endocrinol Metab 2003;88:5593–602.
[52] Terzolo M, Osella G, Alì A, et al. Different patterns of steroid secretion in patients with adrenal incidentaloma. J Clin Endocrinol Metab 1996;81:740–4.
[53] Tsagarakis S, Roboti C, Kokkoris P, et al. Elevated postdexamethasone suppression cortisol concentrations correlate with hormonal alterations of the hypothalamo-pituitary-adrenal axis in patients with adrenal incidentalomas. Clin Endocrinol (Oxf) 1998;49:165–71.
[54] Trainer PJ, Grossman A. The diagnosis and differential diagnosis of Cushing's syndrome. Clin Endocrinol (Oxf) 1991;34:317–30.
[55] Lavoie H, Lacroix A. Partially autonomous cortisol secretion by incidentally discovered adrenal adenomas. Trends Endocrinol Metab 1995;6:191–7.
[56] Huizenga NATM, Koper JW, De Lange P, et al. A polymorphism in the glucocorticoid receptor gene may be associated with an increased sensitivity to glucocorticoids in vivo. J Clin Endocrinol Metab 1988;83:144–51.

[57] Francis IR, Korobkin M, Quint L, et al. Integrated imaging of adrenal disease. Radiology 1992;184:1–13.
[58] Rizza RA, Wahner HW, Spelsberg TC, et al. Visualization of nonfunctioning adrenal adenomas with iodocholesterol: possible relationship to subcellular distribution of tracer. J Nucl Med 1978;19:458–63.
[59] Young WF. Management approaches to adrenal incidentalomas: a view from Rochester, Minnesota. Endocrinol Metab Clin North Am 2000;29:159–85.
[60] Terzolo M, Osella G, Alì A, et al. Adrenal incidentalomas. In: De Herder WW, editor. Functional and morphological imaging of the endocrine system. Endocrine updates, Volume 7. Boston: Kluwer Academic Publishers; 2000. p. 191–211.
[61] Kievit J, Haak HR. Diagnosis and treatment of adrenal incidentaloma: a cost-effectiveness analysis. Endocrinol Metab Clin North Am 2000;29:69–88.
[62] McFarlane SI, Banerji M, Sowers JR. Insulin resistance and cardiovascular disease. J Clin Endocrinol Metab 2001;86:713–8.
[63] Terzolo M, Pia A, Alì A, et al. Adrenal incidentaloma: a new cause of the metabolic syndrome? J Clin Endocrinol Metab 2002;87:998–1003.
[64] Fernandez-Real JM, Ricart EW, Simò R, et al. Study of glucose tolerance in consecutive patients harbouring incidental adrenal tumours. Clin Endocrinol (Oxf) 1998;49:53–61.
[65] Garrapa GGM, Pantanetti P, Arnaldi G, et al. Body composition and metabolic features in women with adrenal incidentaloma or Cushing's syndrome. J Clin Endocrinol Metab 2001; 86:5301–6.
[66] Tauchmanova L, Rossi R, Biondi B, et al. Patients with subclinical Cushing's syndrome due to adrenal adenoma have increased cardiovascular risk. J Clin Endocrinol Metab 2002;87: 4872–8.
[67] Ferranini E, Mari A. How to measure insulin sensitivity. J Hypertens 1998;16:895–906.
[68] Reincke M, Fassnacht M, Vath S, et al. Adrenal incidentalomas: a manifestation of the metabolic syndrome? Endocr Res 1996;22:757–61.
[69] Terzolo M, Bovio S, Pia A, et al. A follow-up evaluation of patients with incidentally discovered adrenal adenoma. A multicentric retrospective in Italy. 12th International Congress of Endocrinology, Lisbon, August 31–September 4, 2004.
[70] Newell-Price J, Trainer P, Perry L, et al. A single sleeping midnight cortisol has 100% sensitivity for the diagnosis of Cushing's syndrome. Clin Endocrinol (Oxf) 1995;43:545–50.
[71] Papanicolaou DA, Yanovski JA, Cutler GB, et al. A single midnight cortisol measurement distinguishes Cushing's syndrome from pseudo-Cushing states. J Clin Endocrinol Metab 1998;83:1163–7.
[72] Raff H, Raff JL, Findling JW. Late-night salivary cortisol as a screening test for Cushing's syndrome. J Clin Endocrinol Metab 1998;83:2681–6.
[73] Alexander CM, Landsman PB, Teutsch SM, et al. NCEP-defined metabolic syndrome, diabetes, and prevalence of coronary heart disease among NHANES III participants age 50 years and older. Diabetes 2003;52:1210–4.
[74] Malik S, Wong ND, Franklin SS, et al. Impact of the metabolic syndrome on mortality from coronary heart disease, cardiovascular disease, and all causes in United States adults. Circulation 2004;110:1245–50.
[75] Barzon L, Scaroni C, Sonino N, et al. Risk factors and long-term follow-up of adrenal incidentalomas. J Clin Endocrinol Metab 1999;84:520–6.
[76] Torlontano M, Chiodini I, Pileri M, et al. Altered bone mass and turnover in female patients with adrenal incidentaloma: the effect of subclinical hypercortisolism. J Clin Endocrinol Metab 1999;84:2381–5.
[77] Chiodini I, Torlontano M, Carnevale V, et al. Bone loss rate in adrenal incidentalomas: a longitudinal study. J Clin Endocrinol Metab 2001;86:5337–41.
[78] Chiodini I, Tauchmanova L, Torlontano M, et al. Bone involvement in eugonadal male patients with adrenal incidentaloma and subclinical hypercortisolism. J Clin Endocrinol Metab 2002;87:5491–4.

[79] Tauchmanova L, Rossi R, Nuzzo V, et al. Bone loss determined by quantitative ultrasonometry correlates inversely with disease activity in patients with endogenous glucocorticoid excess due to adrenal mass. Eur J Endocrinol 2001;145:241–7.

[80] Osella G, Reimondo G, Peretti P, et al. he patients with incidentally discovered adrenal adenoma (incidentaloma) are not at increased risk of osteoporosis. J Clin Endocrinol Metab 2001;86:604–7.

[81] Chiodini I, Guglielmi G, Battista C, et al. Spinal volumetric bone mineral density and vertebral fractures in female patients with adrenal incidentalomas: the effects of subclinical hypercortisolism and gonadal status. J Clin Endocrinol Metab 2004;89:2237–41.

[82] Libè R, Dall'Asta C, Barbetta L, et al. Long-term follow-up study of patients with adrenal incidentalomas. Eur J Endocrinol 2002;147:489–94.

[83] Barry MK, van Heerden JA, Farley DR, et al. Can adrenal incidentalomas be safely observed? World J Surg 1998;22:599–603.

[84] Siren J, Tervahartiala P, Sivula A, et al. Natural course of adrenal incidentalomas: seven-year follow-up study. World J Surg 2000;24:579–82.

[85] Arlt W, Allolio B. Adrenal insufficiency. Lancet 2003;361:1881–93.

[86] Udelsman R. Adrenal. In: Norton JA, Bollinger RR, Chang AE, et al, editors. Surgery: basic science and clinical evidence. New York: Springer-Verlag; 2001. p. 897–917.

[87] Colao A, Pivonello R, Spiezia S, et al. Persistence of increased cardiovascular risk in patients with Cushing's disease after five years of successful cure. J Clin Endocrinol Metab 1999;84: 2664–72.

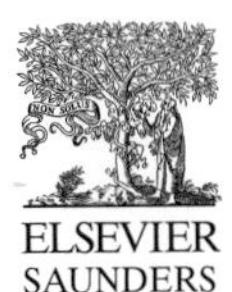

ELSEVIER
SAUNDERS

Endocrinol Metab Clin N Am
34 (2005) 441–458

ENDOCRINOLOGY
AND METABOLISM
CLINICS
OF NORTH AMERICA

Bilateral Adrenal Cushing's Syndrome: Macronodular Adrenal Hyperplasia and Primary Pigmented Nodular Adrenocortical Disease

André Lacroix, MD*, Isabelle Bourdeau, MD

Department of Medicine,
Hôtel-Dieu du Centre Hospitalier de l'Université de Montréal, 3840 Saint-Urbain Street,
Montreal, QC H2W 1T8, Canada

Primary corticotropin (ACTH)-independent adrenal etiologies account for 15% to 20% of endogenous Cushing's syndrome (CS) in adults; they are secondary to unilateral tumors in approximately 90% of cases [1–3]. The incidence of clinical CS secondary to unilateral adrenal adenoma is approximately two cases per million per year [4]. This is close to the 0.6 to 2 cases per million per year for adrenocortical carcinoma, in which hormone secretion occurs in 30% to 60% of cases; excess cortisol production is present in approximately half of them [4–7]. In adults, some series have found that adenomas and carcinomas are equally responsible for adrenal CS, but, in most series, adenomas represent up to 80% of cases [4,8,9]. In contrast, in prepubertal children, primary adrenal causes are responsible for close to 65% of CS; cortisol-secreting adrenal carcinomas are three to four times more frequent than adrenal adenomas in children [4–6]. For unclear reasons, adrenal tumors are more frequent in females than in males, with a ratio of 4:1 for adenomas and 2:1 for carcinomas [4–6]. The increasing identification of subclinical cortisol-secreting adrenal incidentalomas renders the precise estimation of the overall incidence of cortisol-secreting adrenal lesions even more difficult [4,10,11]. Box 1 displays etiologies of adrenal CS.

Approximately 10% of ACTH-independent CS is secondary to bilateral adrenal lesions, and pathophysiology is diverse [1–3]. In rare cases,

This work was supported by a grant from the Canadian Institutes of Health Research (MA-10339).

* Corresponding author.
E-mail address: andre.lacroix@umontreal.ca (A. Lacroix).

doi:10.1016/j.ecl.2005.01.004 **endo.theclinics.com**

Box 1. Etiologies of adrenal Cushing's syndrome

Unilateral tumor

Adrenocortical adenomas
- Unknown etiology
- Ectopic gastric inhibitory polypeptide (GIP)-receptor (food-dependent)
- Aberrant V_1-vasopressin receptor activity (posture-dependent)
- Aberrant luteinizing hormone/human chorionic gonadotrophin (LH/hCG) receptor (pregnancy- or menopause-dependant)
- Other aberrant receptors (eg, interleukin [IL]-1, thyrotropin [TSH], in vitro studies)

Adrenocortical carcinoma
- Unknown etiology
- Li-Fraumeni syndrome (*p53* tumor suppressor gene)
- Beckwith-Wiedemann syndrome, sporadic or familial (insulinlike growth factor [IGF] II overexpression)
- Aberrant β-adrenergic or V_1-vasopressin receptor activity (in vitro studies)

Unilateral adrenocortical hyperplasia (possibly asynchronous ACTH-independent bilateral macronodular adrenal hyperplasia [AIMAH])

Bilateral nodules or hyperplasia

AIMAH
- Unknown etiology
- Ectopic GIP-receptor (food-dependent)
- Ectopic β-adrenergic receptor (catecholamine-dependant)
- Increased activity of V_1-, or ectopic V_2- or V_3-vasopressin receptor (posture-dependent)
- Increased activity of LH/hCG receptor (pregnancy- or menopause-dependant)
- Increased activity of serotonin 5-HT_4 or 5-HT_7 receptor (unknown stimulus)
- Ectopic angiotensin AT-1 receptor (posture-dependent)
- Other aberrant receptors (eg, leptin, TSH)

Bilateral nodular adrenals
- Unknown etiology
- $G_s\alpha$ mutation isolated or with the McCune-Albright syndrome (internodular atrophy)
- Multiple endocrine neoplasia syndrome type 1 (MEN 1; usually nonfunctional)

Primary pigmented adrenocortical disease (PPNAD)
- Sporadic: isolated or with Carney complex
- Familial: isolated or with Carney complex

adrenocortical adenomas or carcinomas can occur in both adrenals. Most cases of ACTH-independent bilateral diseases, however, are secondary to two main types of adrenal nodular hyperplasias that will be reviewed [12,13].

Bilateral macronodular adrenal hyperplasia

ACTH-independent bilateral macronodular adrenal hyperplasia is a rare cause of CS, as it is estimated to represent less than 1% of endogenous cases [1–3,8,9]. In an initial review by Lieberman et al [14] in 1994, only 24 cases had been published, but since then many cases and series have been reported [15–75]. AIMAH has been described by various terms, including massive macronodular adrenocortical disease (MMAD), autonomous macronodular adrenal hyperplasia (AMAH), ACTH-independent massive bilateral adrenal disease (AIMBAD) and giant or huge macronodular adrenal disease [13]. AIMAH should not be confused with diffuse nodular or bilateral macronodular adrenal hyperplasia, which can occur following chronic stimulation by ACTH in Cushing's disease or ectopic ACTH secretion [76,77]. In most of the latter cases, inappropriately normal or elevated plasma ACTH levels identify ACTH-dependent causes. Some cases, however, have been described where chronic stimulation by ACTH induced the growth of adrenal nodules that acquired the capacity to secrete cortisol autonomously and to eventually suppress ACTH levels [78–81]. Administering corticotropin-releasing hormone may produce an increase of ACTH in most of these cases and allow the appropriate diagnosis. In some patients initially suspected of having primary AIMAH, the presence of a corticotroph adenoma and elevated ACTH became evident only following bilateral adrenalectomy [82]. Bilateral adrenal lesions are also present in as many as 10% to 15% of patients who have incidentalomas, and these often can be secondary to subclinical AIMAH, in which ACTH usually is not suppressed fully [23,25,28,57,69,83]; these cases may also be misclassified, as they demonstrate partial suppression to dexamethasone and increases of ACTH and cortisol following CRH administration [69].

Cushing's syndrome associated with McCune-Albright syndrome is a rare particular variant of bilateral macronodular adrenals with suppressed levels of ACTH. In this syndrome, activating mutations of $G_{s\alpha}$ occur in some adrenal cells in a mosaic pattern during early embryogenesis and lead to the formation of adrenal nodules, in which constitutive activation of the cAMP pathway leads to excess cortisol secretion and to ACTH suppression. The internodular adrenal cortex, where the $G_{s\alpha}$ mutation is not present, becomes atrophic, in contrast to AIMAH, where there is usually diffuse hyperplasia between nodules [84,85]. Activating mutations of $G_{s\alpha}$ occasionally have been found in the AIMAH nodules of adult patients who do not have any other features of McCune-Albright syndrome [72].

Bilateral adrenal nodules also have been described as part of MEN 1, which is caused by the tumor suppressor gene menin. In a series of 33 MEN

1 patients, bilateral adrenal enlargement was found in 21%; more than half of the remaining patients also had unilateral adrenal disease [86]. Similarly, in 33 patients from a single kindred who had MEN 1, the overall prevalence of adrenal disease was 36%; bilateral macronodular cortical hyperplasia was present in 6% of patients [87]. In the vast majority of MEN 1 patients who had adrenal lesions, there was no evidence of abnormal hormone secretion.

The possibility of activating mutations of the ACTH receptor (*MC2R*) gene also was examined and found not to be present in most adrenal tumors. In one case of AIMAH, however, a naturally occurring *MC2R* mutation (F278C) was associated with elevated basal cAMP production when compared with wild-type receptor-expressing cell lines. This mutation in the C-terminal tail of the *MC2R* impairs desensitization and internalization of the receptor [88]. Two mutations in the same allele of the *MC2R* gene associated with clinical hypersensitivity to ACTH have been described in a single case report. The presence of both C21R and S247G mutations in the same molecule leads to a receptor with a highly significant elevation in constitutive activity. The coexpression of the normal MC2R allele results in the retention of a normal dose response to ACTH despite the presence of constitutive activity [89].

Clinical manifestations of CS usually occur at a later age in AIMAH compared with unilateral cortisol-secreting adenoma or Cushing's disease; they become evident during the patient's fifth or sixth decade [13,14,90]. In one National Institutes of Health (NIH) series, the mean age of patients who had AIMAH was 51 years, while that of PPNAD was 18 years [20]. AIMAH was reported to have a relatively even gender distribution when compared with Cushing's disease or unilateral adrenal tumors [13,14,90]. It, however, was reported to be more frequent in males in one report [21] or in woman who had GIP-dependent AIMAH [91]. The most frequent clinical presentation of AIMAH is CS. Cases of AIMAH with combinations of gluco–mineralocorticoid [23,26,48], cortisol–estrone secretion [55], or with androgen secretion [71] also have been reported.

Diagnosis of AIMAH almost always is suggested by imaging studies (CT scan or MRI) in a patient who had the biochemical demonstration of ACTH-independent CS. The adrenal glands can be replaced by the presence of numerous nodules up to 4 cm in diameter; in other cases, the adrenal appears diffusely enlarged without macroscopic nodules [22]. On CT, the adrenal nodules are of soft tissue density; on T1-weighted MRI, the signal intensity is equal to muscle, while in T2-weighted images, the intensity can be higher than liver [22]. Combined adrenal weight is usually above 60 g and can reach more than 200 g per adrenal gland [12–14,52]. In some cases, there is asymmetric development of adrenal macronodules, mimicking unilateral disease; the development of contralateral disease can occur several years later [13,14,53]. The nodules are composed of two types of cells, those with clear cytoplasm (lipid-rich) that forms cordon nestlike structures, and those with a compact cytoplasm (lipid-poor) that forms small nest or islandlike structures [13,14,21,56]. Overall, steroid hormone synthesis in AIMAH is an inefficient process. The increased glucocorticoid secretion is the result of a significant increase in the number of adrenocortical cells rather than an augmented synthesis per cell [12–14]. In AIMAH, the MC2R is expressed, although at lower levels compared with the normal adrenal gland [92]. The increase in cortisol following administration of exogenous ACTH is larger than in normal adrenals and reflects the large adrenal cell mass [41]. This can be useful in distinguishing AIMAH from other causes of bilaterally enlarged adrenals such as metastatic or infiltrative diseases, where steroidogenic response to ACTH administration is decreased. Inefficient hormone synthesis in AIMAH results from altered steroidogenic enzymatic pathways. Immunohistochemical studies showed that 3β-HSD2 was expressed only in large clear cells, whereas CYP17 (P450C17) was seen predominantly in small compact cells [30,56,59]. The differential expression of these two steroidogenic enzymes has been observed only in AIMAH and not in other adrenocortical diseases. Immunoreactivities for CYP11A1 (P450scc), CYP21A2 (P450c21), and CYP11B2 (P450C11) are present in both cell types, but the level of expression of several enzymes was found to be decreased [56,58,93,94]. The relative inefficient steroidogenesis in AIMAH is probably responsible for the growing number of cases of AIMAH with subclinical production of cortisol [23,25,28,57,69,83]. These cases usually are found incidentally as bilateral large multinodular adrenals without any clinical symptoms of steroid excess. Urinary free cortisol levels are within the normal range, but there can be a diversity of subtle modifications of the hypothalamic–pituitary–adrenal axis, such as slightly elevated midnight plasma or salivary cortisol, subnormal suppression of cortisol following 1 mg of dexamethasone at midnight (> 50 nmol/L), and partial suppression of plasma ACTH levels. An increase in ACTH following administration of CRH is usually still present; a large increase in cortisol following administration of ACTH and evidence of altered steroidogenic enzymes (elevated 17-hydroxyprogesterone levels) also can be found [83].

The composition of different nodules in AIMAH showed different clonal patterns between glands and within the same gland; in addition, clonality differed between nodules [95–97]. There are polyclonal and monoclonal areas in AIMAH adrenocortical tissue, whereas patients who had ACTH-dependent macronodular adrenal disease had an exclusively polyclonal pattern. This suggests that in AIMAH different stages of a common multistep tumoral process are present in different locations at the same time, as suggested by the heterogeneous clonal pattern [98].

Most cases of AIMAH appear to be sporadic; however, the number of reported patients remains small, and family screening has not been performed systematically [12]. There are seven reports of familial cases of AIMAH with presentation suggesting an autosomal-dominant transmission [54,65,66,68,73–75].

Aberrant hormone receptors in adrenal Cushing's syndrome

The mechanisms by which cortisol is produced in adrenal CS, when ACTH is suppressed, were previously unknown and referred to as being autonomous. Studies by several groups now have shown that a significant proportion of the cortisol-producing adrenal tumors or hyperplasias actually may be under the control of aberrant (ectopic or eutopic) hormone membrane receptors [41,91,98,99]. Cortisol secretion becomes driven by a hormone that escapes cortisol-mediated feedback.

The adrenal expression of GIP receptor causes food-dependent cortisol production, where plasma cortisol levels can be relatively low during fasting and increase transiently following meals [33,34,91,100]. GIP-dependent CS has been identified in several countries in at least 17 patients who had AIMAH [33–38,53,69,91] and in 7 patients with a unilateral adenoma [91,100–104]. GIP receptor is expressed in GIP-dependent adrenal adenomas or AIMAH, but not in the normal adult or fetal adrenal cortex or non-GIP–dependent adrenal CS tissues [35,53,102, 103,105]. Sequence analysis of the full-length cDNA of GIP-dependent adrenals revealed no GIP receptor mutation [102,105]. Ectopic GIP receptor expression was found in the early stages of adrenal hyperplasia [53]. GIP stimulates cAMP production and DNA synthesis in GIP-dependent cortisol-secreting adenoma cells in primary culture [102]; the latter two findings thus suggest a role for ectopic GIP receptors not only in steroid secretion, but also in adrenal cell proliferation [102]. This was supported by the demonstration that bovine adrenal cells transfected with the GIP receptor generate adrenal-like hyperplastic nodules and glucocorticoid excess when injected under the renal capsule of nude mice [106]. GIP-dependent androgen secretion and hirsutism was found in an adrenal adenoma, probably resulting from the GIP-dependent clonal proliferation of a zona reticularis cell [104].

Vasopressin-responsive CS was reported in several patients who had a unilateral adenoma or AIMAH who increase their secretion of cortisol with upright posture or other physiologic stimuli of endogenous vasopressin [15–17,39–42,61,67,75,91,107,108]. In most, cortisol secretion was regulated by the nonmutated V_1-vasopressin receptor expressed either at higher or similar levels in the adrenal tissues of vasopressin-responsive CS patients compared with normal individuals [42,61,67,75,108]. In a retrospective study of 26 patients who had unilateral cortisol-secreting tumors, plasma cortisol increased after lysine-vasopressin testing in 27% of cases (5 adenomas and 2 carcinomas) [108]. Because the V_1-vasopressin receptor normally is expressed in the adrenal cortex and modulates modest in vitro effects on steroidogenesis, this exaggerated steroidogenic responses to vasopressin is secondary to the increased activity or expression of a eutopic receptor-effector system [42,61,67,75,91,107,108]. Recently, ectopic expression of V_2- and V_3-vasopressin receptors was reported in vitro in some

AIMAH cases, but the effect of dDAVP, a preferential V_2-vasopressin receptor agonist, was not studied in vivo [67,75].

The aberrant adrenal expression of β-adrenergic receptors was identified in four patients who had AIMAH and CS who increased their plasma cortisol and aldosterone levels during elevations of endogenous catecholamines (upright posture, insulin-induced hypoglycemia, and exercise) [41,45,52,62]. Isoproterenol infusion stimulated cortisol and aldosterone secretion in these patients, but not in normal subjects. High-affinity binding sites compatible with β_1- or β_2-adrenergic receptors were coupled efficiently to steroidogenesis in the adrenal tissues of such patients, but not in controls, indicating the ectopic nature of this receptor [52,91]. The combined presence of adrenal β-adrenergic receptor and V_1-vasopressin receptor was identified in two women who had AIMAH [41,62]. It was shown that fluctuations of endogenous physiologic levels of vasopressin (water and hypertonic sodium loading) resulted in parallel changes of plasma cortisol levels.

The aberrant adrenal function of LH/hCG receptor first was identified in a woman who had transient CS during sequential pregnancies; persistent CS and AIMAH developed only after the postmenopausal long-term increase of LH [43]. Administration of the long-acting GnRH analog leuprolide acetate led to suppression of endogenous LH and normalization of cortisol production. In the same patient, cisapride and metoclopramide, two serotonin 5-HT_4 receptor agonists, also stimulated plasma cortisol; they were without effect in several other patients who had AIMAH, unilateral adenoma or carcinoma, and CS [41,43]. Other cases of aberrant receptors for LH/hCG or serotonin either alone or in combination have been reported [44,60,109]. In six patients who had CS and aberrant response to cisapride or metoclopramide, adrenal overexpression of 5-HT_4 receptor was found in four adrenals; in the two patients who had normal levels of 5-HT_4 receptor, the molecular mechanism of aberrant response is unclear, as there were no differences in splice variants or in the cDNA sequence of the receptor [47]. Another female patient who had AIMAH had predominant hyperaldosteronism and cyclical CS with aberrant response of cortisol to 5-HT_4 receptor agonists [48]. A 59-year-old virilized woman who had androgen-secreting AIMAH regulated by hCG was shown to express the LH/hCG receptor in one resected adrenal. Suppression of endogenous LH with leuprolide acetate normalized androgen secretion from the contralateral adrenal, avoiding bilateral adrenalectomy [71]. More recently, the ectopic expression of 5-HT_7 receptor was identified in patients who had serotonin-responsive AIMAH and CS [67].

In a patient who had AIMAH and a large increase in plasma aldosterone and cortisol levels during upright posture, short-term oral administration of the AT-1 receptor antagonist candesartan completely inhibited the elevation in cortisol and aldosterone [46]. Chronic treatment of the patient who had an AT-1 receptor antagonist was not attempted, and no in vitro demonstration of the presence of AT-1 receptor has been provided. In vitro stimulation of cortisol secretion by angiotensin-II also was found in patients who had AIMAH and CS and increases in cortisol levels with upright posture [49].

Several other in vitro studies have supported the expression of membrane hormone receptors in human adrenocortical benign and malignant tumors; these include thyrotropin, follicle-stimulating hormone, leptin, and IL-1, in addition to those clearly confirmed in vivo [36,91,98,110]. Another paracrine regulatory mechanism was proposed following the investigation of a patient who had AIMAH and CS (without any aberrant hormone response) in whom an increased adrenocortical expression of proopiomelanocortin/ACTH was found [63].

Investigation protocols have been developed to systematically evaluate patients with adrenal CS for the presence of aberrant adrenal hormone receptors [41,83,91,111–113]. The strategy is to modulate the levels of ligands for the potential aberrant receptors using various physiologic (upright posture, mixed meals) and pharmacologic (gonadotropin-releasing hormone, thyrotropin-releasing hormone, vasopressin, glucagon, and metoclopramide) tests and to examine whether levels of cortisol and other steroids are modified. In a systematic clinical screening of 20 consecutive patients with adrenal CS, all 6 patients with AIMAH had at least one aberrant receptor (2 had GIP receptor, 1 had LH/hCG and 5-HT_4 receptors, 1 had β-adrenergic receptor, 1 had V_1-vasopressin receptor, and 1 had β-adrenergic and V_1-vasopressin receptors) [41]. In patients who had a unilateral adenoma, only 3 of 13 patients had aberrant responses, whereas none was found in one adrenal carcinoma. The French COMET multicenter group also studied 11 patients who had AIMAH and 2 who had bilateral adenomas [112]; no aberrant responses were found in the latter. All 11 AIMAH patients had aberrant responses of cortisol to at least one, and frequently to several stimuli (8 to upright posture, 2 of 4 to lysine-vasopressin, 4 of 10 to combined gonadotropin-releasing hormone/thyrotropin-releasing hormone, 6 of 10 to cisapride or metoclopramide, 2 to food combined with LH/hCG response). In a French multicenter in vitro study, GIP receptor was found in 4 of 8 AIMAH, 1 of 16 unilateral adenomas, and 0 of 14 carcinomas [38].

The expression of aberrant receptors also was found in four of four patients who had incidentally found AIMAH and subclinical CS. Two had combined V_1-vasopressin receptor, LH/hCG receptor, and 5-HT_4 receptor; one had combined V_1-vasopressin and 5-HT_4 receptors, and one had V_1-vasopressin receptor only [83]. Similarly, a Japanese group found an aberrant response to vasopressin in vivo and increased V_1-vasopressin receptor expression in adrenal tissues of five patients who had AIMAH and subclinical CS [64]. In a prospective multicenter French study of 21 patients who had unilateral adrenal adenoma and subclinical or mild CS, all had at least one aberrant cortisol response, and 86% had subclinical CS and multiple aberrant responses (90% to terlipressin [V_1-vasopressin receptor], 81% to cisapride [5-HT_4 receptor], these 2 responses being the most frequent). Four of 21 patients had a response to exogenous glucagon (first report); 4 of 21 patients had a response to a mixed meal, and 3 of 8 had a response to angiotensin-II infusion [113].

In familial cases of AIMAH, the potential presence of aberrant receptors was evaluated only in the most recently studied families; in all of those, aberrant receptors were identified. Aberrant V1-vasopressin receptor and β-adrenergic receptor were found in one family [65], β-adrenergic receptor in another family [73], and V_1-, V_2-, and V_3-vasopressin receptors in a third family [75].

Treatment of macronodular adrenal hyperplasia

Surgical treatment has been recommended for most patients who have CS and AIMAH; it is now questionable whether bilateral adrenalectomy always should be performed. Unilateral adrenalectomy also was found to give good results, although it is expected that, as the cell mass increases in the contralateral adrenal, a second adrenalectomy may become necessary [50,51]. Ketoconazole was able to normalize cortisol production in patients who had AIMAH before performing surgery [39]. In patients who have subclinical AIMAH, the decision for therapy should be based on manifestations of cortisol excess such as hypertension, diabetes, osteoporosis, apparent brain atrophy, or neuropsychologic manifestations. As AIMAH is a benign process that has not been shown to become malignant, follow-up with annual CT scan and biochemical assessment is sufficient.

The identification of aberrant adrenal hormone receptors in AIMAH provides new opportunities to use specific pharmacologic therapies as alternatives to adrenalectomy. Pharmacologic blockade of postprandial release of GIP with octreotide led to clinical and biochemical improvement of CS, but did not persist in the long term, probably because of eventual desensitization of somatostatin receptors in GIP-secreting duodenal K cells [34,101]. In catecholamine-dependent CS and AIMAH, β-adrenergic receptor antagonists were efficient in the long-term control of hypercortisolism [45,52]. In LH/hCG-dependent AIMAH and CS, suppression of endogenous LH levels with long-acting leuprolide acetate controlled steroid secretion and avoided bilateral adrenalectomy [43,71]. It is possible that despite complete blockade of the aberrant receptors, tumor regression would not occur, as other genetic events inducing proliferative gain-of-function mutation (other than aberrant receptors) have accumulated over time [94,98].

Based on current studies, the authors recommend that all patients who have AIMAH and clinical or subclinical CS undergo screening for aberrant receptors, as this may change the therapeutic strategy. For patients who have unilateral lesions and CS, the screening for aberrant receptors still should be conducted in the context of clinical research projects.

Primary pigmented nodular adrenocortical disease

Carney complex (CNC) is a familial multiple neoplasia syndrome with an autosomal dominant mode of transmission [114,115]. CNC was described as the association of myxomas, spotty skin pigmentation, schwannomas, and a variety of endocrine and nonendocrine tumors [13,114,116]. PPNAD is the main endocrine manifestation of CNC. It is observed in 25% of patients who have CNC [13,114]. Growth hormone (GH) secreting pituitary adenoma and acromegaly can occur in 10% of CNC cases [13,114]; slowly progressive macroadenomas can be detected by early evaluations of elevated IGF-1 and nonsuppressible GH levels. Testicular tumors can be found in 30% of affected males and can include large-cell calcifying Sertoli-cell tumors (estrogen production with gynecomastia and precocious puberty), adrenocortical rest, and Leydig-cell tumors. Thyroid follicular benign and malignant neoplasms are also more frequent in CNC. Other tumors include psammomatous melanotic schwannomas, epithelioid blue nevi, and ductal adenomas of the breast. The centrofacial spotty pigmentation of CNC includes irregular and poorly delineated tanned lesions or very dark brown to black well-delineated lesions. Conjunctival pigmented lesions can be found on the lacrimal caruncle, semilunar fold or the sclera. In some patients, pigmented spots are found in the intraoral cavity and in large amounts on female external genitalia. Blue naevi, compound naevi, and café-au-lait spots also can be found [13,114]. Cardiac myxomas can affect all cardiac chambers and occur at multiple sites; they are responsible for a significant morbidity and mortality in CNC. Cutaneous myxomas are more frequent on eyelids and external ear canals [13,114].

Approximately half of the cases of CNC are familial [117]. Putative genetic loci have been identified by linkage analysis at chromosomes 2p16 and 17q22–q24 [118,119]. Recently, the responsible gene on 17q22–q24 was identified as type 1α regulatory subunit of cAMP-dependent protein kinase A (*PRKAR1A*) [120]. Initially, inactivating mutations of this gene were observed in 41% of CNC kindreds; however, they appear to be present in a higher proportion of PPNAD patients [121]. Additional mutations in this gene were described later in other kindreds and in sporadic cases [70, 121,122].

Approximately 50% of PPNAD patients appear to be sporadic, while the other half are familial, usually associated with CNC [13,114,117]. PPNAD may cause classic CS or be atypical with cyclical CS, or simple disturbances of the normal circadian variation of cortisol secretion. Some patients present with osteoporosis, and occasionally myopathy and cachexia, but tend to lack severe obesity, persistent hypertension, moon facies, and other manifestations of CS [114,117].

In PPNAD, the overall size of the adrenal gland often is not enlarged, but occupied by several small black or brown nodules spread in an otherwise atrophic cortex; this can be seen as a string of beads on thinned section high-resolution CT scan [123]. In other patients, one or several larger nodules can be present and mimic unilateral tumors. Bilateral uptake of iodocholesterol was found in most patients studied [116]. Histologically, most nodules are less than 4 mm, unencapsulated, but sharply demarcated from the adjacent atrophic cortex, which lacks the usual adrenal zonation. The cells in the nodules are large and globular with eosinophilic or clear cytoplasm; many of these cells contain coarsely granular brown pigment, identified as lipofuscin [13,114,116]. High synaptophysin expression in PPNAD nodules suggests a neuroendocrine phenotype of these cells [124]. The adrenal medulla appears normal.

In PPNAD, the secretion of cortisol usually is poorly stimulated by exogenous ACTH [116]. A high proportion of patients who have PPNAD respond to the sequential low and high doses of oral dexamethasone tests with a more than 50% increase in urinary free cortisol excretion occurring during the last day of dexamethasone. This delayed paradoxical response can be useful diagnostically to identify otherwise asymptomatic carriers or to distinguish PPNAD from other adrenocortical tumors [125]. This paradoxical response was not associated with the presence of aberrant membrane hormone receptors, and could be reproduced in vitro by incubating PPNAD cells directly with dexamethasone [126]. An important overexpression of the glucocorticoid receptor (GR) was demonstrated by immunohistochemistry and polymerase chain reaction in the micronodules. The increased expression of GR and the modulation of steroidogenesis by glucocorticoids were present in PPNAD patients who had or did not have CNC or PRKARIA mutations; the molecular etiology of GR upregulation remains to be determined [126]. A similar phenomenon may underlie the report of a PPNAD woman, paradoxical response to dexamethasone, but also increased steroidogenesis during pregnancy and the use of contraceptive pills. Increased production of cortisol occurred in vitro following incubation with estrogens, suggesting possible additional overexpression of estrogen receptors [127].

Treatment of primary pigmented nodular adrenocortical disease

Bilateral adrenalectomy has been the most frequently used and successful therapy for PPNAD with CS. In a few selected cases with mild hypercortisolism, however, subtotal or unilateral adrenalectomies have resulted in remission of overt CS. In these patients, there was still evidence of constitutive steroidogenesis. In 8 of 23 patients responding favorably to partial adrenalectomy at the Mayo Clinic, completion of adrenalectomy was eventually necessary [116]. Ketoconazole was found to inhibit excess glucocorticoid secretion efficiently in PPNAD [128]. Therapy of osteoporosis with bisphosphonates and adequate calcium and vitamin D intake are also important. Long-term investigation and follow-up for other manifestations of CNC are described in more details elsewhere [116,117].

Acknowledgments

The authors wish to express their gratitude to Dr. Stavroula Christopoulos for her critical review of this article and to Mrs. Josée Baker for her secretarial assistance in preparing the manuscript.

References

[1] Nieman LK. Cushing's syndrome. In: De Groot LJ, Jameson JL, editors. Endocrinology. Philadelphia: WB Saunders Company; 2001. p. 1691–720.

[2] Stewart PM. The adrenal cortex. In: Larsen PR, Kronenberg HM, Melmed S, et al, editors. Williams textbook of endocrinology. Philadelphia: WB Saunders Company; 2003. p. 491–551.

[3] Newell-Price J, Trainer P, Besser M, et al. The diagnosis and differential diagnosis of Cushing's syndrome and pseudo-Cushing's states. Endocr Rev 1998;19(5):647–72.

[4] Ross NS. Epidemiology of Cushing's syndrome and subclinical disease. Endocrinol Metab Clin North Am 1994;23(3):539–46.

[5] Latronico AC, Chrousos GP. Extensive personal experience: adrenocortical tumors. J Clin Endocrinol Metab 1997;82(5):1317–24.

[6] Bornstein SR, Stratakis CA, Chrousos GP. Adrenocortical tumors: recent advances in basic concepts and clinical management. Ann Intern Med 1999;130(9):759–71.

[7] Schteingart DE, Homan D. Management of adrenal cancer. In: Margioris AN, Chrousos GP, editors. Contemporary endocrinology: adrenal disorders. Totowa (NJ): Humana Press; 2001. p. 231–47.

[8] Samuels MH, Loriaux DL. Cushing's syndrome and the nodular adrenal gland. Endocrinol Metab Clin North Am 1994;23(3):555–69.

[9] Trainer PJ, Grossman A. The diagnosis and differential diagnosis of Cushing's syndrome. Clin Endocrinol (Oxf) 1991;34(4):317–30.

[10] Reincke M. Subclinical Cushing's syndrome. Endocrinol Metab Clin North Am 2000; 29(1):43–56.

[11] Mansmann G, Lau J, Balk E, et al. The clinically inapparent adrenal mass: update in diagnosis and management. Endocr Rev 2004;25:309–40.

[12] Bourdeau I, Stratakis CA. Cyclic AMP-dependent signaling aberrations in macro-nodular adrenal disease. Ann N Y Acad Sci 2002;968:240–55.

[13] Stratakis CA, Kirschner LS. Clinical and genetic analysis of primary bilateral adrenal diseases (micro- and macro-nodular disease) leading to Cushing's syndrome. Horm Metab Res 1998;30:456–63.

[14] Lieberman SA, Eccleshall TR, Feldman D. ACTH-independent massive bilateral adrenal disease (AIMBAD): a subtype of Cushing's syndrome with major diagnostic and therapeutic implications. Eur J Endocrinol 1994;131(1):67–73.

[15] Horiba N, Suda T, Aiba M, et al. Lysine vasopressin stimulation of cortisol secretion in patients with adrenocorticotropin-independent macronodular adrenal hyperplasia. J Clin Endocrinol Metab 1995;80(8):2336–41.

[16] Iida K, Kaji H, Matsumoto H, et al. Adrenocorticotrophin-independent macronodular adrenal hyperplasia in a patient with lysine vasopressin responsiveness but insensitivity to gastric inhibitory polypeptide. Clin Endocrinol (Oxf) 1997;47(6):739–45.

[17] Daidoh H, Morita H, Hanafusa J, et al. In vivo and in vitro effects of AVP and V1a receptor antagonist on Cushing's syndrome due to ACTH-independent bilateral macronodular adrenocortical hyperplasia. Clin Endocrinol (Oxf) 1998;49(3):403–9.

[18] Hashimoto K, Kawada Y, Murakami K, et al. Cortisol responsiveness to insulin-induced hypoglycemia in Cushing's syndrome with huge nodular adrenocortical hyperplasia. Endocrinol Jpn 1986;33(4):479–87.

[19] Lamberts SW, Bons EG, Bruining HA. Different sensitivity to adrenocorticotropin of dispersed adrenocortical cells from patients with Cushing's disease with macronodular and diffuse adrenal hyperplasia. J Clin Endocrinol Metab 1984;58(6):1106–10.
[20] Zeiger MA, Nieman LK, Cutler GB, et al. Primary bilateral adrenocortical causes of Cushing's syndrome. Surgery 1991;110(6):1106–15.
[21] Aiba M, Hirayama A, Iri H, et al. Adrenocorticotropic hormone-independent bilateral adrenocortical macronodular hyperplasia as a distinct subtype of Cushing's syndrome. Enzyme histochemical and ultrastructural study of four cases with a review of the literature. Am J Clin Pathol 1991;96(3):334–40.
[22] Doppman JL, Nieman LK, Travis WD, et al. CT and MR imaging of massive macronodular adrenocortical disease: a rare cause of autonomous primary adrenal hypercortisolism. J Comput Assist Tomogr 1991;15(5):773–9.
[23] Yamada Y, Sakaguchi K, Inoue T, et al. Preclinical Cushing's syndrome due to adrenocorticotropin-independent bilateral adrenocortical macronodular hyperplasia with concurrent excess of gluco- and mineralocorticoids. Intern Med 1997;36(9):628–32.
[24] Swain JM, Grant CS, Schlinkert RT, et al. Corticotropin-independent macronodular adrenal hyperplasia: a clinicopathologic correlation. Arch Surg 1998;133(5):541–5.
[25] Sasao T, Itoh N, Sato Y, et al. Subclinical Cushing's syndrome due to adrenocorticotropic hormone- independent macronodular adrenocortical hyperplasia: changes in plasma cortisol levels during long-term follow-up. Urology 2000;55(1):145.
[26] Hayashi Y, Takeda Y, Kaneko K, et al. A case of Cushing's syndrome due to ACTH-independent bilateral macro-nodular hyperplasia associated with excessive secretion of mineralocorticoids. Endocr J 1998;45(4):485–91.
[27] Suda T. Preclinical Cushing's syndrome and adrenocorticotropic hormone-independent bilateral adrenocortical macronodular hyperplasia. Intern Med 1997;36(9):601–2.
[28] Nemoto Y, Aoki A, Katayama Y, et al. Noncushingoid Cushing's syndrome due to adrenocorticotropic hormone-independent bilateral adrenocortical macro-nodular hyperplasia. Intern Med 1995;34(5):446–50.
[29] Nomata K, Sakai H, Suzuki S, et al. Proliferating cell nuclear antigen in ACTH-independent bilateral macronodular adrenal hyperplasia. Int J Urol 1995;2(3):203–5.
[30] Koizumi S, Beniko M, Ikota A, et al. Adrenocorticotropic hormone-independent bilateral adrenocortical macronodular hyperplasia: a case report and immunohistochemical studies. Endocr J 1994;41(4):429–35.
[31] Gupta S, Chopra P, Sikora S, et al. Macro-nodular adrenal hyperplasia causing Cushing's syndrome: report of two cases and an overview. Surg Today 1992;22(5):456–60.
[32] Shinojima H, Kakizaki H, Usuki T, et al. Clinical and endocrinological features of adrenocorticotropic hormone-independent bilateral macronodular adrenocortical hyperplasia. J Urol 2001;166:1639–42.
[33] Lacroix A, Bolte E, Tremblay J, et al. Gastric inhibitory polypeptide-dependent cortisol hypersecretion—a new cause of Cushing's syndrome. N Engl J Med 1992;327(14):974–80.
[34] Reznik Y, Allali-Zerah V, Chayvalle JA, et al. Food-dependent Cushing's syndrome mediated by aberrant adrenal sensitivity to gastric inhibitory polypeptide. N Engl J Med 1992;327(14):981–6.
[35] Lebrethon MC, Avallet O, Reznik Y, et al. Food-dependent Cushing's syndrome: characterization and functional role of gastric inhibitory polypeptide receptor in the adrenals of three patients. J Clin Endocrinol Metab 1998;83(12):4514–9.
[36] Pralong FP, Gomez F, Guillou L, et al. Food-dependent Cushing's syndrome: possible involvement of leptin in cortisol hypersecretion. J Clin Endocrinol Metab 1999;84(10): 3817–22.
[37] Gerl H, Rohde W, Biering H, et al. [Food-dependent Cushing syndrome of long standing with mild clinical features]. Dtsch Med Wochenschr 2000;125:1565–8.
[38] Groussin L, Perlemoine K, Contesse V, et al. The ectopic expression of the gastric inhibitory polypeptide receptor is frequent in adrenocorticotropin-independent bilateral

macronodular adrenal hyperplasia, but rare in unilateral tumors. J Clin Endocrinol Metab 2002;87(5):1980–5.

[39] Lacroix A, Tremblay J, Touyz RM, et al. Abnormal adrenal and vascular responses to vasopressin mediated by a V1- vasopressin receptor in a patient with adrenocorticotropin-independent macro-nodular adrenal hyperplasia, Cushing's syndrome, and orthostatic hypotension. J Clin Endocrinol Metab 1997;82(8):2414–22.

[40] Yamakita N, Murai T, Ito Y, et al. Adrenocorticotropin-independent macronodular adrenocortical hyperplasia associated with multiple colon adenomas/carcinomas which showed a point mutation in the APC gene. Intern Med 1997;36(8):536–42.

[41] Mircescu H, Jilwan J, N'Diaye N, et al. Are ectopic or abnormal membrane hormone receptors frequently present in adrenal Cushing's syndrome? J Clin Endocrinol Metab 2000;85(10):3531–6.

[42] Campbell KK, Baysdorfer C, Antonini S, et al. V_1 vasopressin receptor sequence and expression in adrenal Cushing's syndrome with abberant response to vasopressin. Presented at the 86th Meeting of the Endocrine Society. New Orleans, Louisiana, June 16–19, 2004.

[43] Lacroix A, Hamet P, Boutin JM. Leuprolide acetate therapy in luteinizing hormone-dependent Cushing's syndrome. N Engl J Med 1999;341(21):1577–81.

[44] Feelders RA, Lamberts SW, Hofland LJ, et al. Luteinizing hormone (LH)-responsive Cushing's syndrome: the demonstration of LH receptor messenger ribonucleic acid in hyperplastic adrenal cells, which respond to chorionic gonadotropin and serotonin agonists in vitro. J Clin Endocrinol Metab 2003;88(1):230–7.

[45] Pignatelli D, Rodrigues E, Barbosa AM, et al. Cushing's syndrome due to the ectopic expression of adrenergic receptors in the adrenal cortex. A case of ACTH-independent macronodular adrenal hyperplasia (AIMAH). Presented at the 86th Meeting of the Endocrine Society. New Orleans, Louisiana, June 16–19, 2004.

[46] Nakamura Y, Son Y, Kohno Y, et al. Case of adrenocorticotropic hormone-independent macronodular adrenal hyperplasia with possible adrenal hypersensitivity to angiotensin II. Endocrine 2001;15(1):57–61.

[47] Cartier D, Lihrmann I, Parmentier F, et al. Overexpression of serotonin 4 receptors in cisapride-responsive adrenocorticotropin-independent bilateral macronodular adrenal hyperplasia causing Cushing's syndrome. J Clin Endocrinol Metab 2003;88(1):248–54.

[48] Yared Z, Antonini S, Lacroix A. Macronodular adrenal hyperplasia with long-term primary hyperaldosteronism and recent cyclical Cushing's syndrome with aberrant response of cortisol to serotonin agonist 5–HT4 R. Presented at the 85th Meeting of the Endocrine Society. Philadelphia, Pennsylvania, June 19–22, 2003.

[49] Bertherat J, Contesse V, Louiset E, et al. Abnormal sensitivity of the adrenocortical tissue to multiple stimuli in ACTH-independent macronodular adrenal hyperplasia (AIMAH) causing Cushing's syndrome: in vivo and in vitro studies. Presented at the 86th Meeting of the Endocrine Society. New Orleans, Louisiana, June 16–19, 2004.

[50] Boronat M, Lucas T, Barcelo B, et al. Cushing's syndrome due to autonomous macronodular adrenal hyperplasia: long-term follow-up after unilateral adrenalectomy. Postgrad Med J 1996;72(852):614–6.

[51] Ogura M, Kusaka I, Nagasaka S, et al. Unilateral adrenalectomy improves insulin resistance and diabetes mellitus in a patient with ACTH-independent macronodular adrenal hyperplasia. Endocr J 2003;50(6):715–21.

[52] Lacroix A, Tremblay J, Rousseau G, et al. Propranolol therapy for ectopic beta-adrenergic receptors in adrenal Cushing's syndrome. N Engl J Med 1997;337(20):1429–34.

[53] N'Diaye N, Hamet P, Tremblay J, et al. Asynchronous development of bilateral nodular adrenal hyperplasia in gastric inhibitory polypeptide-dependent Cushing's syndrome. J Clin Endocrinol Metab 1999;84(8):2616–22.

[54] Minami S, Sugihara H, Sato J, et al. ACTH-independent Cushing's syndrome occurring in siblings. Clin Endocrinol (Oxf) 1996;44(4):483–8.

[55] Malchoff CD, Rosa J, DeBold CR, et al. Adrenocorticotropin-independent bilateral macro-nodular adrenal hyperplasia: an unusual cause of Cushing's syndrome. J Clin Endocrinol Metab 1989;68(4):855–60.
[56] Wada N, Kubo M, Kijima H, et al. Adrenocorticotropin-independent bilateral macronodular adrenocortical hyperplasia: immunohistochemical studies of steroidogenic enzymes and postoperative course in two men. Eur J Endocrinol 1996;134(5):583–7.
[57] Murakami O, Satoh F, Takahashi K, et al. Three cases of clinical or preclinical Cushing's syndrome due to adrenocorticotropic hormone-independent bilateral adrenocortical macronodular hyperplasia: pituitary-adrenocortical function and immunohistochemistry. Intern Med 1995;34(11):1074–81.
[58] Sasano H, Suzuki T, Nagura H. ACTH-independent macronodular adrenocortical hyperplasia: immunohistochemical and in situ hybridization studies of steroidogenic enzymes. Mod Pathol 1994;7(2):215–9.
[59] Morioka M, Ohashi Y, Watanabe H, et al. ACTH-independent macronodular adrenocortical hyperplasia (AIMAH): report of two cases and the analysis of steroidogenic activity in adrenal nodules. Endocr J 1997;44(1):65–72.
[60] Mannelli M, Ferruzzi P, Luciani P, et al. Cushing's syndrome in a patient with bilateral macro-nodular adrenal hyperplasia responding to cisapride: an in vivo and in vitro study. J Clin Endocrinol Metab 2003;88(10):4616–22.
[61] Mune T, Murase H, Yamakita N, et al. Eutopic overexpression of vasopressin V1a receptor in adrenocorticotropin-independent macronodular adrenal hyperplasia. J Clin Endocrinol Metab 2002;87(12):5706–13.
[62] Miyamura N, Tsutsumi A, Senokuchi H, et al. A case of ACTH-independent macronodular adrenal hyperplasia: simultaneous expression of several aberrant hormone receptors in the adrenal gland. Endocr J 2003;50(3):333–40.
[63] Lefebvre H, Duparc C, Chartrel N, et al. Intra-adrenal adrenocorticotropin production in a case of bilateral macro-nodular adrenal hyperplasia causing Cushing's syndrome. J Clin Endocrinol Metab 2003;88(7):3035–42.
[64] Tatsuno I, Uchida D, Tanaka T, et al. Vasopressin responsiveness of subclinical Cushing's syndrome due to ACTH-independent macro-nodular adrenocortical hyperplasia. Clin Endocrinol (Oxf) 2004;60(2):192–200.
[65] Miyamura N, Taguchi T, Murata Y, et al. Inherited adrenocorticotropin-independent macronodular adrenal hyperplasia with abnormal cortisol secretion by vasopressin and catecholamines: detection of the aberrant hormone receptors on adrenal gland. Endocrine 2002;19(3):319–26.
[66] Nies C, Bartsch DK, Ehlenz K, et al. Familial ACTH-independent Cushing's syndrome with bilateral macronodular adrenal hyperplasia clinically affecting only female family members. Exp Clin Endocrinol Diabetes 2002;110(6):277–83.
[67] Louiset E, Contesse V, Cartier D, et al. Pharmacological profile and coupling mechanisms of illegitimate receptors in ACTH-independent macronodular bilateral adrenal hyperplasia causing Cushing's syndrome. Presented at the 86th Meeting of the Endocrine Society. New Orleans, Louisiana, June 16–19, 2004.
[68] Findlay JC, Sheeler LR, Engeland WC, et al. Familial adrenocorticotropin-independent Cushing's syndrome with bilateral macronodular adrenal hyperplasia. J Clin Endocrinol Metab 1993;76(1):189–91.
[69] Croughs RJ, Zelissen PM, Van Vroonhoven THJ, et al. GIP-dependent adrenal Cushing's syndrome with incomplete suppression of ACTH. Clin Endocrinol (Oxf) 2000;52:235–40.
[70] Groussin L, Kirschner LS, Vincent-Dejean C, et al. Molecular analysis of the cyclic AMP-dependent protein kinase A (PKA) regulatory subunit 1A (PRKAR1A) gene in patients with Carney complex and primary pigmented nodular adrenocortical disease (PPNAD) reveals novel mutations and clues for pathophysiology: augmented PKA signaling is associated with adrenal tumorigenesis in PPNAD. Am J Hum Genet 2002;71(6):1433–42.

[71] Goodarzi MO, Dawson DW, Li X, et al. Virilization in bilateral macronodular adrenal hyperplasia controlled by luteinizing hormone. J Clin Endocrinol Metab 2003;88(1):73–7.
[72] Fragoso MC, Domenice S, Latronico AC, et al. Cushing's syndrome secondary to adrenocorticotropin-independent macronodular adrenocortical hyperplasia due to activating mutations of GNAS1 gene. J Clin Endocrinol Metab 2003;88(5):2147–51.
[73] Imohl M, Koditz R, Stachon A, et al. Catecholamine-dependent hereditary Cushing's syndrome—follow-up after unilateral adrenalectomy. Med Klin 2002;97(12):747–53.
[74] Jelcic J, Cacic M, Kastelan D, et al. Screening for p53 and c-kit mutations in patients with familial ACTH-independent adrenal macronodular adrenal hyperplasia. Presented at the 12th International Congress of Endocrinology. Lisbon, Portugal, August 31–September 4, 2004.
[75] Lee S, Jun S, Hong SW, et al. Familial adrenocorticotropin-independent macronodular adrenal hyperplasia: Ectopic expression of vasopressin V1b, V2 receptors in the adrenal gland. Presented at the 86th Meeting of the Endocrine Society. New Orleans, Louisiana, June 16–19, 2004.
[76] Smals AG, Pieters GF, van Haelst UJ, et al. Macronodular adrenocortical hyperplasia in long-standing Cushing's disease. J Clin Endocrinol Metab 1984;58(1):25–31.
[77] Doppman JL, Miller DL, Dwyer AJ, et al. Macronodular adrenal hyperplasia in Cushing's disease. Radiology 1988;166(2):347–52.
[78] Sturrock ND, Morgan L, Jeffcoate WJ. Autonomous nodular hyperplasia of the adrenal cortex: tertiary hypercortisolism? Clin Endocrinol (Oxf) 1995;43(6):753–8.
[79] Hocher B, Bahr V, Dorfmuller S, et al. Hypercortisolism with non-pigmented micronodular adrenal hyperplasia: transition from pituitary-dependent to adrenal-dependent Cushing's syndrome. Acta Endocrinol (Copenh) 1993;128(2):120–5.
[80] Choi Y, Werk EE Jr, Sholiton LJ. Cushing's syndrome with dual pituitary–adrenal control. Arch Intern Med 1970;125(6):1045–9.
[81] Aron DC, Findling JW, Fitzgerald PA, et al. Pituitary ACTH dependency of nodular adrenal hyperplasia in Cushing's syndrome. Report of two cases and review of the literature. Am J Med 1981;71(2):302–6.
[82] Fish HR, Sobel DO, Miegel CA. Macronodular adrenal hyperplasia with hypothalamic-pituitary-adrenal suppression by ultra-high-dose dexamethasone: regression following hypophysectomy. Clin Neuropharmacol 1986;9(3):303–8.
[83] Bourdeau I, D'Amour P, Hamet P, et al. Abberant membrane hormone receptors in incidentally discovered bilateral macronodular adrenal hyperplasia with subclinical Cushing's syndrome. J Clin Endocrinol Metab 2001;86:5534–40.
[84] Weinstein LS, Shenker A, Gejman PV, et al. Activating mutations of the stimulatory G protein in the McCune-Albright syndrome. N Engl J Med 1991;325(24):1688–95.
[85] Boston BA, Mandel S, LaFranchi S, et al. Activating mutation in the stimulatory guanine nucleotide-binding protein in an infant with Cushing's syndrome and nodular adrenal hyperplasia. J Clin Endocrinol Metab 1994;79(3):890–3.
[86] Skogseid B, Larsson C, Lindgren PG, et al. Clinical and genetic features of adrenocortical lesions in multiple endocrine neoplasia type 1. J Clin Endocrinol Metab 1992;75:76–81.
[87] Burgess JR, Harle RA, Tucker P, et al. Adrenal lesions in a large kindred with multiple endocrine neoplasia type 1. Arch Surg 1996;131:699–702.
[88] Swords FM, Baig A, Malchoff DM, et al. Impaired desensitization of a mutant adrenocorticotropin receptor associated with apparent constitutive activity. Mol Endocrinol 2002;16:2746–53.
[89] Swords FM, Noon LA, King PJ, et al. Constitutive activation of the human ACTH receptor resulting from a synergistic interaction between two naturally occurring missense mutations in the MC2R gene. Mol Cell Endocrinol 2004;213:149–54.
[90] Malchoff CD, MacGillivray D, Malchoff DM. Adrenocorticotropic hormone-independent adrenal hyperplasia. Endocrinologist 1996;6:79–85.

[91] Lacroix A, N'Diaye N, Tremblay J, et al. Ectopic and abnormal hormone receptors in adrenal Cushing's syndrome. Endocr Rev 2001;22(1):75–110.
[92] Antonini SR, Hamet P, Tremblay J, et al. Expression of ACTH receptor pathway genes in GIP-dependent Cushing's syndrome (CS). Endocr Res 2002;28:753–4.
[93] Sasano H. Localization of steroidogenic enzymes in adrenal cortex and its disorders. Endocr J 1994;41:471–82.
[94] Bourdeau I, Antonini S, Lacroix A, et al. Gene array analysis of macronodular adrenal hyperplasis confirms clinical heterogeneity and identifies several genes as molecular mediators. Oncogene 2004;26:1575–85.
[95] Gicquel C, Bertagna X, Le Bouc Y. Recent advances in the pathogenesis of adrenocortical tumours. Eur J Endocrinol 1995;133(2):133–44.
[96] Diaz-Cano SJ, de Miguel M, Blanes A. Clonality as expression of distinctive cell kinetics patterns in nodular hyperplasias and adenomas of the adrenal cortex. Am J Pathol 2000; 156(1):311–9.
[97] Beuschlein F, Reincke M, Karl M, et al. Clonal composition of human adrenocortical neoplasms. Cancer Res 1994;54:4927–32.
[98] Lacroix A, Baldacchino V, Bourdeau I, et al. Cushing's syndrome variants secondary to aberrant hormone receptors. Trends Endocrinol Metab 2004;15:375–82.
[99] Hingshaw HT, Ney RL. Abnormal control in the neoplastic adrenal cortex. In: McKerns KW, editor. Hormones and cancer. New York: Academic Press; 1974. p. 309–27.
[100] Hamet P, Larochelle P, Franks DJ, et al. Cushing's syndrome with food-dependent periodic hormonogenesis. Clin Invest Med 1987;10(6):530–3.
[101] de Herder WW, Hofland LJ, Usdin TB, et al. Food-dependent Cushing's syndrome resulting from abundant expression of gastric inhibitory polypeptide receptors in adrenal adenoma cells. J Clin Endocrinol Metab 1996;81(9):3168–72.
[102] Chabre O, Liakos P, Vivier J, et al. Cushing's syndrome due to a gastric inhibitory polypeptide-dependent adrenal adenoma: insights into hormonal control of adrenocortical tumorigenesis. J Clin Endocrinol Metab 1998;83(9):3134–43.
[103] Luton JP, Bertagna X. Membrane receptors and endocrine tumors: expression of vasopressin receptor V1 modulates the pharmacologic phenotype of adrenocortical tumors. Bull Acad Natl Med 1998;182(2):299–309.
[104] Tsagarakis S, Tsigos C, Vassiliou V, et al. Food-dependent androgen and cortisol secretion by a gastric inhibitory polypeptide-receptor expressive adrenocortical adenoma leading to hirsutism and subclinical Cushing's syndrome: in vivo and in vitro Studies. J Clin Endocrinol Metab 2001;86(2):583–9.
[105] N'Diaye N, Tremblay J, Hamet P, et al. Adrenocortical overexpression of gastric inhibitory polypeptide receptor underlies food-dependent Cushing's syndrome. J Clin Endocrinol Metab 1998;83(8):2781–5.
[106] Longo-Mazzuco T, Chabre O, Feige JJ, et al. Démonstration du potentiel transformant du gène du récepteur du GIP dans les cellules du cortex surrénalien: un pas vers l'étiologie du syndrome de Cushing lié à l'alimentation [Demonstration of transforming potential of GIP receptor gene in adrenocortical cells: a step towards the etiology of food-dependent Cushing's syndrome]. Ann Endocrinol (Paris) 2004;65:267 [in French].
[107] Perraudin V, Delarue C, de Keyzer Y, et al. Vasopressin-responsive adrenocortical tumor in a mild Cushing's syndrome: in vivo and in vitro studies. J Clin Endocrinol Metab 1995; 80(9):2661–7.
[108] Arnaldi G, Gasc JM, de Keyzer Y, et al. Variable expression of the V1 vasopressin receptor modulates the phenotypic response of steroid-secreting adrenocortical tumors. J Clin Endocrinol Metab 1998;83(6):2029–35.
[109] Bugalho MJ, Li X, Rao CV, et al. Presence of a Gs alpha mutation in an adrenal tumor expressing LH/hCG receptors and clinically associated with Cushing's syndrome. Gynecol Endocrinol 2000;14(1):50–4.

[110] Willenberg HS, Stratakis CA, Marx C, et al. Aberrant interleukin-1 receptors in a cortisol-secreting adrenal adenoma causing Cushing's syndrome. N Engl J Med 1998;339(1):27–31.
[111] Lacroix A, Mircescu H, Hamet P. Clinical evaluation of the presence of abnormal hormone receptors in adrenal Cushing's syndrome. Endocrinologist 1999;9:9–15.
[112] Bertherat J, Barrande G, Lefebvre H, et al. Illegitimate membrane receptors are frequent and often multiple in bilateral ACTH-independent macronodular adrenal hyperplasia. Presented at the 85th Meeting of the Endocrine Society. Philadelphia, Pennsylvania, June 19–22, 2003.
[113] Reznik Y, Lefebvre H, Rohmer V, et al. Aberrant sensitivity to multiple ligands in unilateral adrenal incidentaloma: a prospective study. Clin Endocrinol (Oxf) 2004;61(3):311–9.
[114] Carney JA, Gordon H, Carpenter PC. The complex of myxomas, spotty pigmentation, and endocrine overactivity. Medicine (Baltimore) 1985;64(4):270–83.
[115] Carney JA, Hruska LS, Beauchamp GD, et al. Dominant inheritance of the complex of myxomas, spotty pigmentation, and endocrine overactivity. Mayo Clin Proc 1986;61(3): 165–72.
[116] Carney JA, Young WF Jr. Primary pigmented nodular adrenocortical disease and its associated conditions. Endocrinologist 1992;2:6–21.
[117] Stratakis CA, Kirschner LS, Carney JA. Clinical and molecular features of the Carney complex: diagnostic criteria and recommendations for patient evaluation. J Clin Endocrinol Metab 2001;86(9):4041–6.
[118] Stratakis CA, Carney JA, Lin JP, et al. Carney complex, a familial multiple neoplasia and lentiginosis syndrome. Analysis of 11 kindreds and linkage to the short arm of chromosome 2. J Clin Invest 1996;97(3):699–705.
[119] Casey M, Mah C, Merliss AD, et al. Identification of a novel genetic locus for familial cardiac myxomas and Carney complex. Circulation 1998;98(23):2560–6.
[120] Kirschner LS, Carney JA, Pack SD, et al. Mutations of the gene encoding the protein kinase A type I-alpha regulatory subunit in patients with the Carney complex. Nat Genet 2000; 26(1):89–92.
[121] Kirschner LS, Sandrini F, Monbo J, et al. Genetic heterogeneity and spectrum of mutations of the PRKAR1A gene in patients with the Carney complex. Hum Mol Genet 2000;9(20): 3037–46.
[122] Casey M, Vaughan CJ, He J, et al. Mutations in the protein kinase A R1alpha regulatory subunit cause familial cardiac myxomas and Carney complex. J Clin Invest 2000;106(5): R31–8.
[123] Doppman JL, Travis WD, Nieman L, et al. Cushing's syndrome due to primary pigmented nodular adrenocortical disease: findings at CT and MR imaging. Radiology 1989;172(2): 415–20.
[124] Stratakis CA, Carney JA, Kirschner LS, et al. Synaptophysin immunoreactivity in primary pigmented nodular adrenocortical disease: neuroendocrine properties of tumors associated with Carney complex. J Clin Endocrinol Metab 1999;84(3):1122–8.
[125] Stratakis CA, Sarlis N, Kirschner LS, et al. Paradoxical response to dexamethasone in the diagnosis of primary pigmented nodular adrenocortical disease. Ann Intern Med 1999; 131(8):585–91.
[126] Bourdeau I, Lacroix A, Schurch W, et al. Primary pigmented nodular adrenocortical disease: paradoxical responses of cortisol secretion to dexamethasone occur in vitro and are associated with increased expression of the glucocorticoid receptor. J Clin Endocrinol Metab 2003;88(8):3931–7.
[127] Caticha O, Odell WD, Wilson DE, et al. Estradiol stimulates cortisol production by adrenal cells in estrogen-dependent primary adrenocortical nodular dysplasia. J Clin Endocrinol Metab 1993;77(2):494–7.
[128] Oelkers W, Bahr V, Hensen J, et al. Primary adrenocortical micronodular adenomatosis causing Cushing's syndrome. Effects of ketoconazole on steroid production and in vitro performance of adrenal cells. Acta Endocrinol (Copenh) 1986;113(3):370–7.

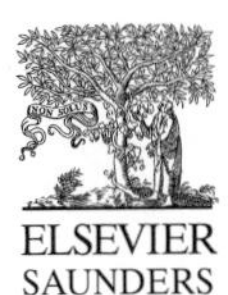

ELSEVIER
SAUNDERS

Endocrinol Metab Clin N Am
34 (2005) 459–478

ENDOCRINOLOGY
AND METABOLISM
CLINICS
OF NORTH AMERICA

Pituitary Surgery and Postoperative Management in Cushing's Disease

Andrea L. Utz, MD, PhD[a,b],
Brooke Swearingen, MD[a,c],
Beverly M.K. Biller, MD[a,b,*]

[a]*Harvard Medical School, Boston, MA, USA*
[b]*Neuroendocrine Unit, Massachusetts General Hospital, 55 Fruit Street, Bulfinch 457, Boston, MA 02114, USA*
[c]*Department of Neurosurgery, Massachusetts General Hospital, 15 Parkman Street, WACC 331, Boston, MA 02114, USA*

Transsphenoidal pituitary surgery is the primary therapy for Cushing's disease because of its potential to produce a lasting remission without long-term drug or hormone replacement therapy. Surgical therapy has been a treatment for basophil adenomas since Cushing's original description in 1932. He performed a craniotomy, a subtemporal decompression for presumed hydrocephalus, on one of his index cases, Minnie G [1]. Although no tumor was found, the underlying concept that surgery would be effective in removing the pituitary source of corticotropin (ACTH) overproduction was proven correct some 30 years later, when Hardy described the first successful removal of a pituitary microadenoma [2]. In the interim, treatment aimed at controlling the hypercortisolemia by adrenalectomy became possible after the introduction of cortisol replacement in the early 1950s [3,4], although this approach was complicated by the risk of unrestrained growth of the untreated pituitary adenoma resulting in Nelson's syndrome [5–11]. Since then, advances have been made in diagnostic evaluation and surgical technique. Operative centers that specialize in pituitary surgery have emerged throughout the world, and reports from these expert centers show successful transsphenoidal removal of ACTH-producing pituitary adenomas and remission of Cushing's disease in most cases.

* Corresponding author. Department of Neurosurgery, Massachusetts General Hospital, 55 Fruit Street, Bulfinch 457, Boston, MA 02114.
E-mail address: bbiller@partners.org (B.M.K. Biller).

0889-8529/05/$ - see front matter
doi:10.1016/j.ecl.2005.01.007 ***endo.theclinics.com***

Preoperative evaluation

The diagnosis of Cushing's disease is described in detail in the article by Lindsay and Nieman elsewhere in this issue. Hormonal testing must confirm that the patient has ACTH-dependent hypercortisolemia from a pituitary source. Because basophil adenomas are often below the resolution of high-field strength MR imaging, confirmation by endocrine testing of a pituitary, rather than an ectopic, source of ACTH hypersecretion is necessary to justify transsphenoidal pituitary exploration [12,13]. The inferior petrosal sinus sampling (IPSS) procedure is the most definitive test in determining the location of ACTH production [14,15], although it is not infallible [16,17].

Anesthetic considerations

Patients who have hypercortisolemia are prone to several medical comorbidities as described elsewhere in this issue; these may complicate surgical and anesthetic management. Patients who have Cushing's disease can present with refractory hypertension and unrecognized coronary artery disease, which increases their anesthetic risk. Many have diabetes or insulin resistance and may be more prone to perioperative infection from their relatively immunocompromised state. The risk of postoperative venous thrombosis is increased with the hypercoagulability associated with hypercortisolemia. Central obesity can complicate airway management and increase the incidence of postoperative pulmonary complications.

Surgical technique

The transsphenoidal approach to the sella remains the most effective and least invasive means of exploring the pituitary gland. The pituitary is located within the bony sella turcica (Turkish saddle), extending into the sphenoid sinus, and bounded laterally by the carotid arteries within the cavernous sinuses, posteriorly by the dorsum sella, and superiorly by the suprasellar cistern, through which pass the optic nerves and chiasm. There are three routes to the sphenoid and sella in use today. The traditional approach employed by Cushing was by means of a sublabial incision, identifying the nasal spine, and fracturing and displacing the nasal septum. This approach gives a relatively wide exposure, as the opening of the leaves of the nasal speculum is not limited by the size of the nostril, but has the disadvantage of a painful gingival incision and possible postoperative numbness of the front teeth. Most neurosurgeons now use a variation of the transnasal approach to the sphenoid, working directly through the nostril. An incision can be made at the intersection of the posterior septum and the face of the sphenoid, entering directly into the sphenoid sinus, or the sphenoid os can be enlarged. This approach minimizes the need for postoperative nasal packing if there is no extensive mucosal dissection. Alternatively, a mucosal incision can be made along the anterior margin of the nasal mucosa and a submucosal tunnel created back along the septum to the face of the sphenoid.

After the sphenoid sinus has been entered, the sella usually can be visualized. Following removal of the floor of the sella, the dura is opened and the gland entered. If the MRI has demonstrated the presumed adenoma, that region of the gland is explored first. If no adenoma was seen on preoperative imaging, the gland is explored systematically, using the lateralization data from the IPSS as guidance. Multiple frozen section biopsies are taken and reviewed intraoperatively by the pathologist. If adenoma is found, that portion of the gland is removed. If not, despite careful exploration of both sides of the gland, many surgeons empirically perform a hemi-hypophysectomy based upon IPSS lateralization, which is correctly predictive about 70% of the time [18].

The tumor bed then is packed with fat, typically harvested from a small subcutaneous abdominal incision, and the sella floor reconstructed with bone previously removed from the nasal septum, if available, or with titanium mesh. A watertight repair is critical to prevent a postoperative cerebrospinal fluid leak, especially if extensive dissection was required, with damage to the diaphragma sella.

Complications

Transsphenoidal surgery is safe and effective for the treatment of Cushing's disease. The incidence of complications after transsphenoidal surgery generally correlates with the experience of the surgeon [19,20]. Postoperative complications include those resulting in pituitary hormonal insufficiency, new neurologic deficits, or other medical problems. Patients who have Cushing's disease are more prone to systemic complications caused by inherent metabolic and cardiovascular abnormalities associated with the disorder. In particular, perioperative deep venous thrombosis was reported in approximately 4% of cases [21]. Additional complications include diabetes insipidus, syndrome of inappropriate antidiuretic hormone, cerebrospinal fluid rhinorrhea, meningitis, optic nerve injury, other cranial nerve palsies, vascular injury, nasal septum perforations, epistaxis, sinusitis, and graft site dehiscence. The perioperative mortality ranges from 0% to 2% [21–23].

Defining postoperative remission

Following surgical resection for Cushing's disease, there are three possible outcomes: complete and lasting remission or cure, remission with future return of hypercortisolism, or persistent postoperative hypercortisolism. Appropriate classification of postoperative outcome is dependent on biochemical assessment of endogenous cortisol production. There is no consensus, however, concerning the timing, choice of biochemical tests, or threshold values to define remission [24]. Thus, a gold standard for classifying patients in the postoperative period has not yet been established. The most commonly used tests are serum cortisol and 24-hour urinary cortisol. Table 1 summarizes outcome data for transsphenoidal resection for Cushing's disease from medical centers with expertise in pituitary surgery. Remission was achieved in approximately 70% to 90% of cases. Notably, the criteria for remission vary significantly between studies (Table 2). Surgeons without significant pituitary surgery experience may not attain this high level of success.

In most patients who obtain cure or remission, there is a period of severe hypoadrenalism following adenoma resection, likely because of the suppression of normal pituitary corticotroph function by previous hypercortisolemia [25]. These patients often display undetectable or extremely low serum and urine cortisol in the early postoperative period. Following a period of hypoadrenalism, the hypothalamic–pituitary–adrenal (HPA) axis typically recovers, with a time to recovery of approximately 11 to 14 months [25–28]. Exogenous steroid replacement is required to treat adrenal insufficiency during this recovery phase. Cushing's disease cure should be accompanied by resolution of the clinical features of hypercortisolism. Over time, the normal cortisol response to hypoglycemia and cosyntropin stimulation recovers in most patients, allowing withdrawal of glucocorticoid replacement, and typically there is a return of the diurnal pattern of cortisol secretion [29,30].

Patients who have persistent hypercortisolemia following surgery are considered surgical failures. Early identification of such patients allows expedient secondary intervention. Benefits of early cortisol status assessment include shorter exposure to a high cortisol state, potentially easier secondary surgical approach [31], and earlier radiation treatment.

The postoperative cortisol dynamics of a number of patients lie between the two extremes of very low endogenous cortisol and persistent hypercortisolemia. In this population, debate has arisen about the definition of remission and appropriate course of further intervention. Although these patients do not have overt hypercortisolism in the early postoperative period, the absence of adrenal insufficiency raises concern for subsequent relapse of Cushing's disease. A lack of complete or near complete cortisol suppression in the early postoperative period is considered an indication of residual adenoma and thus absence of a true remission [30,32]. Some patients, however, have normal cortisol levels in the immediate postoperative period that subsequently remain stable during long-term follow-up. In others, levels may decline in the early postoperative period [33,34].

Studies of postoperative cortisol status generally have reported biochemical test results from the 1- to 2-week period following transsphenoidal surgery. Immediate postoperative cortisol levels during the first 24 hours also have been used [35]. Others suggest that testing after 6 to 12 weeks prevents misclassification of patients who have a delayed decline in

Table 1
Efficacy of transsphenoidal surgery for Cushing's disease

First author, year [Ref. no.]	N	Follow-up time range in mo (mean) {median}	% Remission[a]	Relapse after remission[b]	Time to relapse in mo (mean) {median}
Hardy, 1982 [80]	75	ND	84 (63/75)	3 (2/63)	10–30 (20)
Boggan, 1983 [81]	100	20–110 (55)	78 (78/100)	5 (4/78)	(26)
Fahlbusch, 1986 [82]	101	8–168 (38)	71 (72/101)	7 (5/72)	6–50 (26) {23}
Chandler, 1987 [83]	33	ND	73 (24/33)	ND	ND
Nakane, 1987 [84]	100	(38)	86 (86/100)	9 (8/86)	19–82 (44)
Schrell, 1987 [85]	30	8–38 (20)	73 (22/30)	5 (1/22)	25
Guilhaume, 1988 [42]	60	3–84 {24}	70 (42/60)	14 (6/42)	24–36 {36}
Mampalam, 1988 [86]	212	12–156 (47)	81 (171/212)	5 (9/171)	(46)
Pieters, 1989 [44]	27	18–90 {54}	59 (16/27)	25 (4/16)	24–60 (42)
Arnott, 1990 [43]	28	3–56 (22)	86 (24/28)	13 (3/24)	14–42 (29)
Burke, 1990 [26]	54	6–156 (56) {39}	81 (44/54)	5 (2/44)	19–64 (42)
Tindall, 1990 [87]	53	2–142 (58)	85 (45/53)	2 (1/45)	34
Ludecke, 1991 [88]	103	ND	90	ND	ND
Robert, 1991 [89]	73	12–216 (77)	77 (56/73)	11 (5/47)	36–120 (60)
Lindholm, 1992 [90]	46	4–110 {34}	80 (36/45)	3 (1/34)	ND
Tahir, 1992 [91]	45	12–180 (70)	76 (34/45)	21 (7/34)	29–62 (40)
McCance, 1993 [9]	41	1–144 (59)	46 (19/41)	0 (0/19)	ND
Trainer, 1993 [32]	48	ND	67 (32/48)	ND	ND
Ram, 1994 [31]	222	ND	87 (193/222)	ND	ND
Bochicchio, 1995 [23]	668	(46)	76 (510/668)	13 (65/510)	6–104 (39) {33}
Bakiri, 1996 [92]	50	(92)	72 (36/50)	8 (3/36)	12–60 (40)
Knappe, 1996 [93]	310	(43)	85 (265/310)	11 (29/264)	ND
Sonino, 1996 [41]	103	24–192 {72}	77 (79/103)	26[c]	24–192 {72}
Blevins, 1998 [38]	96	8–218	85 (82/96)	16 (13/82)	8–142
Invitti, 1999 [28]	236	6–180	69	17	6–84
Semple, 1999 [21]	105	ND	75 (79/105)	ND	ND
Swearingen, 1999 [22]	161	12–240 {96}	85 (137/161)	7 (10/136)	12–132 (68) {48}
Barbetta, 2001 [52]	68	12–252 {58}	90 (61/68)	21 (13/61)	8–84 (36)
Chee, 2001 [29]	61	7–211 {88}	79 (48/61)	15 (7/48)	22–158 (76)
Estrada, 2001 [30]	109	6–198 (61)	69 (75/109)	21 (16/75)	12–110
Rees, 2002 [37]	53	6–252 {72}	77 (41/53)	5 (2/41)	13–36 (25)
Shimon, 2002 [94]	74	(50)	78 (58/74)	5 (3/58)	4–60 (44)
Yap, 2002 [40]	89	6–348 (92) {38}	69 (61/89)	11 (7/61)	6–60 (36)
Chen, 2003 [49]	174	60	82 (142/174)	14 (19/132)	6–48
Pereira, 2003 [33]	78	12–288 {86}	72 (56/78)	9 (5/56)	12–240 (84) {48}
Hammer, 2004 [36]	289	7–289 {133}	82 (236/289)	9 (13/150)	13–133 {59}
Rollin, 2004 [48]	48	4–170 (58)	88 (42/48)	5 (2/42)	54–66 (60)

Abbreviation: ND, no data available.

[a] Remission as defined in Table 2.

[b] Represents number of patients who relapsed following initial remission as assessed by urinary cortisol or low-dose dexamethasone suppression in the majority of studies.

[c] Kaplan-Meier probability of relapse at 10 y.

Data are from studies since 1980 with N > 25. *N* represents the number of patients that underwent transsphenoidal surgery with at least an initial report of postoperative endocrine evaluation. Data for micro- and macroadenomas have been combined. Definition of cure and relapse vary between studies and thus could affect outcome statistics.

Table 2
Biochemical criteria for Cushing's disease remission

First author, year [Ref. no.]	Timing of postoperative test	Biochemical tests	Remission cutoff value[a]
Hardy, 1982 [80]	ND	Cortisol	Normal
		Urinary 17-OHCS ***or***	Normal
		UFC	Normal
Boggan, 1983 [81]	6 wk	ACTH	Normal
		Cortisol	Normal
		LD-DST	Normal suppression
Fahlbusch, 1986 [82]	5–6 d	LD-DST (2 or 3 mg) ***or***	< 2 μg/dL
		Adrenal insufficiency	ND
Chandler, 1987 [83]	Within 1 wk	Cortisol	< 20.5 μg/dL
		UFC	< 130 μg/d
Nakane, 1987 [84]	ND	Cortisol	< 20 μg/dL
		ACTH	< 100 pg/mL
Schrell, 1987 [85]	7–10 d	AM ACTH	< 50 pg/mL
		AM cortisol	< 21 μg/dL
		LD-DST (2 mg)	Normal suppression
Guilhaume, 1988 [42]	3–6 mo	UFC	< 90 μg/d
		8 PM cortisol	< 100 ng/mL
Mampalam, 1988 [86]	ND	Cortisol	Normal
		ACTH	Normal
		LD-DST	Normal suppression
Pieters, 1989 [44]	1 d	AM cortisol	< 7 μg/dL
Arnott, 1990 [43]	1–4 wk	UFC	< 490 nmol/d
Burke, 1990 [26]	4 wk	UFC	< 280 nmol/d
		12 AM cortisol	< 280 nmol/L
Tindall, 1990 [87]	1–24 wk	Cortisol	Normal
		UFC	Normal
Ludecke, 1991 [88]	16 h	Cortisol	Subnormal
		ACTH	Subnormal
Robert, 1991 [89]	ND	ND	ND
Lindholm, 1992 [90]	ND	UFC ***or***	< 235 nmol/d
		ACTH stimulation of cortisol	Low
Tahir, 1992 [91]	ND	ND	ND
McCance, 1993 [9]	1–14 d	AM cortisol	< 550 nmol/L
		LD-DST (2 mg)	< 60 nmol/L
		UFC	< 330 nmol/d
Trainer, 1993 [32]	1 d	AM cortisol	< 50 nmol/L
Ram, 1994 [31]	ND	AM cortisol	< 5 μg/dL
		UFC	< 90 μg/d
Bochicchio, 1995 [23]	Within 6 mo	LD-DST	Normal suppression
Bakiri, 1996 [92]	ND	Circadian cortisol rhythm	Normal
		LD-DST	Normal suppression
Knappe, 1996 [93]	ND	ND	ND
Sonino, 1996 [41]	5–15 d	UFC	< 248 nmol/d
		LD-DST	Normal suppression
Blevins, 1998 [38]	6 mo	Cortisol ***or***	< 5 μg/dL
		UFC ***and***	< 15 μg/d
		LD-DST	Normal suppression

Table 2 (*continued*)

First author, year [Ref. no.]	Timing of postoperative test	Biochemical tests	Remission cutoff value[a]
Invitti, 1999 [28]	ND	UFC	Low/normal
		AM cortisol	Low/normal
		AM ACTH	Low/normal
Semple, 1999 [21]	ND	ND	ND
Swearingen, 1999 [22]	1–10 d	AM cortisol	< 138 nmol/L
		UFC	< 55 nmol/d
Barbetta, 2001 [52]	1 mo	Cortisol	Normal
		UFC	Normal
Chee, 2001 [29]	2 wk	AM cortisol	Normal
		12 AM cortisol	< 200 nmol/L
		LD-DST (2 mg)	Cortisol ≤ 100 nmol/L *and* ACTH ≤ 5 ng/L
Estrada, 2001 [30]	8–12 d	Cortisol every 6 hours ×4	Normal
		UFC	< 331 nmol/d
Rees, 2002 [37]	1–7 d	AM cortisol	< 50 nmol/L
Shimon, 2002 [94]	4–6 wk	UFC	Normal
		LD-DST (2 mg)	< 5 μg/dL
Yap, 2002 [40]	3–4 d	AM cortisol	< 50 nmol/L
Chen, 2003 [49]	2 d	LD-DST (1 mg)	< 8 μg/dL
Pereira, 2003 [33]	6 mo	LD-DST (1 mg)	< 100 nmol/L
		UFC ×2	Normal
Hammer, 2004 [36]	1 wk	AM cortisol ***or***	≤ 5 μg/dL
	Within 6 mo	LD-DST (1 mg) ***or***	≤ 5 μg/dL
		UFC	Normal
Rollin, 2004 [48]	1–12 d	Cortisol	< 5 μg/dL
		LD-DST (1 mg)	< 3 μg/dL

Abbreviations: LD-DST, low-dose dexamethasone suppression test (cutoff value represents AM cortisol level); ND, no data available; UFC, 24-hour urinary cortisol; 17-OHCS, 17-hydroxy-corticosteroids.

[a] Cortisol (nmol/L) = cortisol (μg/dL) × 27.59.

postoperative cortisol levels [33,34]. Another potential confounder during postoperative assessment is the choice of steroid replacement and the timing of steroid discontinuation before biochemical measurement.

Cortisol dynamics after transsphenoidal resection for Cushing's disease can follow several patterns. Although certain biochemical results are more suggestive of remission or surgical failure, none has been proven to be completely accurate. Therefore, a postoperative approach that combines several tests at regular follow-up intervals is most likely to define outcome correctly and guide need for future intervention.

Factors that predict early remission

Adenoma size/extension

Most studies suggest that remission is more likely with smaller adenomas, whereas surgical failure is more common with macroadenomas and with extrasellar extension [36–39]. Not all studies, however, suggest that there is a correlation between size and surgical success [23,29].

Preoperative imaging

There are conflicting data regarding whether preoperative radiologic localization of an adenoma increases the chance of early surgical success. In studies by Yap et al and Invitti et al, 63% to 70% of those with, and 63% to 67% of those without an abnormality noted on imaging entered remission [12,28,40]. Others have reported a significant correlation between radiologic visualization of a lesion and chance of remission [23], with rates of 100% versus 69% in positive and negative scans, respectively [37].

Endocrine assessment

Rees et al showed that baseline preoperative ACTH was correlated indirectly with the likelihood of remission [37,39]; however, this was not seen in all studies [23,41–43]. There is no correlation between preoperative urinary cortisol level and surgical success [42,43]. Surgical failure is more likely in patients who do not respond to corticotropin-releasing hormone (CRH) infusion with an elevation in ACTH and cortisol preoperatively [23,44]. A paradoxical rise in cortisol after thyrotropin-releasing hormone (TRH) or luteinizing hormone-releasing hormone (LHRH) infusion has been reported to predict surgical failure [44]. A decline in intraoperative ACTH level did not prove to be a useful tool for predicting remission [45].

Intraoperative visual tumor identification

Visualization of adenomatous tissue by the surgeon is not required to bring about cure of hypercortisolism [46]. A higher remission rate, 73% versus 33%, however, has been reported when adenomatous tissue was identified [29].

Pathology

The pathologic assessment of resected pituitary tissue cannot be used definitively to predict immediate or long-term remission. In some series, remission rates were higher (75% to 78% versus 24% to 36%) when an adenoma was noted on pathology [28,42]. Others, however, show no correlation between positive histology for adenoma and likelihood of remission [12,30,37,40,46]. In a report by Burke et al, 53% of biopsies showed a corticotroph adenoma; 20% demonstrated corticotroph hyperplasia, and 27% showed normal anterior pituitary tissue. Interestingly, remission rates were 89%, 67%, and 82%, respectively. This suggests that remission is not dependent on finding an abnormality on pathology [26].

This discrepancy may result from destruction of the microscopic specimen during resection or processing.

Early management following transsphenoidal surgery for Cushing's disease

Operative centers that specialize in pituitary surgery have emerged throughout the world. Although each center has an individualized approach to perioperative management, several important principles are universal in caring for this population of patients.

In the early postoperative period, severe adrenal insufficiency may occur. Some clinicians preempt this development by providing intraoperative or early postoperative glucocorticoid replacement. Others withhold steroid replacement until clinical signs and symptoms or biochemical data confirm hypocortisolism and thus prove the need for replacement therapy. In the latter case, vigilant monitoring is necessary to avert the adverse hemodynamic consequences of adrenal insufficiency. The choice of replacement glucocorticoid also varies between practitioners. Dexamethasone does not interfere with standard serum and urine assays of endogenous cortisol production, but its potent corticotroph suppressive effect may affect early tests for assessing remission and may suppress subsequent HPA axis recovery. Hydrocortisone, prednisone, and metabolites interfere with cortisol assays; therefore, a delay of at least 24 hours after the last dose of replacement glucocorticoid is recommended before measurement of endogenous cortisol levels.

The rapid decline in cortisol level that often occurs following corticotroph adenoma resection can produce steroid withdrawal symptoms of headache, fatigue, malaise, or myalgia. Providing a glucocorticoid taper during the initial postoperative days, starting above the physiologic replacement dose, can alleviate these symptoms. Subsequently, patients who are in remission should be maintained on replacement doses during HPA axis recovery. Assessment of recovery is recommended every 3 to 6 months by measurement of morning serum cortisol level or response to cosyntropin stimulation after withholding exogenous glucocorticoids for 24 hours. Replacement therapy can be discontinued safely when a cortisol level above 19 μg/dL (525 nmol/L) is obtained for either test [47].

Relapse of hypercortisolism

Because Cushing's disease can relapse many years after initial remission, long-term studies are most accurate in predicting the risk of a recurrence. Table 1 shows the percentage of patients in several long-term studies with relapse following an initial remission. Relapse in these studies usually was defined by development of an elevated 24-hour urinary cortisol or failure to suppress adequately on low-dose dexamethasone testing. The risk of relapse is approximately 10% to 15%. The relapse percentage represents the minimum rate, as recurrence rates would be expected to increase as follow-up time is extended. Thus the Kaplan-Meier statistical method best predicts relapse risk. A 10-year risk of approximately 25% has been reported [23,41]. With stratification by tumor size, the 10-year risk of relapse was 7% and 45% for micro- and macroadenomas, respectively [22]. Late relapses have been reported at 16 and 20 years after surgery [33,41]. This highlights the importance of lifelong monitoring for return of hypercortisolism.

Predicting return of hypercortisolism

Knowing which patients will experience a relapse of hypercortisolism might allow early planning of secondary treatment options and heighten awareness for symptoms and biochemical evidence of hypercortisolism. Box 1 lists biochemical tests that have been examined for their usefulness in predicting relapse of hypercortisolism following initial remission; however, no test has proven to be completely reliable.

Measurement of morning cortisol in the early period following pituitary resection has been evaluated for predicting future relapse. Several studies [32,44,46] demonstrated that undetectable or subnormal postoperative serum cortisol levels offered the best chance for sustained remission. The duration of glucocorticoid replacement therapy is related inversely to the risk of relapse, with 5-year relapse risks of 3%, 24%, and 47% for greater than 1 year, less than 1 year, and no replacement, respectively [23]. Although postoperative hypoadrenalism is associated with a lower risk of relapse, this is not absolute, and several studies have shown return of hypercortisolism following a period of adrenal insufficiency [23,40,48]. Estrada et al reported

Box 1. Biochemical tests for defining or predicting relapse

Commonly used tests
Morning serum cortisol
24-hour urinary cortisol
Low-dose dexamethasone cortisol suppression

Other testing techniques
CRH stimulation of ACTH or cortisol
Metyrapone stimulation of serum 11-deoxycortisol
Desmopressin stimulation ACTH or cortisol
Loperamide suppression of ACTH or cortisol
Diurnal cortisol variation
Cortisol response to hypoglycemia
Serum ACTH

that 10% of patients who have initial hypocortisolism relapsed within 5 years. This percentage ultimately may be higher as further years of follow-up are examined [30]. Similarly, Pereira showed that 14% of patients who have 2- and 12-week postoperative cortisol levels less than 50 nmol/L (1.8 μg/dL) ultimately relapsed [33].

The timing of the measurement can obscure determination of the nadir of serum cortisol following surgery. For example, in a study by Pereira et al, six patients had a normal serum cortisol in the first several weeks after surgery, followed by the later development of hypocortisolism. Five of these patients had macroadenomas, and none had relapse during an average follow-up period of 4 years [33]. Toms et al showed that a cortisol level less than 35 nmol/L (1.3 μg/dL) at 6 to 12 weeks postoperatively predicted persistent remission, and these cortisol values were, on average, lower than those obtained at 1 to 2 weeks after surgery [34]. These data suggest that there may be gradual resolution of adrenal autonomy in some patients following corticotroph adenoma resection. Alternatively, delayed adenoma necrosis following surgery could account for the gradual decline in cortisol during the early postoperative period.

Patients who lack the early hypoadrenalism phase, but do not have hypercortisolism as assessed by urinary cortisol or low-dose dexamethasone testing, are at significantly increased risk of relapse [23]. Estrada et al showed that patients who had cortisol levels in the normal range postoperatively had a relapse risk of 65% within 3 years after surgery. Kaplan-Meier probability in this population suggests a recurrence rate of 77% by 5 years and 88% by 10 years. It is important to note, however, that 35% had not recurred during follow-up assessment, ranging from 6 to 103 months [30]. Therefore, the risk of relapse is high, but may not be absolute, in this population. Lifelong, periodic follow-up is warranted in patients who have normal serum cortisol levels in the immediate postoperative period.

Low-dose dexamethasone suppression testing

A study by Chen et al showed that a 1 mg overnight dexamethasone test performed on postoperative day 3 could predict risk of relapse. Cortisol suppression to less than 3 μg/dL (83 nmol/L) was associated with a 93% chance of 5-year remission, but a level greater than 3 μg/dL predicted inevitable relapse [49].

Corticotropin-releasing hormone stimulation testing

Corticotropin-releasing hormone stimulates the release of ACTH and subsequently cortisol; this release typically is increased in the setting of a corticotroph adenoma [50]. Presumably, patients destined to relapse have residual corticotroph adenoma present following surgery. Although these remaining tumor cells do not produce enough ACTH to elevate serum cortisol to pathologic levels, they may respond more vigorously than normal corticotrophs to CRH stimulation, and thus distinguish patients who have residual tumor. Avgerinos et al showed that in 23 patients who had subnormal ACTH and cortisol responses to CRH, there were no relapses in 6 to 42 months of follow-up. In contrast, three of the six who had normal responses to CRH experienced relapse [27]. Other studies have reported similar results with the CRH stimulation test [28,51–53].

Metyrapone testing

Metyrapone stimulation has been evaluated as a predictor of future relapse. In a study of 29 postoperative patients, significantly elevated serum 11-deoxycortisol levels (> 350 nmol/L) following metyrapone administration in the early postoperative period were found in patients who failed surgery. Seventy-five percent of those who had intermediate elevation and none who had low levels of 11-deoxycortisol (< 150 nmol/L) after metyrapone had relapsed during a median follow-up of 46 months [54].

Desmopressin testing

Desmopressin activates V2 and V3 receptors on pituitary corticotrophs to stimulate the release of ACTH and thus cortisol. Postoperative remission generally is associated with a lack of ACTH and cortisol response to desmopressin infusion. Conversely, a positive response has been linked to an increased incidence of relapse [52,55,56].

Other testing strategies

Loperamide, an opioid agonist, normally suppresses ACTH and cortisol. Relapse has been associated with inadequate suppression [52]. Abnormal diurnal cortisol variation and blunted cortisol response to hypoglycemia after the initial hypoadrenalism phase predict relapse [30]. A direct correlation between basal postoperative ACTH levels and risk of relapse has been reported [28]. The role of salivary cortisol measurement in the postoperative patient has not been determined.

Risk of hypopituitarism after surgery

An inherent risk of transsphenoidal pituitary surgery is the possibility of pituitary hormone deficiency. The degree or risk of hypopituitarism is correlated with the extent of pituitary resection [32,37,57]. Compared with other anterior pituitary tumors, corticotroph adenomas often can be small and undetectable by radiologic techniques and visual inspection. Additionally, a subset of Cushing's disease is caused by diffuse corticotroph hyperplasia. These factors increase the complexity of surgery and may lead to increased tissue resection in an attempt to produce cure. This is supported by a higher frequency of hypopituitarism in patients who do not have an obvious adenoma on imaging [37].

The following rates of pituitary hormone deficiency after transsphenoidal surgery have been reported: thyrotropin 13% to 45% [22,26,29,32,37,40,46,57], gonadotropin 3% to 48% [22,26,29,32,37,40,46,57], long-term (> 3 years) corticotropin 3% to 53% [22,26,46,57], somatotropin 53% to 93% [37,57], and vasopressin 0% to 46% [22,26,29,32,37,40,46,57]. Thus, postoperative management of patients who have Cushing's disease includes testing and treatment for pituitary hormone deficiencies.

Treatment options for persistent/relapsed hypercortisolism

Treatment strategies for persistent or relapsed Cushing's disease include repeat transsphenoidal adenoma resection, pituitary radiation, medical therapy, and bilateral adrenal resection. Each therapeutic modality is accompanied by risks and benefits. Although a single technique can be effective in some individuals, patients may need multi-modality therapy following initial transsphenoidal surgery.

Repeat transsphenoidal surgery

Repeat transsphenoidal surgery for persistent or recurrent hypercortisolemia induces remission in approximately 70% of patients. The identification of an adenoma during the first surgery or on imaging studies predicts increased success during the subsequent operation. Failure to identify an adenoma during the second surgery often leads to a more extensive surgical resection, remission rates of approximately 20% to 40%, and an increased risk of hypopituitarism [31,58].

Pituitary radiation

Radiation therapy is an alternative treatment for persistent or recurrent Cushing's disease. Radiotherapy options include conventional fractionated radiation and stereotactic radiosurgery with protons or photons (gamma knife; linear-accelerator [LINAC]). Advantages of radiotherapy include efficacy in controlling hypercortisolism and the noninvasive nature of the treatment. A major disadvantage of pituitary radiotherapy for Cushing's disease is the significant delay that exists between radiation delivery and subsequent decline of hypercortisolemia. This delay often necessitates the use of cortisol-lowering medications in the interim. The risk of delayed hypopituitarism is also significant. Other less common potential adverse effects of radiation include optic nerve atrophy with visual impairment, secondary tumor development, and cognitive dysfunction [59].

Details regarding radiation therapy for Cushing's disease are provided by Vance elsewhere in this issue.

Medical therapy

The most commonly used medical treatments for hypercortisolemia inhibit adrenal steroidogenesis. These include ketoconazole, metyrapone, mitotane, aminoglutethimide, trilostane, and etomidate. Drugs to decrease ACTH release have been effective in a small percentage of patients and include bromocriptine, cabergoline, cyptoheptadine, valproate, and octreotide [60,61]. The peroxisome proliferator activated receptor γ (PPAR-γ) agonist, rosiglitazone [62], and the somatostatin analog, SOM230 [63], are under investigation for their potential to decrease ACTH release. The steroid receptor antagonist RU-486 also may be effective in some patients [64]. Because of the potential to produce adrenal insufficiency with these medications, careful dose titration or complete blockade with the addition of glucocorticoid replacement is indicated [61].

Ketoconazole is a commonly used medical therapy for Cushing's disease because of its relative effectiveness, twice daily dosing, and favorable adverse effect profile. Ketoconazole blocks the adrenal side-chain cleavage complex, 17,20-lyase, and 11-β- and 17-α-hydroxylase, leading to decreased steroidogenesis. A proposed additional benefit of ketoconazole is a lack of compensatory increase in ACTH release, suggesting that it also may change hypothalamic-pituitary responsiveness to cortisol or impair ACTH release [65]. The average dose of ketoconazole in pituitary-dependent Cushing's is 400 to 800 mg/d in divided doses, titrated based on urinary cortisol levels. In a study by Sonino et al [66], ketoconazole was very effective at lowering urinary cortisol in 28 Cushing's disease patients from a mean of 1073 ± 125 nmol/24 h to 200 ± 21 nmol/24 h (389 ± 45µg/24 h to 72 ± 8 µg/24 h). Transaminase elevation is the most likely adverse effect; therefore periodic liver function testing during therapy is indicated. Additional adverse effects include gastrointestinal (GI) disturbances, rash, and gynecomastia [66].

Metyrapone has been used effectively in Cushing's disease patients. In a study with 53 subjects, mean serum cortisol declined from 654 to 373 nmol/L (23.7 to 13.5 µg/dL) by 2 to 3 months, with 75% of patients having levels in the normal range. Adverse effects included hypoadrenalism, edema, hirsutism, rash, dizziness, and minor GI upset [67]. Mitotane blocks adrenal steroidogenesis at several enzymatic steps, and at high doses, it is adrenolytic. At an elevated dose, approximately 8 g/d, normalization of urinary cortisol was achieved in 38 of 46 (83%) patients who had Cushing's disease [68]. At these high doses, however, GI and neurologic adverse effects are common. Aminoglutethimide is most effective when given as combination therapy with the medications described above [61].

Bilateral adrenalectomy

Bilateral adrenalectomy usually provides definitive cure of the hypercortisolism of Cushing's disease [69]. An advantage of adrenalectomy is the potential to spare the patient from other pituitary hormone deficiencies that may occur following aggressive pituitary surgery or radiation therapy. The disadvantages of adrenalectomy, however, include the necessity of lifelong glucocorticoid and mineralocorticoid replacement and the potential for development of Nelson's syndrome. Nelson's syndrome is uninhibited growth of pituitary corticotroph adenomas caused by loss of cortisol negative feedback on adenoma growth [5–11]. In addition, there is a rare risk of recurrent hypercortisolism from ACTH stimulation of ectopic adrenal tissue or postsurgical adrenal remnants [70].

The risk of Nelson's syndrome following bilateral adrenalectomy has been reported to be as high as 20% to 35% [28,41,60]. Conflicting data exist concerning the risk of Nelson's syndrome as a function of age at adrenalectomy, with younger, [71], older [72] and no age correlation [41] all being reported. Several studies have reported that previous pituitary radiation did not decrease the risk of Nelson's syndrome after adrenalectomy [41,73]. Jenkins et al, however, saw a 50% reduction in the incidence of Nelson's in those who underwent prophylactic radiation treatment [8].

Monitoring for Nelson's syndrome after bilateral adrenalectomy includes regular physical examination for evidence of hyperpigmentation, ACTH measurements, and pituitary MRI scans. Evidence of rapid ACTH increase or adenoma growth necessitates consideration of pituitary radiation therapy or surgical adenoma resection.

Searching for rare causes of hypercortisolism

The primary cause of persistent hypercortisolism following transsphenoidal surgery is incomplete removal of a discrete corticotroph adenoma. In some cases, however, surgical failure or relapse may represent an inaccurate preoperative localization of the source of ACTH overproduction. Before additional pituitary intervention, a search for an ectopic source of ACTH should be considered if pathology did not confirm an ACTH-staining adenoma [74]. Evaluation for carcinoid or other ectopic source of ACTH may include high-resolution CT or MRI scanning of the neck, chest, abdomen, and pelvis, and whole-body radiolabeled octreotide scanning [24].

In rare cases, excess ACTH may originate from the pituitary gland but be stimulated by ectopic CRH production by a neoplasm elsewhere [75–78]. This possibility should be considered in the presence of diffuse corticotroph hyperplasia on pituitary pathology [79]. If CRH levels are elevated, a radiologic search can be undertaken to locate a potential ectopic CRH-producing neoplasm.

Summary

Transsphenoidal surgery is an effective treatment for Cushing's disease, with initial remission rates of approximately 70% to 90% when performed by an experienced pituitary surgery. Controversy concerning the specific definition of remission, however, affects determination of surgical success. Most cured patients experience a transient postoperative phase of hypocortisolism, requiring initiation of glucocorticoid replacement therapy for approximately a year. With long-term follow-up, the rate of relapse of hypercortisolism is approximately 10% to 15%. Biochemical tests to predict future relapse are not definitive; thus long-term monitoring for the development of cortisol elevation is necessary. Additionally, evaluation for hypopituitarism may reveal other hormonal deficiencies. For persistent or recurrent hypercortisolism, secondary interventions include repeat transsphenoidal surgery, pituitary radiation, medical therapy, and bilateral adrenalectomy.

References

[1] Cushing H. The basophil adenomas of the pituitary body and their clinical manifestations. Bull Johns Hopkins Hosp 1932;50:137–95.
[2] Hardy J. L'exerese des adenomes hypophysiares par voie transsphenoidale. Union Med Can 1962;91:933–45.
[3] Plotz D, Knowlton AL, Ragan C. The natural history of Cushing's disease. Am J Med 1952; 13:597–614.
[4] Orth DN, Liddle GW. Results of treatment of 108 patients with Cushing's syndrome. N Engl J Med 1971;285:243–7.
[5] Favia G, Boscaro M, Lumachi F, et al. Role of bilateral adrenalectomy in Cushing's disease. World J Surg 1994;18:462–6.
[6] Glenn F, Horwith M, Peterson RE, Mannix H. Total adrenalectomy for Cushing's disease. Ann Surg 1972;175:948–55.
[7] Grabner P, Hauer-Jensen M, Jervell J, et al. Long-term results of treatment of Cushing's disease by adrenalectomy. Eur J Surg 1991;157:461–4.
[8] Jenkins PJ, Trainer PJ, Plowman PN, et al. The long-term outcome after adrenalectomy and prophylactic pituitary radiotherapy in adrenocorticotropin-dependent Cushing's syndrome. J Clin Endocrinol Metab 1994;80:165–71.
[9] McCance DR, Russell CF, Kennedy TL, et al. Bilateral adrenalectomy: low mortality and morbidity in Cushing's disease. Clin Endocrinol (Oxf) 1993;39:315–21.
[10] O'Riordain DS, Farley DR, Young WFJ, et al. Long-term outcome of bilateral adrenalectomy in patients with Cushing's syndrome. Surgery 1994;116:1088–93.
[11] Welbourn RB. Survival and causes of death after adrenalectomy for Cushing's disease. Surgery 1985;97:16–20.
[12] Booth GL, Redelmeier DA, Grosman H, et al. Improved diagnostic accuracy of inferior petrosal sinus sampling over imaging for localizing pituitary pathology in patients with Cushing's disease. J Clin Endocrinol Metab 1998;83:2291–5.
[13] Anonymous. Transsphenoidal surgery for Cushing's disease: outcome in patients with a normal magnetic resonance imaging scan. Neurosurgery 2000;46:553–8.
[14] Findling JW, Kehoe ME, Shaker JL, et al. Routine inferior petrosal sinus sampling in the differential diagnosis of adrenocorticotropin (ACTH)-dependent Cushing's syndrome: early recognition of the occult ectopic ACTH syndrome. J Clin Endocrinol Metab 1991;73: 408–13.
[15] Oldfield EH, Doppman JL, Nieman LK, et al. Petrosal sinus sampling with and without corticotropin-releasing hormone for the differential diagnosis of Cushing's syndrome. N Engl J Med 1991;325:897–905.

[16] Calao A, Faggiano A, Pivonello R, et al. Inferior petrosal sinus sampling in the differential diagnosis of Cushing's syndrome: results of an Italian multi-center study. Eur J Endocrinol 2001;144:499–507.

[17] Swearingen B, Katznelson L, Miller K, et al. Diagnostic errors after inferior petrosal sinus sampling. J Clin Endocrinol Metab 2004;89:3752–63.

[18] Oldfield EH, Chrousos GP, Schulte HM, et al. Preoperative lateralization of ACTH-secreting pituitary microadenomas by bilateral and simultaneous inferior petrosal venous sinus sampling. N Engl J Med 1985;312:100–3.

[19] Barker FGN, Klibanski A, Swearingen B. Transsphenoidal surgery for pituitary tumors in the United States, 1996–2000: mortality, morbidity, and the effects of hospital and surgeon volume. J Clin Endocrinol Metab 2003;88:4709–19.

[20] Ciric I, Ragin A, Baumgartner C, et al. Complications of transsphenoidal surgery: results of a national survey, review of the literature, and personal experience. Neurosurgery 1997;40: 225–36.

[21] Semple PL, Laws ERJ. Complications in a contemporary series of patients who underwent transsphenoidal surgery for Cushing's disease. J Neurosurg 1999;91:175–9.

[22] Swearingen B, Biller BM, Barker FGN, et al. Long-term mortality after transsphenoidal surgery for Cushing's disease. Ann Intern Med 1999;130:821–4.

[23] Bochicchio D, Losa M, Buchfelder M. Factors influencing the immediate and late outcome of Cushing's disease treated by transsphenoidal surgery: a retrospective study by the European Cushing's Disease Survey Group. J Clin Endocrinol Metab 1995;80:3114–20.

[24] Arnaldi G, Angeli A, Atkinson AB, et al. Diagnosis and complications of Cushing's syndrome: a consensus statement. J Clin Endocrinol Metab 2003;88:5593–602.

[25] Fitzgerald PA, Aron DC, Findling JW, et al. Cushing's disease: transient secondary adrenal insufficiency after selective removal of pituitary microadenomas; evidence for a pituitary origin. J Clin Endocrinol Metab 1982;54:413–22.

[26] Burke CW, Adams CBT, Esiri MM, et al. Transsphenoidal surgery for Cushing's disease: does what is removed determine the endocrine outcome? Clin Endocrinol (Oxf) 1990;33: 525–37.

[27] Avgerinos PC, Chrousos GP, Nieman LK, et al. The corticotropin-releasing hormone test in the postoperative evaluation of patients with Cushing's syndrome. J Clin Endocrinol Metab 1987;65:906–13.

[28] Invitti C, Giraldi FP, De Martin M, et al. Diagnosis and management of Cushing's syndrome: results of an Italian multi-centre study. J Clin Endocrinol Metab 1999;84:440–8.

[29] Chee GH, Mathias DB, James RA, et al. Transsphenoidal pituitary surgery in Cushing's disease: can we predict outcome? Clin Endocrinol (Oxf) 2001;54:617–26.

[30] Estrada J, Garcia-Uria JL, Lamas C, et al. The complete normalization of the adrenocortical function as the criterion of cure after transsphenoidal surgery for Cushing's disease. J Clin Endocrinol Metab 2001;86:5695–9.

[31] Ram Z, Nieman LK, Cutler GBJ, et al. Early repeat surgery for persistent Cushing's disease. J Neurosurg 1994;80:37–45.

[32] Trainer PJ, Lawrie HS, Verhelst JA, et al. Transsphenoidal resection in Cushing's disease: undetectable serum cortisol as the definition of successful treatment. Clin Endocrinol (Oxf) 1993;38:73–8.

[33] Pereira AM, van Aken MO, van Dulken H, et al. Long-term predictive value of postsurgical cortisol concentrations for cure and risk of recurrence in Cushing's disease. J Clin Endocrinol Metab 2003;88:5858–64.

[34] Toms GC, McCarthy MI, Niven MJ, et al. Predicting relapse after transsphenoidal surgery for Cushing's disease. J Clin Endocrinol Metab 1993;76:291–4.

[35] Simmons NE, Alden TD, Thorner MO, et al. Serum cortisol response to transsphenoidal surgery for Cushing's disease. J Neurosurg 2001;95:1–8.

[36] Hammer GD, Tyrrell JB, Lamborn KR, et al. Transsphenoidal microsurgery for Cushing's disease: initial outcome and long term results. J Clin Endocrinol Metab 2004;89:6348–57.

[37] Rees DA, Hanna FWF, Davies JS, et al. Long-term follow-up results of transsphenoidal surgery for Cushing's disease in a single centre using strict criteria for remission. Clin Endocrinol (Oxf) 2002;56:541–51.
[38] Blevins LSJ, Christy JH, Khajavi M, et al. Outcomes of therapy for Cushing's disease due to adrenocorticotropin-secreting pituitary macro-adenomas. J Clin Endocrinol Metab 1998;83: 63–7.
[39] Cannavo S, Almoto B, Dall'Asta C, et al. Long-term results of treatment in patients with ACTH-secreting pituitary macro-adenomas. Eur J Endocrinol 2003;149:195–200.
[40] Yap LB, Turner HE, Adams CB, et al. Undetectable postoperative cortisol does not always predict long-term remission in Cushing's disease: a single centre audit. Clin Endocrinol (Oxf) 2002;56:25–31.
[41] Sonino N, Zielezny M, Fava GA, et al. Risk factors and long-term outcome in pituitary-dependent Cushing's disease. J Clin Endocrinol Metab 1996;81:2647–52.
[42] Guilhaume B, Bertagna X, Thomsen M, et al. Transsphenoidal pituitary surgery for the treatment of Cushing's disease: results in 64 patients and long term follow-up studies. J Clin Endocrinol Metab 1988;66:1056–64.
[43] Arnott RD, Pestell RG, McKelvie PA, et al. A critical evaluation of transsphenoidal pituitary surgery in the treatment of Cushing's disease: prediction of outcome. Acta Endocrinol (Copenh) 1990;123:423–30.
[44] Pieters GFFM, Hermus ARMM, Meijer E, et al. Predictive factors for initial cure and relapse rate after pituitary surgery for Cushing's disease. J Clin Endocrinol Metab 1989;69: 1122–6.
[45] Graham KE, Samuels MH, Raff H, et al. Intraoperative adrenocorticotropin levels during transsphenoidal surgery for Cushing's disease do not predict cure. J Clin Endocrinol Metab 1997;82:1776–9.
[46] McCance DR, Gordon DS, Fannin TF, et al. Assessment of endocrine function after transsphenoidal surgery for Cushing's disease. Clin Endocrinol (Oxf) 1993;38:79–86.
[47] Grinspoon S, Biller BMK. Laboratory assessment of adrenal insufficiency. J Clin Endocrinol Metab 1994;79:923–31.
[48] Rollin GAFS, Ferreira NP, Junges M, et al. Dynamics of serum cortisol levels after transsphenoidal surgery in a cohort of patients with Cushing's disease. J Clin Endocrinol Metab 2004;89:1131–9.
[49] Chen JC, Amar AP, Choi S, Singer P, et al. Transsphenoidal microsurgical treatment of Cushing's disease: postoperative assessment of surgical efficacy by application of an overnight low-dose dexamethasone suppression test. J Neurosurg 2003;98:967–73.
[50] Chrousos GP, Schulte HM, Oldfield EH, et al. The Corticotropin-releasing factor stimulation test. An aid in the evaluation of patients with Cushing's syndrome. N Engl J Med 1984;310:622–6.
[51] Vignati F, Berselli ME, Loli P. Early postoperative evaluation in patients with Cushing's disease: usefulness of ovine corticotropin-releasing hormone test in the prediction of recurrence of disease. Eur J Endocrinol 1994;130:235–41.
[52] Barbetta L, Dall'Asta C, Tomei G, et al. Assessment of cure and recurrence after pituitary surgery for Cushing's disease. Acta Neurochir (Wien) 2001;143:477–81.
[53] Nishizawa S, Oki Y, Ohta S, et al. What can predict postoperative endocrinological cure in Cushing's disease? Neurosurgery 1999;45:239–44.
[54] van Aken MO, de Herder WW, van der Lely AJ, et al. Postoperative metyrapone test in the early assessment of outcome of pituitary surgery for Cushing's disease. Clin Endocrinol (Oxf) 1997;47:145–9.
[55] Losa M, Mortini P, Dylgjeri S, et al. Desmopressin stimulation test before and after pituitary surgery in patients with Cushing's disease. Clin Endocrinol (Oxf) 2001;55:61–8.
[56] Colombo P, Dall'Asta C, Barbetta L, et al. Usefulness of the desmopressin test in the postoperative evaluation of patients with Cushing's disease. Eur J Endocrinol 2000;143: 227–34.

[57] Semple CG, Thomson JA, Teasdale GM. Transsphenoidal microsurgery for Cushing's disease. Clin Endocrinol (Oxf) 1984;21:621–9.
[58] Friedman RB, Oldfield EH, Nieman LK, et al. Repeat transsphenoidal surgery for Cushing's disease. J Neurosurg 1989;71:520–7.
[59] Plowman PN. Pituitary adenoma radiotherapy—when, who, and how? Clin Endocrinol (Oxf) 1999;51:265–71.
[60] Miller JW, Crapo L. The Medical treatment of Cushing's syndrome. Endocr Rev 1993;14: 443–58.
[61] Nieman LK. Medical therapy of Cushing's disease. Pituitary 2002;5:7–82.
[62] Alevizaki M, Philippou G, Zapanti L, et al. Significant improvement of recurrent pituitary-dependent Cushing's syndrome after administration of a PPAR-gamma agonist [abstract]. Endocrine Society Meeting 2004;P2–453.
[63] Hofland LJ, van der Hoek J, Van Koetsveld PM, et al. The novel somatostatin analog SOM230 has a broad spectrum of inhibitory action on hormone release by human somatotroph, corticotroph and PRL-secreting pituitary adenomas in vitro [abstract]. Endocrine Society Meeting 2004. Chevy Chase (MD): The Endocrine Society Press; 2004. P2–449.
[64] Chu JW, Matthias DF, Belanoff J, et al. Successful long-term treatment of refractory Cushing's disease with high-dose mifepristone (RU-486). J Clin Endocrinol Metab 2001;86: 3568–73.
[65] Tabarin A, Navarrane A, Guerin J, et al. Use of ketoconazole in the treatment of Cushing's disease and ectopic ACTH syndrome. Clin Endocrinol (Oxf) 1991;34:63–9.
[66] Sonino N, Boscaro M, Paoletta A, et al. Ketoconazole treatment in Cushing's syndrome: experience in 34 patients. Clin Endocrinol (Oxf) 1991;35:347–52.
[67] Verhelst JA, Trainer PJ, Howlett TA, et al. Short- and long-term responses to metyrapone in the medical management of 91 patients with Cushing's syndrome. Clin Endocrinol (Oxf) 1991;35:169–78.
[68] Luton JP, Mahoudeau JA, Bouchard P, et al. Treatment of Cushing's disease by O, p'DDD. Survey of 62 cases. N Engl J Med 1979;300:459–64.
[69] Zeiger MA, Fraker DL, Pass HI, et al. Effective reversibility of the signs and symptoms of hypercortisolism by bilateral adrenalectomy. Surgery 1993;114:1138–43.
[70] Kemink L, Hermus A, Pieters G, et al. Residual adrenocortical function after bilateral adrenalectomy for pituitary-dependent Cushing's syndrome. J Clin Endocrinol Metab 1992; 75:1211–4.
[71] Kemink L, Pieters G, Hermus A, et al. Patient's age is a simple predictive factor for the development of Nelson's syndrome after total adrenalectomy for Cushing's disease. J Clin Endocrinol Metab 1994;79:887–9.
[72] Kelly WF, MacFarlane IA, Longson D, et al. Cushing's disease treated by total adrenalectomy: long-term observations of 43 patients. Q J Med 1983;52:224–31.
[73] Moore TJ, Dluhy RG, Williams GH, et al. Nelson's syndrome: frequency, prognosis, and effect of prior pituitary irradiation. Ann Intern Med 1976;85:731–4.
[74] Wajchenberg BL, Mendonca BB, Liberman B, et al. Ectopic adrenocorticotropic hormone syndrome. Endocr Rev 1994;15:752–87.
[75] Carey RM, Varma SK, Drake CRJ, et al. Ectopic secretion of corticotropin-releasing factor as a cause of Cushing's syndrome. a clinical, morphologic, and biochemical study. N Engl J Med 1984;311:13–20.
[76] Asa SL, Kovacs K, Tindall GT, et al. Cushing's disease associated with an intrasellar gangliocytoma producing corticotrophin-releasing factor. Ann Intern Med 1984;50:461–5.
[77] Belsky JL, Cuello B, Swanson LW, et al. Cushing's syndrome due to ectopic production of corticotropin-releasing factor. J Clin Endocrinol Metab 1985;60:496–500.
[78] Schteingart DE, Lloyd RV, Akil H, et al. Cushing's syndrome secondary to ectopic corticotropin-releasing hormone-adrenocorticotropin secretion. J Clin Endocrinol Metab 1986;63:770–5.

[79] Young WFJ, Scheithauer BW, Gharib H, et al. Cushing's syndrome due to primary multinodular corticotrope hyperplasia. Mayo Clin Proc 1988;63:256–62.
[80] Hardy J. L'exerese des adenomes hypophysiares par voie transsphenoidale. Union Med Can 1962;91:933–45.
[81] Boggan JE, Tyrrell B, Wilson CB. Transsphenoidal microsurgical management of Cushing's disease. J Neurosurg 1983;59:195–200.
[82] Fahlbusch R, Buchfelder M, Muller OA. Transsphenoidal surgery for Cushing's disease. J R Soc Med 1986;79:262–9.
[83] Chandler WF, Schteingart DE, Lloyd RV, et al. Surgical treatment of Cushing's disease. J Neurosurg 1987;66:204–12.
[84] Nakane T, Kuwayama A, Watanabe M, et al. Long-term results of transsphenoidal adenectomy in patients with Cushing's disease. Neurosurgery 1987;21:218–22.
[85] Schrell U, Fahlbusch R, Buchfelder M, et al. Corticotropin-releasing hormone stimulation test before and after transsphenoidal selective microadenomectomy in 30 patients with Cushing's disease. J Clin Endocrinol Metab 1987;64:1150–9.
[86] Mampalam TJ, Tyrrell B, Wilson CB. Transsphenoidal microsurgery for Cushing's disease. Ann Intern Med 1988;109:487–93.
[87] Tindall GT, Herring CJ, Clark RV, et al. Cushing's disease: results of transsphenoidal microsurgery with emphasis on surgical failures. J Neurosurg 1990;72:363–9.
[88] Ludecke DK. Transnasal microsurgery of Cushing's disease 1990. Pathol Res Pract 1991; 187:608–12.
[89] Robert F, Hardy J. Cushing's disease: a correlation of radiological, surgical and pathological findings with therapeutic results. Pathol Res Pract 1991;187:617–21.
[90] Lindholm J. Endocrine function in patients with Cushing's disease before and after treatment. Clin Endocrinol (Oxf) 1992;36:151–9.
[91] Tahir AH, Sheeler LR. Recurrent Cushing's disease after transsphenoidal surgery. Arch Intern Med 1992;152:977–81.
[92] Bakiri F, Tatai S, Aouali R, et al. Treatment of Cushing's disease by transsphenoidal, pituitary microsurgery: Prognosis factors and long-term follow-up. J Endocrinol Invest 1996;19:572–80.
[93] Knappe UJ, Ludecke DK. Persistent and recurrent hypercortisolism after transsphenoidal surgery for Cushing's disease. Acta Neurochir Suppl (Wien) 1996;65:31–4.
[94] Shimon I, Ram Z, Cohen ZR, et al. Transsphenoidal surgery for Cushing's disease: endocrinological follow-up monitoring of 82 patients. Neurosurgery 2002;51:57–62.

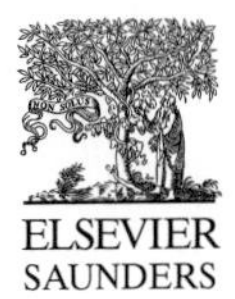

ELSEVIER
SAUNDERS

Endocrinol Metab Clin N Am
34 (2005) 479–487

ENDOCRINOLOGY AND METABOLISM CLINICS OF NORTH AMERICA

Pituitary Radiotherapy

Mary Lee Vance, MD

University of Virginia Health System, Old Medical School Building, 5th Floor, Room 5840, P.O. Box 800601, Charlottesville, VA 22908, USA

Radiotherapy to the pituitary gland for a variety of pituitary lesions has been employed for over 50 years in an attempt to reduce tumor size, to prevent tumor growth, and to reduce hormone hypersecretion to normal in patients who have a secretory pituitary adenoma. Pituitary radiotherapy is used most commonly as adjunctive therapy after unsuccessful pituitary surgery. Evaluation of the effects of pituitary radiation must include effects on tumor size; hormone hypersecretion (if present); development of new pituitary hormone deficiency; and effects on clinical symptoms and signs, on vision, on cognition, on second tumor formation, and on mortality. Although pituitary radiation may prevent tumor growth and control hormone hypersecretion, there is always a risk of adverse effects with any type of radiation delivery. This article includes general comments about pituitary radiation, outcomes in patients who have Cushing's disease and adverse effects of treatment.

Types of pituitary radiotherapy

The most common type of pituitary radiation has been conventional fractionated radiotherapy, in which radiation is delivered by means of two or three ports (bitemporal, or bitemporal and frontal) in a small dose daily over 4 or 5 weeks. A newer method of delivering radiation is stereotactic focused radiation, including a linear accelerator (LINAC)-based system, Gamma Knife, X knife, Cyber knife (a robotic arm attached to a linear accelerator), fractionated stereotactic radiation therapy, heavy charged particles (proton or helium beam radiotherapy), and implantation of radioactive seeds (yttrium, gold; not commonly in use now). These stereotactic methods of radiotherapy most commonly involve a single treatment with delivery of a high dose of radiation to a small focused target

E-mail address: mlv@virginia.edu

0889-8529/05/$ - see front matter
doi:10.1016/j.ecl.2005.01.005

endo.theclinics.com

resulting in decreased radiation exposure to the brain, particularly to the temporal and frontal lobes. Stereotactic delivery of radiation to the pituitary gland may be described as radiosurgery. This nomenclature reflects the fact that it may involve surgical placement of a stereotactic frame to the head. Regardless of the terminology, all types of radiation delivery are pituitary radiotherapy. There may be limitations concerning suitable candidates for stereotactic radiation. A patient who has a large tumor that is near the optic chiasm or an optic nerve is at risk for damage to vision because of radiation scatter. For example, in patients treated with Gamma knife radiosurgery, a distance of 5 mm between the tumor margin and optic chiasm or an optic nerve is recommended to reduce the risk of visual complications.

Unfortunately, there is a dearth of direct comparisons of the efficacy and complications among the various types of radiation delivery. Thus, discussion of these issues will rely on published information on different methods of radiation delivery without direct comparison of efficacy or complications.

Radiation therapy

Cushing's disease

Assessment of treatment outcomes

Remission. There are several methods to assess the efficacy of treatment for Cushing's disease. With pituitary surgery, in some centers, patients are not given a glucocorticoid before, during, or after surgery, thus allowing a prompt assessment of the surgical results. A postoperative decline in serum cortisol to less than 2 or 3 μg/dL, in conjunction with symptoms of adrenal insufficiency requiring steroid replacement, is considered remission. In other centers, a glucocorticoid is administered routinely before and after surgery, thus requiring assessment after surgical recovery and after a period of steroid withdrawal.

If a patient does not achieve remission after surgery and undergoes pituitary radiation, the paradigm for assessing the response to radiation also varies among centers. Because pituitary radiation causes a gradual reduction in pituitary corticotropin (ACTH) secretion and consequent cortisol production, investigators have considered a normal 24-hour urine-free cortisol (UFC) concentration or a suppressed (< 2 or 3 μg/dL) serum cortisol response to a 1 mg overnight dexamethasone suppression test as indicative of remission. Consistent lowering of the plasma ACTH is an indirect indication of a beneficial effect of radiation, but it is not adequate to assess remission, because many patients who have Cushing's disease have a normal serum ACTH before any treatment. A single ACTH measurement does not reflect overall corticotrophin activity; measurement of the 24-hour urine-free cortisol concentration provides an integrated measure of the effect of pituitary ACTH production. Similarly, adequate suppression of serum cortisol after 1 mg of oral dexamethasone reflects normal physiology and is adequate to determine remission. Improvement in symptoms and signs of Cushing's disease is a necessary part of the assessment of the effect of any treatment. In summary, the best biochemical measures of response to pituitary radiation are a normal 24-hour urine-free cortisol concentration or a normal serum cortisol response (< 2 or 3 μg/dL) to the 1 mg overnight dexamethasone test.

Hypopituitarism. Patients who undergo pituitary radiation must be followed regularly for development of new pituitary deficiency or deficiencies (with administration of appropriate hormone replacements as indicated). There is no way to predict if or when a patient will develop secondary hypothyroidism, secondary adrenal insufficiency, secondary hypogonadism, or growth hormone deficiency. It is prudent to evaluate a patient every 6 months for development of new pituitary hormone deficiency or deficiencies. A subnormal morning serum cortisol is usually adequate to diagnose adrenal insufficiency, but a normal value does not assess the response to stress or pituitary ACTH reserve. The most definitive test to determine hypothalamic–pituitary–adrenal (HPA) function is the insulin hypoglycemia test (insulin tolerance test, ITT). This test requires supervision by a physician and frequent blood glucose measurements. It is contraindicated in patients who have a history of coronary artery disease, seizure disorder, or generalized debility. Unfortunately, the less stressful test, ACTH administration (cosyntropin stimulation test), only measures the adrenal response to ACTH and may not be reliable, because it is not known exactly how much ACTH production prevents adrenal atrophy and causes a subnormal cortisol response to exogenous ACTH. A patient who has impaired, but not absent, ACTH production may have a normal serum cortisol response to exogenous ACTH but may not be able to respond adequately to stress, thus giving a false assurance of normal HPA function. The discordance between the cortisol response to hypothalamic stimulation with metyrapone or insulin hypoglycemia compared with the ACTH test was 34% in 32 patients who recently had undergone pituitary surgery or were treated recently with a glucocorticoid. Eleven patients had a normal cortisol response to exogenous ACTH but a subnormal response to metyrapone; four patients also received insulin and had a subnormal cortisol response when the response to ACTH was normal [1]. In a study of 90 patients who had confirmed or suspected HPA dysfunction, however, there was very close correlation ($r = 0.92$) between the cortisol response to hypoglycemia and exogenous ACTH [2]. The diagnosis of secondary hypothyroidism is more straightforward; a subnormal serum-free T4 concentration is adequate for this diagnosis. The serum thyrotropin (TSH) may be, and usually is, normal in patients who have pituitary disease, resulting in a misdiagnosis of normal thyroid function if only serum TSH is measured. Secondary hypogonadism in premenopausal women is characterized by irregular menses or amenorrhea, a low serum estradiol level, and serum luteinizing hormone (LH) and follicle-stimulating hormone (FSH) levels in the normal range. Menstrual function is the best indicator of gonadotropin deficiency or sufficiency in premenopausal women who have pituitary disease. Men who have secondary hypogonadism usually have diminished libido, erectile dysfunction, and a low serum testosterone; the LH and FSH levels are usually in the normal range. The diagnosis of growth hormone (GH) deficiency usually requires a GH stimulation test (insulin hypoglycemia, GH-releasing hormone plus arginine, or arginine). Patients who had three pituitary hormone deficiencies had a 96% probability of being GH deficient, and those who had four pituitary hormone deficits had a 99% probability of this diagnosis [3]. Currently, many third-party payers require a GH stimulation test to confirm the diagnosis of GH deficiency in patients who have other pituitary hormone deficiencies. Diabetes insipidus (DI) is not a usual effect of pituitary radiation (usually occurs after pituitary surgery), and this is more common in patients who have a lesion that involves the pituitary stalk such as a craniopharyngioma or Rathke's cleft cyst, or an infiltrative disease (sarcoidosis, granulomatous disease, lymphocytic hypophysitis). New-onset DI requires a pituitary MRI study to determine if there has been regrowth of a pituitary lesion that is impairing transport of hypothalamic antidiuretic hormone (vasopressin) to the posterior pituitary.

Other adverse effects of pituitary radiation. All forms of pituitary radiation may cause damage to vision or ocular motor function. All patients should have a thorough ophthalmologic evaluation, including visual field testing, before pituitary radiation and regular follow-up examinations to determine if there is any change over time. Pituitary radiation uncommonly causes damage to brain tissue, most often resulting in temporal lobe necrosis that may cause temporal lobe epilepsy. The MRI study usually shows an area of hyperintensity in the area of radiation damage. Ocular nerve dysfunction most commonly involves the third or sixth cranial nerves, resulting in ptosis and diplopia with a third nerve palsy or diplopia with a sixth nerve palsy. The effects of cranial radiation on cognitive function have not been studied well. Some clinicians, however, have observed a decline in cognitive and neurologic function in patients treated with pituitary radiation. Second tumor formation has been reported with conventional fractionated radiation and stereotactic radiation; this appears to be dose-dependent with conventional radiation, but this is less defined with stereotactic delivery.

Hypopituitarism from surgery and conventional fractionated radiation therapy has been associated with an increased risk of premature cardiovascular disease and premature mortality [4,5]. This risk has been attributed to growth hormone deficiency, because patients received hormone replacements other than growth hormone. An epidemiologic study of 344 Swedish patients who had hypopituitarism (304 patients [88%] received conventional fractionated pituitary radiation), however, found increased cerebrovascular mortality in this cohort. The standardized mortality ratio (SMR) for death from cerebrovascular disease was 3.39; 95% confidence interval (CI) 2.27 to 4.99, while the cardiac disease SMR was 1.4; 95% CI 1.04 to 1.88 [6]. A review of risk factors for premature mortality in patients who had acromegaly found that conventional radiotherapy was associated with an increased risk of premature mortality, with cerebrovascular disease the predominant cause of death. The SMR for cerebrovascular disease was 4.42 (range 1.09 to 7.22, $P = 0.005$) [7]. These epidemiologic studies raise the question regarding the long-term effect of radiation on brain vasculature and its consequences. To date, there have been no reports of increased risk of cerebrovascular mortality in patients treated with stereotactic radiation, but the experience and duration of follow-up with this method are less extensive.

Efficacy of pituitary radiation

Pituitary radiation is an effective treatment to reduce cortisol hypersecretion to normal. No form of radiation delivery, however, is effective immediately. Because Cushing's disease causes a great deal of morbidity, medical therapy to reduce cortisol production should be administered while awaiting a beneficial effect of radiation. Medical therapy with ketoconazole effectively lowers cortisol production; the dose required to achieve a normal 24-hour UFC level usually ranges between 400 to 1200 mg per day in divided doses [8]. Serum liver enzymes should be measured before this drug is administered and followed at regular intervals, because ketoconazole may cause elevation of serum aspartate aminotransferase (AST), alanine aminotransferase (ALT), and alkaline phosphatase. If this occurs, the drug should be discontinued and liver enzymes repeated at a later time.

Conventional radiotherapy

Adults. In a review the results of 10 studies involving 255 patients, remission occurred in 53% to 100% of patients followed from 3.5 to 17.8 years. The time to remission ranged from 4 months to 26 months; development of new pituitary hormone deficiency or deficiencies occurred in 14% to 56% of patients [9]. The response to conventional fractionated radiation appears to be dose-dependent, because the relapse rate was about 50% when patients were given a total dose of 20 Gy in eight fractions compared with a total dose of 40 to 50 Gy [10,11]. Control of tumor growth occurred in 79% to 100% of patients [9]. Estrada et al's study of 30 adults (included in the article by Mahmoud-Ahmed elsewhere in this issue) found that 25 patients (83%) achieved remission from 6 to 60 months after treatment. Post-radiation hormone deficiencies included growth hormone deficiency in 57% of patients, gonadotropin deficiency in 33% of patients, TSH deficiency in 13% of patients, and ACTH deficiency in 3% of patients [12].

Children. In a 1977 report of 15 children and adolescents (7.9 to 18.7 years) treated with conventional fractionated pituitary radiotherapy (total dose 35 to 49.5 Gy), 12 achieved remission within 18 months of treatment, with 10 achieving remission within 9 months. The three children who did not achieve remission subsequently underwent bilateral adrenalectomy. Linear growth resumed in 12 children, and all had normal puberty and gonadal function. No change in personality or intelligence was observed, but formal testing was not performed. No visual abnormalities occurred during the follow-up period that ranged from 1 to 18.25 years [13]. In seven children treated with conventional radiation after unsuccessful pituitary surgery, all achieved remission with a mean time of 11.3 months (range 3–34 mo). One boy experienced premature puberty and six patients (86%) developed growth hormone deficiency. No patient had recurrence of Cushing's disease [14].

Stereotactic radiotherapy

Adults. Focused radiation delivery using the Gamma knife is an effective treatment for Cushing's disease, but as with any form of radiation delivery, it is not effective immediately. In 29 patients who had Cushing's disease treated with the Gamma knife and followed for 3 to 9 years, 76% achieved remission. Eight patients required two to four Gamma knife treatments. The time to remission was 1 year in 12 patients and within 3 years in the remaining 10 patients. Development of new pituitary hormone deficiency occurred in 55% of the 22 patients who achieved remission [15]. In 43 patients (44 Gamma knife treatments) followed for 18 to 113 months (mean 39 months), remission occurred in 27 (63%). The average time to remission was 12.1 months (range 3 to 48 months); three patients had a relapse 19, 37, and 38 months after treatment. Seven patients (16%) developed new pituitary hormone deficiency; tumor size decreased in 33 patients (77%), and there was no growth in the remaining 11 patients. One patient developed a superior temporal visual defect [16].

Children. Eight children and adolescents, aged 6 to 18 years, underwent Gamma knife radiation; seven achieved clinical and biochemical remission with a follow-up of 2.6 to 6.8 years. One patient required bilateral adrenalectomy after two Gamma knife treatments. All patients developed growth failure and growth hormone deficiency; two developed secondary hypothyroidism, and three developed secondary hypogonadism. There were no studies of cognitive function [17].

Complications of pituitary radiation

Expected effects of all types of pituitary radiation are the loss of pituitary function and need for hormone replacement(s); this may not be considered by some as a complication, but it is an untoward effect. Less common adverse effects include development of a second tumor (astrocytoma) [18], temporal lobe necrosis, and temporal lobe epilepsy [19] after conventional radiation. Four of 46 patients treated with conventional radiation developed central nervous system (CNS) necrosis within 6 years of treatment; three of the patients who developed necrosis had Cushing's disease, leading the authors to suggest that the metabolic disturbance of Cushing's disease may reduce tolerance to radiation [20]. There are no studies in large numbers of patients who have Cushing's disease, however, to determine if these patients have greater morbidity from pituitary radiation than patients with other types of pituitary lesions.

Personal comments

In general, I think that pituitary radiation has a role as a part of the treatment regimen for selected patients with pituitary lesions. Pituitary radiation is not usually the best first treatment; it should be recommended in specific patients who have persistent hormone hypersection after surgery, for patients who do not respond to medical treatment, and for patients who have lesions that cannot be resected completely and that have increased probability of aggressiveness and growth (eg, silent ACTH adenoma). After more than 20 years of caring for patients who have pituitary disorders, it is apparent to me that every type of treatment has success, failure, and complications. The patients who are treatment failures or who develop complications are the most memorable. The 15-year-old girl who had conventional radiation for Cushing's disease at the age of 12 and who developed severe neurologic dysfunction and subsequently died; the 30-year-old man who had post-operative residual craniopharyngioma and underwent conventional pituitary radiation at 21 years is now marginally functional and continues to deteriorate neurologically and mentally; and the 46-year-old physician who had acromegaly and developed temporal lobe necrosis and epilepsy after Gamma knife radiosurgery make me think very carefully about recommending postoperative pituitary radiation (most commonly stereotactic Gamma Knife radiation). There are definite risks with any type of pituitary radiation, although low. These risks cannot be ignored and should be considered carefully and explained thoroughly to the patient before he or she undergoes this treatment. The concern about hypopituitarism, in my opinion, is not a significant issue, because all pituitary hormones can be replaced physiologically. This is a very important concern, however, for many patients who are apprehensive about having to take life-long replacements. The desire for fertility requires more work, time, and expense. I think it is necessary to achieve control of pituitary hormone hypersecretion before fertility treatment is instituted. Both men and women have the potential to achieve fertility with gonadotropin therapy, presuming that the reproductive organs are normal. If fertility is a concern, men should be encouraged to have a semen analysis and to bank sperm (if the sperm count and motility are acceptable) before any treatment for a pituitary tumor.

In the end, the decision to recommend pituitary radiation must be made based on a careful assessment of the potential benefits and risks, and treatment should be given only to a patient who is fully informed of these issues.

Summary

Pituitary radiation has a definite and defined role for treating patients who have Cushing's disease. Ideally, pituitary surgery by an accomplished pituitary neurosurgeon obviates the need for additional treatment. This is not the outcome in approximately 20% to 25% of patients, however. The morbidity and risk of premature cardiovascular mortality associated with uncontrolled Cushing's disease makes it imperative that disease control be achieved as rapidly as possible. It does not appear that one form of radiation is superior to another in achieving remission from Cushing's disease, nor does the reported incidence of new pituitary deficiency differ. The method of radiation delivery differs regarding the amount of radiation to brain, particularly the frontal and temporal lobes, with greater exposure with conventional fractionated therapy than with stereotactic delivery. The choice of the method of radiation delivery is determined by availability, by the size and location of the lesion, and by patient preference. The issue of damage to the cerebral vasculature and increased risk of cerebrovascular mortality must continue to be addressed to determine if all methods of radiation delivery pose this risk.

References

[1] Cunningham SK, Moore A, McKenna TJ. Normal cortisol response to corticotrophin in patients with secondary adrenal failure. Arch Intern Med 1983;143:2275–9.

[2] Lindholm J, Kehlet H, Blichert-Toft M, et al. Reliability of the 20-minute ACTH test in assessing hypothalamic-pituitary-adrenal function. J Clin Endocrinol Metab 1978;47:272–4.

[3] Hartman ML, Crowe BJ, Biller BMK, et al. Which patients do not require a GH stimulation test for the diagnosis of adult GH deficiency? J Clin Endocrinol Metab 2002;87:477–85.

[4] Markussis V, Beshyah SA, Fisher C, et al. Detection of premature atherosclerosis by high-resolution ultrasonography in symptom-free hypopituitary adults. Lancet 1992;340: 1188–92.

[5] Rosen T, Bengtsson BA. Premature mortality due to cardiovascular disease in hypopituitarism. Lancet 1990;336:285–8.

[6] Bulow B, Hagmar L, Mikoczy Z, et al. Increased cerebrovascular mortality in patients with hypopituitarism. Clinical Endocrinology 1997;46:75–81.

[7] Ayuk J, Clayton RN, Holder G. Growth hormone and pituitary radiotherapy, but not serum insulin-like growth factor-I concentrations, predict excess mortality in patients with acromegaly. J Clin Endocrinol Metab 2004;89:1613–7.

[8] Sonino N, Boscaro M, Paoletta A, et al. Ketoconazole treatment in Cushing's syndrome: experience in 3 patients. Clin Endocrinol 1991;35:347–52.

[9] Mahmoud-Ahmed AS, Suh JH. Radiation therapy for Cushing's disease: a review. Pituitary 2002;5:175–80.

[10] Ahmed SR, Shalet SM, Beardwell CG, et al. Treatment of Cushing's disease with low-dose radiation therapy. Br Med J (Clin Res Ed) 1984;289(6446):643–6.
[11] Littley MD, Shalet SM, Beardwell CG, et al. Long-term follow-up of low-dose external pituitary irradiation for Cushing's disease. Clin Endocrinol (Oxf) 1990;33(4):445–55.
[12] Estrada J, Boronat M, Mielgo M, et al. The long-term outcome of pituitary irradiation after unsuccessful transsphenoidal surgery in Cushing's disease. N Engl J Med 1997;336:172–7.
[13] Jennings AS, Liddle GW, Roth DN. Results of treating childhood Cushing's disease with pituitary irradiation. N Engl J Med 1977;297:957–62.
[14] Storr HL, Plowman PN, Carroll PV, et al. Clinical and endocrine response to pituitary radiotherapy in pediatric Cushing's disease: an effective second-line treatment. J Clin Endocrinol Metab 2003;88:34–7.
[15] Degerblad M, Rahn T, Bergstrand G, et al. Long-term results of stereotactic radiosurgery to the pituitary gland in Cushing's disease. Acta Endocrinol (Copenh) 1986;112:310–4.
[16] Sheehan JM, Vance ML, Sheehan JP, et al. Radiosurgery for Cushing's disease after failed transsphenoidal surgery. J Neurosurg 2000;93(5):738–42.
[17] Thoren M, Rahn T, Hallengren B, et al. Treatment of Cushing's disease in childhood and adolescence by stereotactic pituitary radiation. Acta Paediatr Scand 1986;75(3):388–95.
[18] Kitanaka C, Shitara N, Nakagomi T, et al. Postradiation astrocytoma. J Neurosurg 1989; 70:469–74.
[19] Woo E, Lam K, Yu YL, et al. Temporal lobe and hypothalamic-pituitary dysfunctions after radiotherapy for nasopharyngeal carcinoma: a distinct clinical syndrome. J Neurol Neurosurg Psychiatry 1988;51:1302–7.
[20] Grattan-Smith PJ, Morris JG, Langlands AO. Delayed radiation necrosis of the central nervous system in patients irradiated for pituitary tumors. J Neurol Neurosurg Psychiatry 1992;55:949–55.

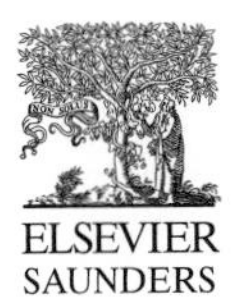
ELSEVIER
SAUNDERS

Endocrinol Metab Clin N Am
34 (2005) 489–499

ENDOCRINOLOGY
AND METABOLISM
CLINICS
OF NORTH AMERICA

Laparoscopic Adrenalectomy for Patients Who Have Cushing's Syndrome

William F. Young, Jr, MD[a,*], Geoffrey B. Thompson, MD[b]

[a]*Divisions of Endocrinology, Diabetes, Metabolism, Nutrition, and Internal, Medicine Mayo Clinic, 200 First Street Southwest, Rochester, MN 55905, USA*
[b]*Division of Gastroenterologic and General Surgery, Mayo Clinic, Rochester, MN, USA*

Since its description in 1992 [1,2], laparoscopic adrenalectomy rapidly has become the procedure of choice for unilateral adrenalectomy when the adrenal mass is less than 8 cm in size and there are no frank signs of malignancy (eg, invasion of contiguous structures) [3]. The postoperative recovery time and long-term morbidity associated with laparoscopic adrenalectomy are reduced significantly when compared with open adrenalectomy [3].

Among 2550 laparoscopic adrenalectomy procedures reported in the literature, the most frequent adrenal disorder operated laparoscopically was aldosterone-producing adenoma (36.2%), followed by cortisol-producing cortical adenoma (19.1%), apparent nonfunctioning cortical adenoma (18.2%), and pheochromocytoma (18.0%) [3]. However, patients who have corticotropin (ACTH)-dependent Cushing's syndrome who have experienced failed attempts to remove the ACTH-secreting tumor (pituitary or ectopic) are also ideal candidates for one-stage bilateral laparoscopic adrenalectomy [4,5]. The types of Cushing's syndrome that can be treated with laparoscopic unilateral or bilateral adrenalectomy are summarized in Box 1.

Advantages of the laparoscopic approach

The introduction of laparoscopy has revolutionized the surgical approach to adrenalectomy. Although laparoscopic adrenalectomy is technically more demanding to perform than conventional posterior adrenalectomy, it is

* Corresponding author.
E-mail address: young.william@mayo.edu (W.F. Young).

0889-8529/05/$ - see front matter
doi:10.1016/j.ecl.2005.01.006

Box 1. Spectrum of Cushing's syndrome disorders that may be treated laparoscopically

- Unilateral adrenalectomy
  - Cortisol-producing adenoma
- Bilateral partial adrenalectomy
  - Bilateral cortisol-secreting adenomas
- Bilateral adrenalectomy
  - ACTH-dependent Cushing's syndrome that failed attempts at removal of ACTH-secreting tumor (pituitary or ectopic)
  - ACTH-independent Cushing's syndrome caused by primary pigmented nodular adrenal disease or bilateral adrenal macronodular hyperplasia

associated with shorter hospitalization, less morbidity, and earlier return to daily activities [3,6–12]. Conventional open adrenalectomy by means of the anterior or posterior approach requires a large incision to gain access to a relatively small gland. Moreover, the incision used for posterior adrenalectomy, with its associated 12th rib resection and subcostal (T12) nerve retraction, has been associated with various incisional and musculoskeletal problems that may persist long after the operation [6,13]. These incisional problems are especially pronounced and severe in patients who have Cushing's syndrome because of poor wound healing, laxity of the abdominal wall, obesity, and musculoskeletal complaints associated with the condition [14–17]. Fig. 1 shows an abdominal CT scan of an adrenal cortical adenoma in a typical patient who had Cushing's syndrome treated with unilateral laparascopic adrenalectomy.

Bilateral laparoscopic adrenalectomy

Bilateral laparoscopic adrenalectomy is an excellent treatment option for ACTH-dependent Cushing's syndrome after failed pituitary surgery for Cushing's disease or when the ACTH source cannot be resected or localized, as in ectopic ACTH syndrome. Bilateral laparoscopic subtotal adrenalectomy is indicated in patients who have bilateral cortisol-secreting adenomas. Compared with the open approach, bilateral laparoscopic adrenal surgery is associated with much less tissue injury in patients who are immunocompromised or are predisposed to delayed wound healing. In addition, because of the magnification, there is better visibility of the surgical field, thus decreasing the risk for retained remnants and adrenal rests.

Although transsphenoidal surgery for resection of an ACTH-secreting pituitary tumor is the standard of therapy for Cushing's disease, this surgery

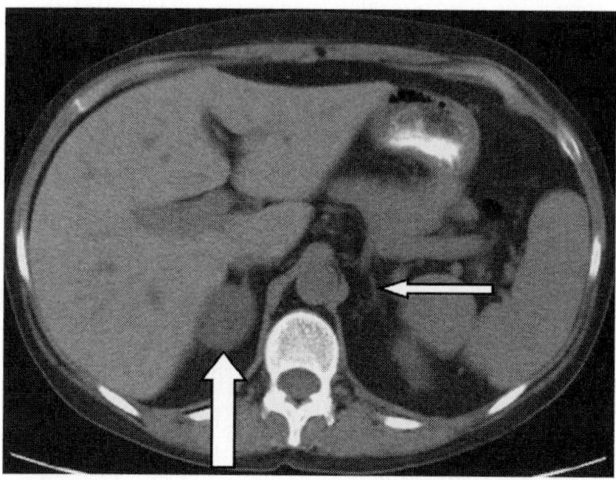

Fig. 1. Abdominal CT scan from a 34-year-old woman who presented with osteoporosis, easy bruising, proximal muscle weakness, and poor wound healing. Laboratory studies showed elevated serum cortisol concentrations that lacked diurnal variation, undetectable serum ACTH, increased level of 24-hour urinary-free cortisol (393 μg; normal = 5–55 μg). CT scan of the adrenal glands showed a 3.0 × 3.5–cm right adrenal mass (*large arrow*), and the left adrenal gland appeared atrophic (*small arrow*). At laparoscopic right adrenalectomy, a 3.6 × 3.0 × 2.4–cm cortical adenoma was found. Two days after surgery, the serum cortisol concentration was undetectable. The patient was dismissed from the hospital on the second postoperative day on temporary glucocorticoid replacement, and her signs and symptoms of Cushing's syndrome slowly resolved.

is not always successful [18–20]. Such tumors may invade contiguous structures such as the cavernous sinuses, thus precluding complete resection. Other ACTH-secreting pituitary tumors may be so small that they escape detection and resection at the time of surgery. For these reasons, transsphenoidal surgery is associated with a 20% to 40% failure rate, even for experienced surgeons [21–24]. Reoperation carries an increased risk of inducing panhypopituitarism in conjunction with the treatment difficulties and complications associated with the hypercortisolism. Therefore, bilateral adrenalectomy has an important therapeutic role in a significant subset of patients who have Cushing's disease, in whom transsphenoidal surgery has failed, placing them at high risk of panhypopituitarism with additional cranial surgery.

Sellar radiation therapy is not an optimal therapy for Cushing's disease, because its onset of action is slow, and its failure rate is unacceptably high [25]. Some degree of pituitary insufficiency is a relatively common adverse effect, and the mean onset of action is 18 months [26]. Therefore, primary treatment with irradiation is not optimal in patients who have clinically significant hypercortisolism and its numerous comorbidities. Because bilateral laparoscopic adrenalectomy results in immediate cure of hypercortisolism, the role of pituitary irradiation in Cushing's disease in these patients is limited to the treatment of the small subset of patients who have large pituitary tumors (Nelson's syndrome). In patients who have enlarging pituitary tumors, sellar radiation therapy or gamma knife radiosurgery is used to prevent a locally invasive pituitary tumor from further encroaching on surrounding structures.

Patients who have the syndrome of ectopic ACTH secretion often have an unresectable or occult source of ACTH secretion [27,28]. The metabolic manifestations of cortisol excess appear suddenly and progress rapidly. In these situations, adrenalectomy offers long-term relief from the symptoms associated with cortisol excess. In the authors' experience, most patients who have clinically evident ectopic ACTH syndrome have more indolent tumors, such as bronchial or thymic carcinoid tumors, islet cell tumors, or medullary carcinoma of the thyroid [28]. In contrast to the typical patient who has ectopic ACTH syndrome, carcinoid tumors that secrete ACTH may not be apparent even with careful radiologic investigation and may take up to 20 years to localize [28] (Fig. 2). When the source of ACTH is unresectable or occult, bilateral laparoscopic adrenalectomy is a life-saving treatment option because of the minimal morbidity associated with the procedure, especially when compared with conventional adrenalectomy. Laparoscopic adrenalectomy is also superior to medical therapy in regard to tolerance, efficacy, and safety. The procedure can treat the symptoms of cortisol excess successfully in patients who have malignancy, and thus it offers improved quality of life and effective palliation of symptoms even in patients who have disseminated, untreatable malignancy (Fig. 3).

The adrenal enzyme inhibitors, aminoglutethimide, metyrapone, and ketoconazole, are used most commonly to treat Cushing's syndrome medically. Complete blockade of adrenal steroid synthesis is achieved only transiently, however; ACTH levels increase and override the blockade, requiring additional increases in the dosage of enzyme inhibitor. Furthermore, the incidence of patient intolerance and adverse effects (eg, liver enzyme abnormalities) of these

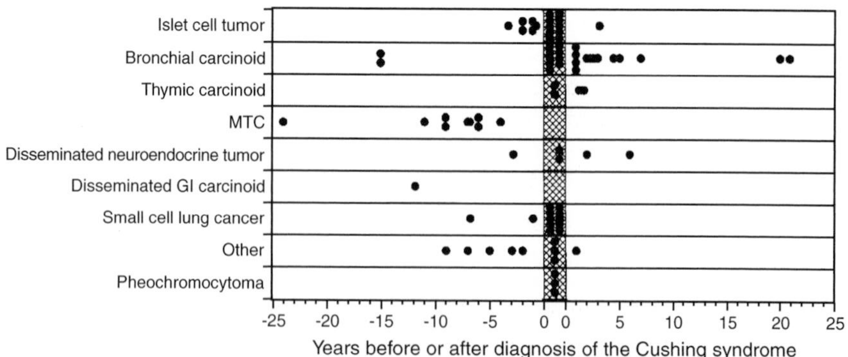

Fig. 2. The temporal relationship between the diagnosis of the Cushing's syndrome and the diagnosis of the responsible neoplasm is shown. GI, gastrointestinal; MTC, medullary thyroid carcinoma. (*From* Aniszewski JP, Young WF Jr, Thompson GB, et al. Cushing Syndrome due to ectopic adrenocorticotropic hormone secretion. World J Surg 2001;25;934–40; with permission.)

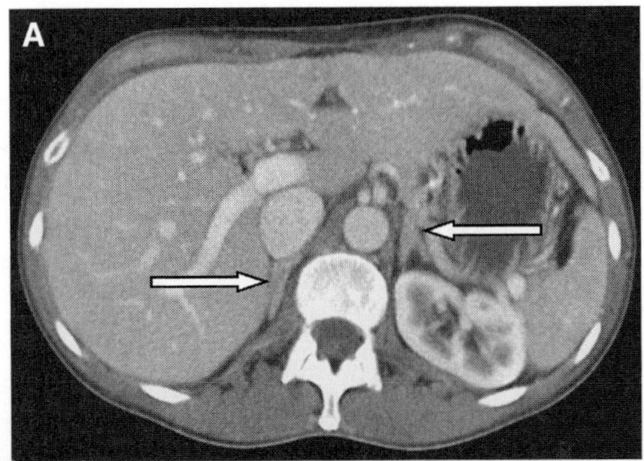

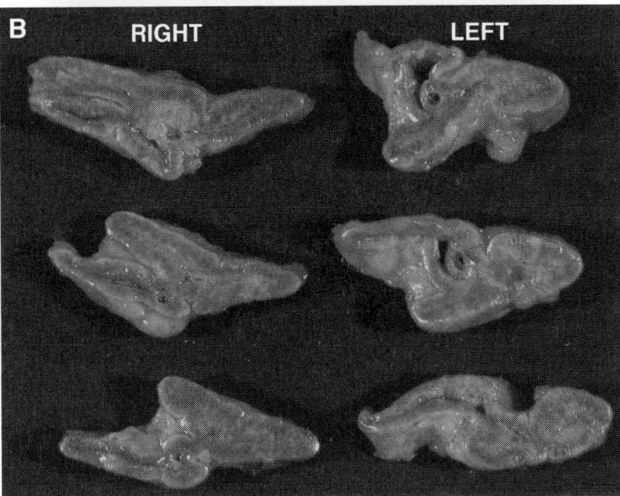

Fig. 3. Images from a 50-year-old woman who had an ACTH-secreting metastatic medullary thyroid carcinoma (MTC). Although she was known to have widely metastatic MTC dating back to 1987, it was not until early 2003 that she started to develop signs and symptoms of Cushing's syndrome. Laboratory studies in early 2004 showed elevated serum cortisol concentrations that lacked diurnal variation, increased serum ACTH concentration (123 pg/mL; normal = 10–60 pg/mL), increased level of 24-hour urinary-free cortisol (730 μg; normal = 5–55 μg). (*A*) CT scan of the abdomen showed bilaterally enlarged adrenal glands (*arrows*). Because the source of ectopic ACTH production could not be removed, the patient was treated with bilateral laparoscopic adrenalectomy. (*B*) Cut sections of the right and left adrenal glands showed cortical hyperplasia. The postoperative serum cortisol concentration was undetectable. The patient was dismissed from the hospital on the second postoperative day on permanent glucocorticoid and mineralocorticoid replacement, and her signs and symptoms of Cushing's syndrome slowly resolved.

medications is high. Few patients are able to tolerate long-term therapy with aminoglutethimide, metyrapone, or ketoconazole. Also, to prevent an Addisonian crisis in patients receiving adrenal enzyme inhibitors, glucocorticoid and mineralocorticoid replacement may be necessary.

Since the description of laparoscopic adrenalectomy in 1992 [1,2], various groups have described their experience with bilateral laparoscopic adrenalectomy for treating Cushing's syndrome [3–5,29–35]. Increased experience with the technique has resulted in a decreased conversion rate to open adrenalectomy and a decreased incidence of pancreatitis and perioperative hemorrhage. None of these complications was observed in the authors' initial series of 16 patients, and biochemical cure of Cushing's syndrome was achieved in all patients [5]. There have been two reported cases of partial hormonal recurrence, which may be related to accessory adrenal gland tissue or intraoperative fragmentation of the adrenal gland [36,37]. It also has been reported that the operative time is longer in bilateral laparoscopic versus bilateral open adrenalectomy, and this may be a limitation in high-risk patients [38].

Contraindications to laparoscopic adrenalectomy in Cushing's syndrome patients

There are three situations when the laparoscopic approach to the adrenal may not or should not be the procedure of choice for patients who have Cushing's syndrome:

1. Adrenocortical carcinomas that invade surrounding structures should be resected en bloc by means of an open anterior abdominal incision.
2. Very large tumors (eg, greater than 10 to 12 cm in diameter) may be difficult to remove laparoscopically. The risk of adrenocortical carcinoma increases proportionate to size, as does the risk of capsular disruption.
3. Malignant ACTH-secreting pheochromocytoma, especially if lymphadenopathy is found on computerized imaging, should be resected en bloc by means of an open anterior abdominal incision.

Surgical approaches to the adrenal gland

Until the development of laparoscopic adrenalectomy, the open posterior retroperitoneal approach was favored by many adrenal surgeons [39]. The open posterior approach, when compared with the open anterior approach, caused less pain, ileus, and other complications [39]. For laparoscopic adrenalectomy, the lateral transabdominal approach, developed by Higashihara et al in Tokyo (1992) and Gagner et al in Montreal (1992) remains the preference of most surgeons. The lateral decubitus position of the patient and the medial rotation of the viscera allow gravity to keep the liver, bowel, and spleen away from the surgical field. The posterior retroperitoneal and lateral retroperitoneal approaches for laparoscopic adrenalectomy have the disadvantage of poor exposure, and, in general, they have not been found to be superior to the lateral transabdominal approach. These approaches may be indicated in patients who have had prior upper abdominal surgery. It should be noted that some surgeons prefer the retroperitoneal laparoscopic adrenalectomy approach for left-sided adrenal tumors because of shorter operating time, reduced blood loss, reduced risk of injury to the viscera, and lack of interference from previous abdominal surgery [40]. Regardless of the approach, the keys to successful laparoscopic adrenalectomy are knowledge of the anatomy, delicate tissue handling, and meticulous hemostasis. Because clinical outcomes are similar among the different approaches for laparoscopic adrenalectomy [41], the choice of the approach is dependent upon surgeon preference and other practical considerations.

Laparoscopic technique

The key steps in the lateral transabdominal approach to laparoscopic adrenalectomy include:

- General endotracheal anesthesia
- Lateral decubitus position, with the affected adrenal gland placed in the upper position
- Operating table placed in the flexed position, so that the patient's flank is maximally exposed in the extended position
- A skin incision 1 cm in length and 2 cm below and parallel to the costal margin; a pneumoperitoneum is established with carbon dioxide.
- Placement of three to four 10 mm trocar ports; the laparoscope initially is placed through the most anterior trocar and working instruments through the other ports, but camera and instruments are interchangeable throughout the dissection.
- The right adrenal gland approach: mobilization of the lateral attachments of the liver for medial rotation and elevation; inferior retraction of the kidney; exposure of adrenal vein and vena cava. Arterial tributaries are divided with ultrasonic dissection.
- The left adrenal gland approach: mobilization of the left colon along its attachments to the spleen; mobilization of the spleen and pancreas to allow a medial position; exposure of left adrenal vein/inferior phrenic vein junction; mobilization of the adrenal gland along Gerota's fascia
- The main adrenal vein identified, clipped, and transected; the adrenal gland and tumor are resected and placed in a retrieval pouch and delivered by means of a port site. The adrenal vein may be transected early or late in the dissection depending on the ease of exposure.

Most patients begin a clear liquid diet the evening of surgery and a regular diet the next day. Patients are encouraged to ambulate the evening of surgery. Most patients undergoing unilateral adrenalectomy may be dismissed from the hospital on postoperative day 1 or 2. Bilateral adrenalectomy patients and patients who have severe Cushing's syndrome may require more than a 2-day hospitalization.

Efficacy of laparoscopic adrenalectomy

No prospective human randomized controlled trial comparing laparoscopic adrenalectomy to any of the open surgical approaches has been performed [3]. In a prospective randomized study done at the Mayo Clinic, the authors examined the acute-phase response and wound healing in laparoscopic adrenalectomy versus open adrenalectomy in a cushingoid porcine model [17]. Nitrogen balance, wound scores, and tensile strength at 24 hours and 1 week were more favorable in the laparoscopic adrenalectomy group than in the open adrenalectomy group. Since 1995, 20 case–control retrospective comparative studies have evaluated the efficacy of laparoscopic adrenalectomy [3]. All of the studies reported less analgesia requirement, less blood loss, lower complication rate, and shorter hospital stay for laparoscopic than open adrenalectomy [3]. At Mayo Clinic, the authors performed a matched case–control study comparing 50 patients having laparoscopic adrenalectomy with 50 patients having adrenalectomy through the open posterior approach [6]. The authors found that laparoscopic adrenalectomy, compared with open adrenalectomy, was associated significantly with shorter hospital stay, less postoperative narcotic use, more rapid return to normal activity, increased patient satisfaction, and less late morbidity. The late morbidity associated with posterior open adrenalectomy includes chronic pain, severe laxity involving the oblique muscles, and bothersome flank numbness [6]. The average conversion rate to open adrenalectomy in 2550 patients from 28 reports was 3.6% [3]. The reasons for conversion included bleeding, adhesions, difficulty of dissection, unexpected malignancy, large size of tumor, vascular invasion, inadvertent pancreatic injury, damage to the pleura, failure to identify the adrenal tumor, and unsuspected Bochdalek hernia [6,36,42–44].

Risks of laparoscopic adrenalectomy

When performing laparoscopic adrenalectomy, the surgeon sacrifices some tactile sensation, when compared with open surgery, and the small, flat, friable adrenal gland is manipulated with instruments in a two-dimensional plane. The overall complication rate associated with laparoscopic adrenalectomy from a summary of 2550 procedures was 9.5% [3]. Some complications of laparoscopic adrenalectomy include conversion to open adrenalectomy, bleeding, gland fragmentation, wound hematomas, organ injury, port site incisional hernia [45], and port site pain [46]. Nerve root pain has been reported with the posterior laparoscopic adrenalectomy approach [41]. There is risk of violating the tumor capsule and organ parenchyma during manipulation with the laparoscopic instruments. In one large series involving 88 patients [36], there was a 12% postoperative complication rate (eg, deep venous thrombosis, hematomas, and anemia), a 3% conversion rate to open adrenalectomy, and no mortality. If any viable cortical cells are left behind in the patient who has ACTH-dependent Cushing's syndrome, the procedure will fail [4]. Recurrent adrenocortical carcinoma following laparoscopic adrenalectomy has been reported [47,48]; it is not known if the laparoscopic adrenalectomy approach is related to the recurrent disease. An additional concern about laparoscopic adrenalectomy for malignant adrenal disease is tumor seeding at the level of the port incision. The mean mortality rate for 2550 procedures was 0.2% [3]. Four of the seven deaths occurred in Cushing's disease patients who underwent bilateral laparoscopic adrenalectomy [3].

Summary

Laparoscopic adrenalectomy is safe, effective, and curative, and it shortens hospitalization and convalescence. Laparoscopic adrenalectomy is the procedure of choice for the surgical management of Cushing's syndrome patients who have cortisol-producing adenomas (unilateral or bilateral), ACTH-dependent Cushing's syndrome and failed surgery for the removal of the source of ACTH, bilateral primary pigmented nodular adrenal disease, and ACTH-independent bilateral adrenal macronodular hyperplasia. Contraindications for laparoscopic adrenalectomy include adrenocortical carcinomas, very large tumors (eg, greater than 10 cm in diameter), and patients who have malignant ACTH-secreting pheochromocytomas. The keys to successful laparoscopic adrenalectomy are appropriate patient selection, knowledge of anatomy, delicate tissue handling, meticulous hemostasis, and experience with advanced laparoscopic surgery.

References

[1] Gagner M, Lacroix A, Bolte E. Laparoscopic adrenalectomy in Cushing's syndrome and pheochromocytoma [letter]. N Engl J Med 1992;327:1033.

[2] Higashihara E, Tanaka Y, Horie S, et al. A case report of laparoscopic adrenalectomy. Nippon Hinyokika Gakkai Zasshi 1992;83:1130–3.

[3] Assalia A, Gagner M. Laparoscopic adrenalectomy. Br J Surg 2004;91:1259–74.

[4] Chapuis Y, Chastanet S, Dousset B, et al. Bilateral laparoscopic adrenalectomy for Cushing's disease. Br J Surg 1997;84:1009.

[5] Vella A, Thompson GB, Grant CS, et al. Laparoscopic adrenalectomy for adrenocorticotropin-dependent Cushing's syndrome. J Clin Endocrinol Metab 2001;86:1596–9.

[6] Thompson GB, Grant CS, van Heerden JA, et al. Laparoscopic versus open posterior adrenalectomy: a case–control study of 100 patients. Surgery 1997;122:1132–6.

[7] Korman JE, Ho T, Hiatt JR, et al. Comparison of laparoscopic and open adrenalectomy. Am Surg 1997;63:908–12.

[8] Guazzoni G, Montorsi F, Bocciardi A, et al. Transperitoneal laparoscopic versus open adrenalectomy for benign hyperfunctioning adrenal tumors: a comparative study. J Urol 1995;153:1597–600.

[9] Prinz RA. A comparison of laparoscopic and open adrenalectomies. Arch Surg 1995;130: 489–94.

[10] MacGillivray DC, Shichman SJ, Ferrer FA, et al. A comparison of open vs laparoscopic adrenalectomy. Surg Endosc 1996;10:987–90.
[11] Hansen P, Bax T, Swanstrom L. Laparoscopic adrenalectomy: history, indications, and current techniques for a minimally invasive approach to adrenal pathology. Endoscopy 1997;29:309–14.
[12] Horgan S, Sinanan M, Helton WS, et al. Use of laparoscopic techniques improves outcome from adrenalectomy. Am J Surg 1997;173:371–4.
[13] Buell JF, Alexander HR, Norton JA, et al. Bilateral adrenalectomy for Cushing's syndrome. Anterior versus posterior surgical approach. Ann Surg 1997;225:63–8.
[14] van Heerden JA, Young WF Jr, Grant CS, et al. Adrenal surgery for hypercortisolism: surgical aspects. Surgery 1995;117:466–72.
[15] Watson RG, van Heerden JA, Northcutt RC, et al. Results of adrenal surgery for Cushing's syndrome: 10 years experience. World J Surg 1986;10:531–8.
[16] O'Riordain DS, Farley DR, Young WF Jr, et al. Long-term outcome of bilateral adrenalectomy in patients with Cushing's syndrome. Surgery 1994;116:1088–93.
[17] Kollmorgen CF, Thompson GB, Grant CS, et al. Laparoscopic versus open posterior adrenalectomy: Comparison of acute-phase response and wound healing in the cushingoid porcine model. World J Surg 1998;22:613–20.
[18] Swearingen B, Biller BM, Barker FG, et al. Long-term mortality after transsphenoidal surgery for Cushing's disease. Ann Intern Med 1999;130:821–4.
[19] Mampalam TJ, Tyrrell JB, Wilson CB. Transsphenoidal microsurgery for Cushing disease: a report of 216 cases. Ann Intern Med 1988;109:487–93.
[20] Chee GH, Mathias DB, James RA, et al. Transsphenoidal pituitary surgery in Cushing's disease: can we predict outcome? Clin Endocrinol (Oxf) 2001;54:617–26.
[21] Invitti C, Giraldi FP, de Martin M, et al. Diagnosis and management of Cushing's syndrome: results of an Italian multi-centre study. Study Group of the Italian Society of Endocrinology on the Pathophysiology of the Hypothalamic-Pituitary-Adrenal Axis. J Clin Endocrinol Metab 1999;84:440–8.
[22] McCance DR, Russell CF, Kennedy TL, et al. Bilateral adrenalectomy: low mortality and morbidity in Cushing's disease. Clin Endocrinol (Oxf) 1993;39:315–21.
[23] Tahir AH, Sheeler LR. Recurrent Cushing's disease after transsphenoidal surgery. Arch Intern Med 1992;152:977–81.
[24] Toms GC, McCarthy MI, Niven MJ, et al. Predicting relapse after transsphenoidal surgery for Cushing's disease. J Clin Endocrinol Metab 1993;76:291–4.
[25] Orth DN, Liddle GW. Results of treatment in 108 patients with Cushing's syndrome. N Engl J Med 1972;285:243–7.
[26] Estrada J, Boronat M, Mielgo M, et al. The long-term outcome of pituitary irradiation after unsuccessful transsphenoidal surgery in Cushing's disease. N Engl J Med 1997;336:172–7.
[27] Limper AH, Carpenter PC, Scheithauer B, et al. The Cushing's syndrome induced by bronchial carcinoid tumors. Ann Intern Med 1992;117:209–14.
[28] Aniszewski JP, Young WF Jr, Thompson GB, et al. Cushing's syndrome due to ectopic adrenocorticotropic hormone secretion. World J Surg 2001;25:934–40.
[29] Chapuis Y. Laparoscopic versus Young-Mayor open posterior adrenalectomy: a case–control study of 100 patients. Chirurgie 1998;123:322–3.
[30] Chapuis Y, Pitre J, Conti F, et al. Role and operative risk of bilateral adrenalectomy in hypercortisolism. World J Surg 1996;20:775–9.
[31] Ferrer FA, MacGillivray DC, Malchoff CD, et al. Bilateral laparoscopic adrenalectomy for adrenocorticotropic dependent Cushing's syndrome. J Urol 1997;157:16–8.
[32] Bax TW, Marcus DR, Galloway GO, et al. Laparoscopic bilateral adrenalectomy following failed hypophysectomy. Surg Endosc 1996;10:1150–3.
[33] Lanzi R, Montorsi F, Losa M, et al. Laparoscopic bilateral adrenalectomy for persistent Cushing's disease after transsphenoidal surgery. Surgery 1998;123:144–50.

[34] Acosta E, Pantoja JP, Famino R, et al. Laparoscopic versus open adrenalectomy in Cushing's syndrome and disease. Surgery 1999;126:1111–6.
[35] Hawn MT, Cook D, Deveney C, et al. Quality of life after laparoscopic bilateral adrenalectomy for Cushing's disease. Surgery 2002;132:1064–9.
[36] Gagner M, Pomp A, Haeniford BT, et al. Laparoscopic adrenalectomy: lessons learned from 100 consecutive procedures. Ann Surg 1997;226:238–47.
[37] Kebebew E, Siperstein AE, Duh QY. Laparoscopic adrenalectomy: the optimal surgical approach. J Laparoendosc Adv Surg Tech A 2001;11:409–13.
[38] Porpiglia F, Fiori C, Bovio S, et al. Bilateral adrenalectomy for Cushing's syndrome: a comparison between laparoscopy and open surgery. J Endocrinol Invest 2004;27:654–8.
[39] Proye CA, Huart JY, Cuvillier XD, et al. Safety of the posterior approach in adrenal surgery: experience in 105 cases. Surgery 1993;114:1126–31.
[40] Miyake O, Yoshimura K, Yoshioka T, et al. Laparoscopic adrenalectomy. Comparison of the transperitoneal and retroperitoneal approach. Eur Urol 1998;33:303–7.
[41] Duh QY, Siperstein AE, Clark OH, et al. Laparoscopic adrenalectomy. Comparison of the lateral and posterior approaches. Arch Surg 1996;131:870–6.
[42] Higashihara E, Baba S, Nakagawa K, et al. Learning curve and conversion to open surgery in cases of laparoscopic adrenalectomy and nephrectomy. J Urol 1998;159:650–3.
[43] Bonjer HJ, Lange JF, Kazemier G, et al. Comparison of three techniques for adrenalectomy. Br J Surg 1997;84:679–82.
[44] Shen WT, Kebebew E, Clark OH, et al. Reasons for conversion from laparoscopic to open or hand-assisted adrenalectomy: review of 261 laparoscopic adrenalectomies from 1993 to 2003. World Journal of Surgery 2004;28:1176–9.
[45] Rutherford JC, Stowasser M, Tunny TJ, et al. Laparoscopic adrenalectomy. World J Surg 1996;20:758–61.
[46] Vargas HI, Kavoussi LR, Bartlett DL, et al. Laparoscopic adrenalectomy: a new standard of care. Urology 1997;49:673–8.
[47] Hofle G, Gasser RW, Lhotta K, et al. Adrenocortical carcinoma evolving after diagnosis of preclinical Cushing's syndrome in an adrenal incidentaloma. A case report. Horm Res 1998; 50:237–42.
[48] Hamoir E, Meurisse M, Defechereux T. Is laparoscopic resection of a malignant cortico-adrenaloma feasible? Report of a case of early, diffuse and massive peritoneal recurrence after attempted laparoscopic resection. Ann Chir 1998;52:364–8.

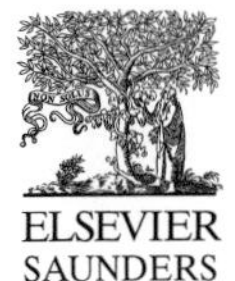

ELSEVIER SAUNDERS

Endocrinol Metab Clin N Am 34 (2005) 501–519

ENDOCRINOLOGY AND METABOLISM CLINICS OF NORTH AMERICA

Index

Note: Page numbers of article titles are in **boldface** type.

doi:10.1016/S0889-8529(05)00057-5

endo.theclinics.com

B

C

D

G

H

N

S